Integrative Cardiology

Massimo Fioranelli
Editor

Integrative Cardiology

A New Therapeutic Vision

Springer

Editor
Massimo Fioranelli
Department of Nuclear Physics
Guglielmo Marconi University
Rome, Italy

ISBN 978-3-319-40008-2 ISBN 978-3-319-40010-5 (eBook)
DOI 10.1007/978-3-319-40010-5

Library of Congress Control Number: 2016946610

Printed on acid-free paper

This Springer imprint is published by Springer Nature
The registered company is Springer International Publishing AG Switzerland

Foreword

I've always been a little afraid of cardiology as a medical specialty. It always seemed to me a too delicate and, at the same time, "explosive" subject to be addressed by complementary medicine. Therefore, it is something to be handled with care, otherwise risking the health of a vital organ, and that of the patient.

It is a "dangerous" topic in which the general practitioner does not intervene if not carrying out the wishes of the specialist, as the complementary medicine practitioner does most of the time, often renouncing from the start to provide possible indications for natural substances useful in improving the clinical situation of patients with heart problems.

We often intervene in circulatory disorders and, in particular, in changes in blood pressure so frequently now, even when people are in their prime, but when it comes to real heart problems we proceed with caution, often fearfully, avoiding interference with conventional therapies prescribed to the patient as much as possible.

Yet, the heart is not only the vital organ par excellence, but it is also central to the holistic vision, which is the basis for the practice of complementary medicine.

On this issue, I allow myself to digress briefly before commenting. It is precisely the vital organs, with their function and physiology, that express more clearly the correspondence between the inner man, or the psychic and spiritual sphere of the person, and the outer man, the physical body with its organs and systems. Some organs and functions are related to the emotional side of the person, such as the heart and liver, and, on the other hand, some organs are connected to personal aspects, such as the digestive system (the stomach and intestines) and kidneys. The stomach, in fact, receives food and the intestine assimilates it, absorbing what is good for the body and rejecting what is dangerous or toxic, just as the intellect introjects what it considers true and eliminates the false.

The heart and circulatory system carry oxygen and nourishment to the tissues and they do not choose or select anything, holding for themselves only the minimum necessary for subsistence, distributing to the tissues as required according to their needs. What the heart receives from the pulmonary circulation is then donated. For this reason, we speak of a "person of heart" and the reference is a mother's love, unconditional love. For this correspondence, emotions such as love, hate, fear, or courage are felt in the heart and therefore, the health of this organ; its integrity becomes essential for the continuation of life.

To take care of the heart, and all vital organs, is to take care of the whole person and coincides with the preservation of life. This concept emerges strongly when reading this book as a whole and in many of its parts.

Another important aspect of this book consists of the quality and the great expertise of each of the authors, starting with the curator Massimo Fioranelli. In this case, the reader can not only enjoy the fruits of experience gained in the field over decades of clinical activity, but also receive the teaching of true masters, each in their own discipline. The editorial proposal is therefore more of a real professional training manual than a book about unconventional therapies in cardiology.

We live in an age where information in all fields, but especially on health issues, come from a thousand different sources, primarily via social networks. None or very few of these are scientifically verified or evaluated based on the experience of competent professionals.

How then to judge the appropriateness of the treatment choices proposed? How to decide which path to take in the plethora of news that is often based on a desire for intellectual provocation or a need for glamour rather than on evidence for effectiveness?

Another aspect is the content of this text, which is based on three fundamental elements: the authority and expertise of the authors, the completeness of the information, and an updated bibliography.

We have already mentioned the authority of the masters, but equally important in the evaluation of text quality is the completeness of the information provided. These not only concern the range of possible interventions with the different complementary therapies—acupuncture, homeopathy, homotoxicology, herbal medicine, medicinal mushrooms, in addition to nutrition and meditation—but also the complex relationships between the cardiovascular system and the endocrine system, or the microbiota, interpreting the function of this system in the context of psycho-neuro-endocrine immunology (PNEI).

Moreover, it is not only a theoretical text. The clear aim is to train doctors and provide useful tools for their therapeutic intervention in extremely complex pathological situations such as cardiovascular disease. Thus, valuable indications for the prevention and treatment of dyslipidemia, hypertension, but also of arrhythmias, coronary heart disease, heart failure and even the cardiac protection that is so important in cancer disease and its treatment, particularly in chemotherapy.

Obviously, this text is not opposed to conventional therapy but represents its natural complement. This does not mean, however, that, for some situations and settings, it may not be the first choice of treatment for the cardiologist.

How many are, in fact, the situations of suffering for which conventional medicine does not provide satisfactory answers, because it is ineffective in that specific case, or because it is poorly tolerated owing to the adverse effects produced by standard drugs?

As this book demonstrates, and especially from now on, the lack of integration of complementary therapies in cardiology in appropriate situations and settings can only be explained by the lack of knowledge and the resistance to change of most conservative conventional medicine practitioners.

In the future, this resistance will certainly be overcome, but it is very important that the future begins now, immediately. Not as a matter of principle, but namely the affirmation of the freedom of therapeutic choice, but for the patient's benefit.

Finally, I would like to sincerely acknowledge all the authors who participated in this project, which is important for our world and marks a point of no return for the development of a higher level of integration of complementary medicine into mainstream medicine.

Elio G. Rossi
Responsabile Ambulatorio di omeopatia
ASL Toscana Nordovest Lucca
Centro di riferimento regionale
toscano per l'omeopatia
Lucca, Italy

Foreword

A book can synthesize a shared knowledge or open a new territory in a scientific field.

The book *Integrative Cardiology* by Massimo Fioranelli encompasses both aspects.

Integrative medicine is a combination of conventional medicine and traditional healing modalities, not commonly taught in Western medical schools. Nutrition, low-dose therapy, herbal medicine, metabolic cardiology, acupuncture, psycho-neuro-endocrine immunology (PNEI), immunomodulation through the intervention on microbioma, and attention to mind–body influences cover many aspects of integrative cardiology.

Many medical conditions, such as hypertension, coronary artery disease, congestive heart failure, arrhythmias, and cardiac surgery can benefit from this natural approach.

This book translates this holistic strategy into the treatment of cardiovascular diseases.

The main merit of the Editor is to have collected the experience of eminent scholars in the field of integrative medicine and to highlight a new pathway in the treatment of cardiovascular diseases. This book is something very new in the publishing field that will be helpful to practitioners seeking to translate various bodies of knowledge into the clinical field.

Along with traditional therapy, in accordance with the current guidelines, I believe that there is space in the clinical field to integrate conventional medical treatment with nonconventional therapies.

My best wishes to Massimo Fioranelli for this new achievement in a field of medicine that deserves larger diffusion into the scientific community.

Serafino Ricci
Faculty of Medicine and Surgery
University La Sapienza University
Rome, Italy

Contents

Part I

The Basis of Integration

Herbal Medicine in Cardiology

1

Ivo Bianchi

All over the world, herbs are currently used in the treatment of cardiovascular disease. Ample evidence shows that heart diseases can be prevented or even reversed with traditional medicine using ethnobotanical remedies. Diet and lifestyle are a fundamental part of a strategy that is effective in the fight again atherosclerosis, the underlying cause of most cases of heart disease. There are few but very effective and well-studied herbs and herbal derivatives useful for pathological heart conditions; we describe the most important, some of which have been or are currently used in conventional medical practice [1–4]:

1. *Allium sativum* (garlic)
2. *Arnica montana*
3. *Astragalus membranaceus*
4. *Camelia sinensis* (green tea)
5. *Commiphora mukul* (guggul)
6. *Convallaria majalis*
7. *Crataegus oxyacantha* (hawthorn)
8. *Cytisus scoparius*
9. *Digitalis purpurea*
10. *Gelsemium sempervirens* (Carolina yellow jasmine)
11. *Ginkgo biloba*
12. *Hibiscus sabdariffa* (roselle)
13. *Leonurus cardiaca* (motherwort)
14. Nattokinase (fermented soybeans)
15. *Plectranthus barbatus* (forskolin)
16. *Rauvolfia serpentina*
17. *Ruscus aculeatus* (butcher's broom)
18. *Salvia miltiorrhiza* (danshen)
19. *Scilla maritima*
20. *Strophanthus kombe*
21. *Terminalia arjuna*
22. *Viscum album*

1.1 Primary Cardiological Herbs

1. *Arnica montana*
2. *Convallaria majalis*
3. *Crataegus oxyacantha* (hawthorn)
4. *Cytisus scoparius*
5. *Digitalis purpurea*
6. *Scilla maritima*
7. *Strophanthus kombe*
8. *Terminalia arjuna*

1.2 Metabolic Herbs

1. *Allium sativum* (garlic)
2. *Astragalus*
3. *Camelia sinensis* (green tea)

I. Bianchi (✉)
University Guglielmo Marconi, Rome, Italy
e-mail: dr.ivobianchi@gmail.com

M. Fioranelli (ed.), *Integrative Cardiology*, DOI 10.1007/978-3-319-40010-5_1

4. *Commiphora mukul* (guggul)
5. Nattokinase (fermented soybeans)

1.3 Nervous Sedation and Neurovegetative Herbs

1. *Crataegus oxyacantha* (hawthorn)
2. *Gelsemium sempervirens* (Carolina yellow jasmine)
3. *Leonurus cardiaca* (motherwort)
4. *Plectranthus barbatus* (forskolin)
5. *Rauvolfia serpentina*
6. *Salvia miltiorrhiza* (danshen)

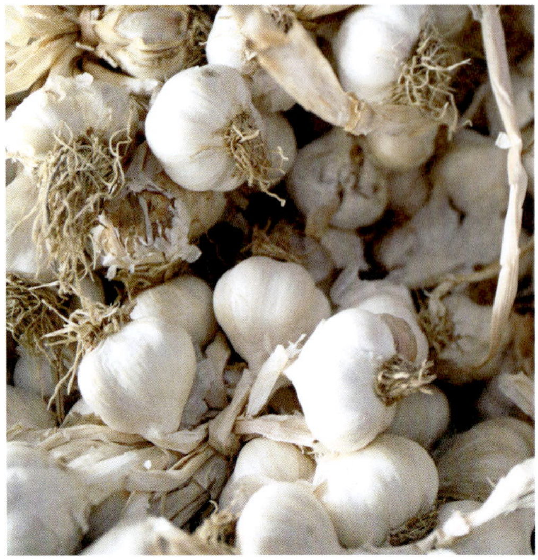

Fig. 1.1 *Allium sativum*

1.4 *Allium sativum* (Garlic)

Garlic is a perennial odiferous bulb containing 10–20 cloves, is native to the northern hemisphere, and belongs to the Liliaceae family. Its virtues were described in inscriptions on the Great Pyramid of Cheops. The pharmacologically active compound is allicin, which also gives crushed garlic its characteristic pungent odor (Fig. 1.1).

Allium sativum exerts **antiaggregatory effects** by inhibiting the adenosine diphosphate pathway; its mechanisms of action are comparable with those of conventional drugs [5]. Treatment with garlic tablets standardized to deliver 0.6% allicin, the active ingredient of garlic, produced a significantly greater **reduction in total cholesterol** and low-density lipoprotein (LDL) cholesterol and a moderate increase in high-density lipoprotein (HDL) cholesterol compared with placebo, whereas it has no significant effect on serum triglyceride levels.

Garlic supplements have shown promise in the treatment of uncontrolled **hypertension**, lowering blood pressure (BP) by about 10 mmHg systolic and 8 mmHg diastolic, similar to standard BP medication. Modern garlic extract, which contains S-allylcysteine as the bioactive sulfur compound, is particularly standardizable and highly tolerable, with little or no known harmful interaction when taken with other BP-reducing or blood-thinning medications. Garlic-derived polysulfides stimulate the production of the vascular hydrogen sulfide (H_2S) and enhance the regulation of endothelial nitric oxide (NO), which induces **smooth muscle cell relaxation**, vasodilation, and BP reduction. Normally, several dietary and genetic factors influence the efficiency of the H_2S and NO signaling pathways and may contribute to the development of hypertension. Sulfur deficiency may play a part in the etiology of hypertension and could be alleviated with supplementation of organosulfur compounds derived from garlic. The available data suggest that garlic might be of value in either the prevention or treatment of atherosclerotic diseases [6–12].

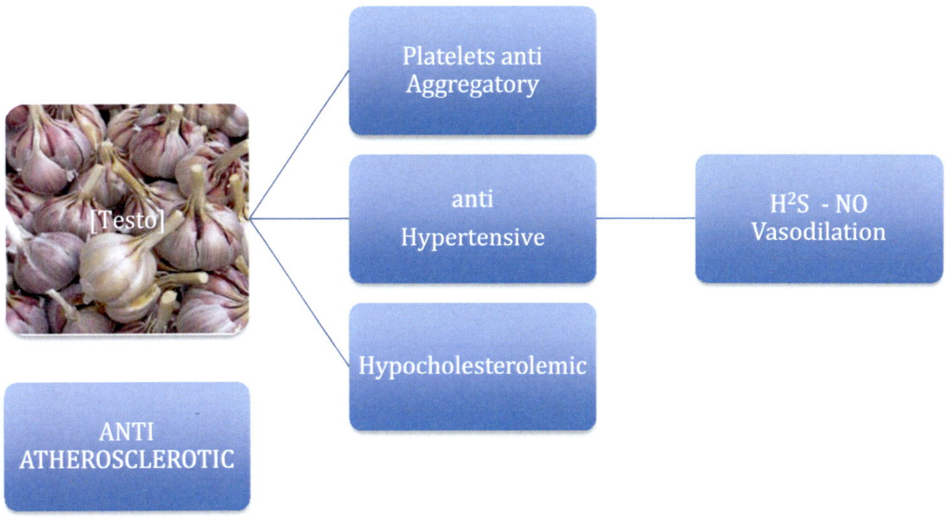

1.5 *Arnica montana*

Arnica is a perennial herb native to the mountainous regions of Europe and southern Russia and belong to the Asteraceae family. *Arnica* flowers contain helenanolide-type sesquiterpene lactones, flavonoids (isoquercetin, astragalin, etc.), volatile oils, and coumarins. Goethe recommended it for coronary heart disease and acute treatment of angina pectoris. Although *Arnica* can improve coronary circulation in much the same manner as *Crataegus*, it has a more rapid onset of action. Therefore, *Arnica* is preferred for **acute** and *Crataegus* for long-term treatment of **coronary heart disease** [7–9, 13, 14] (Fig. 1.2).

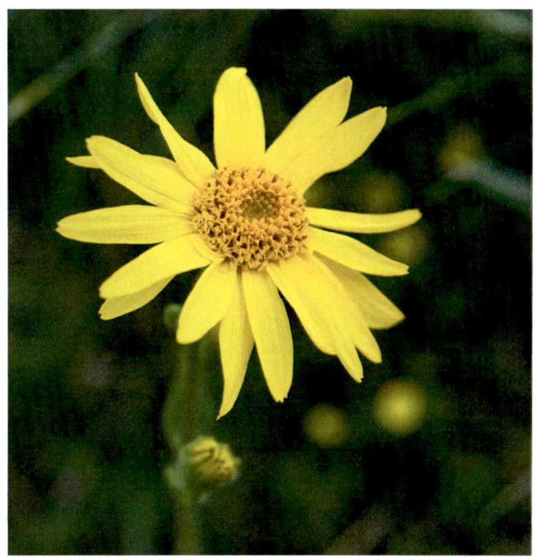

Fig. 1.2 *Arnica montana*

1.6 *Astragalus membranaceus*

Astragalus is a small shrub native to temperate regions of the northern hemisphere and belongs to the Fabaceae family. Use of *Astragalus* roots is very old and well known in traditional Chinese medicine, employed principally as a tonic and for the treatment of diabetes and kidney diseases. *Astragalus* root contains a series of cycloartane triterpene glycosides named astragalosides I to VII. Several saponins based on the oleanane skeleton have also been reported. *Astragalus* saponins demonstrated a positive **inotropic action**, improving walking distance and quality of life in patients with chronic heart failure. Oral administration of extracts of the root countered the rise in blood pressure and plasma renin activity in a hypertensive model. Astragaloside IV improved **homocysteine-**induced endothelial dysfunction in rat aortic rings via antioxidant activity and exhibited vasodilatory effects. Oral administration of *Astragalus* has an **inhibitory effect on left ventricular hypertrophy** induced

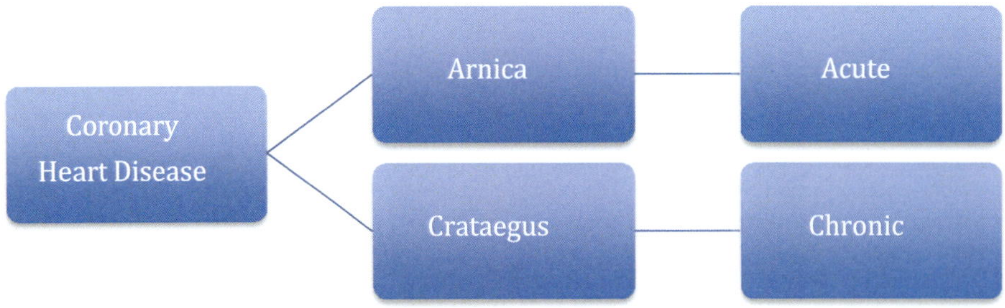

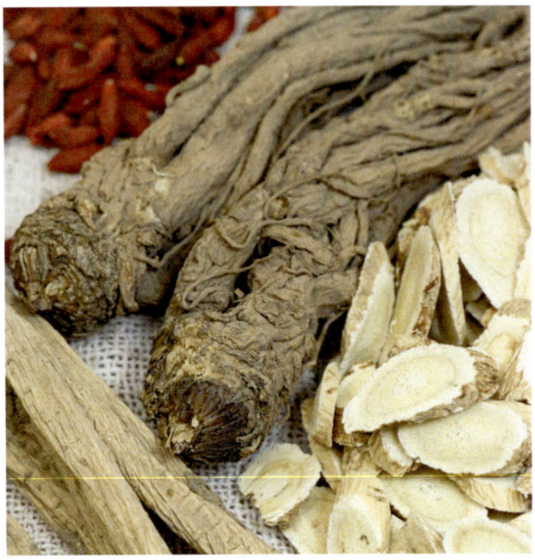

Fig. 1.3 *Astragalus membranaceus*

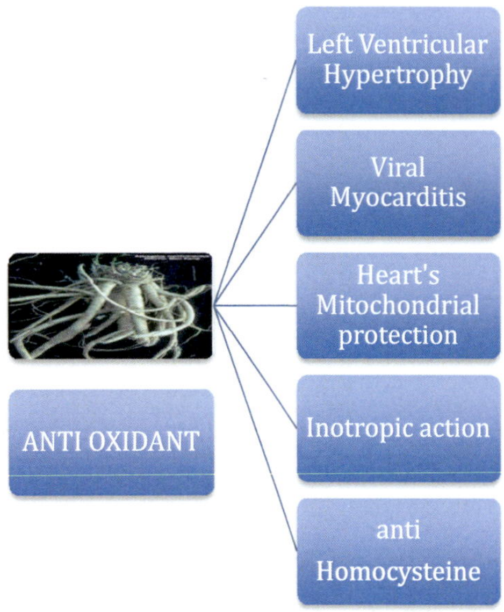

by pressure overload in rats. After acute myocardial infarction, there is an anti-free radical effect and amelioration of left ventricular function. *Astragalus* increases the survival rate and improves some abnormal electrophysiological parameters in **acute viral myocarditis**. Routine therapy combined with oral administration of *Astragalus* in these patients significantly enhanced immune parameters compared with patients receiving routine therapy alone. **Heart mitochondria** are also **protected** by toxic insult experimentally produced with daunorubicin [13, 15–18] (Fig. 1.3).

1.7 Berberine

Berberine is a quaternary ammonium salt derived from protoberberine, and belongs to the isoquinoline alkaloid family. This molecule is found in the roots, rhizomes, stems, and bark of plants such as *Berberis aquifolium* and *vulgaris*, *Hydrastis canadensis*, *Xanthorhiza simplicissima*, *Tinospora cordifolia*, and *Eschscholzia californica*. A detailed review concluded that berberine possesses a range of cardiovascular properties, including **positive inotropic, negative chronotropic, anti-arrhythmic, and vasodilatory activities**. In experiments, berberine prevented the development of pressure overload induced by **left ventricular hypertrophy** in vivo after aortic banding. Oral administration of 10 mg/kg decreased left ventricular, **diastolic pressure,** and **plasma levels of adrenaline and noradrenaline**. In a rat model of hypertension, 5–10 mg/kg of berberine improved cardiac contractility and inhibited left ventricular remodeling and global **myocardial fibrosis**. Such effects might be

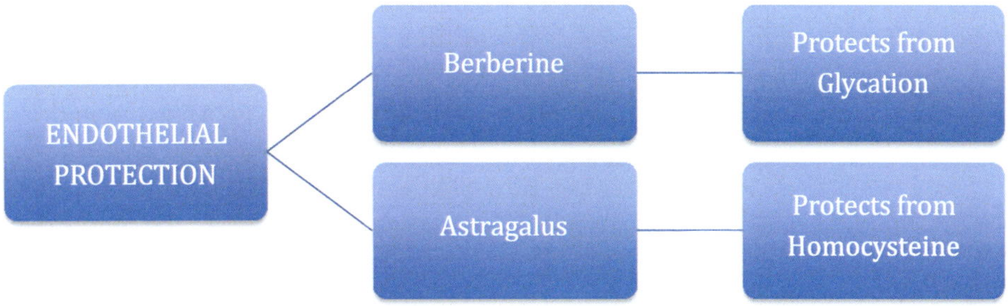

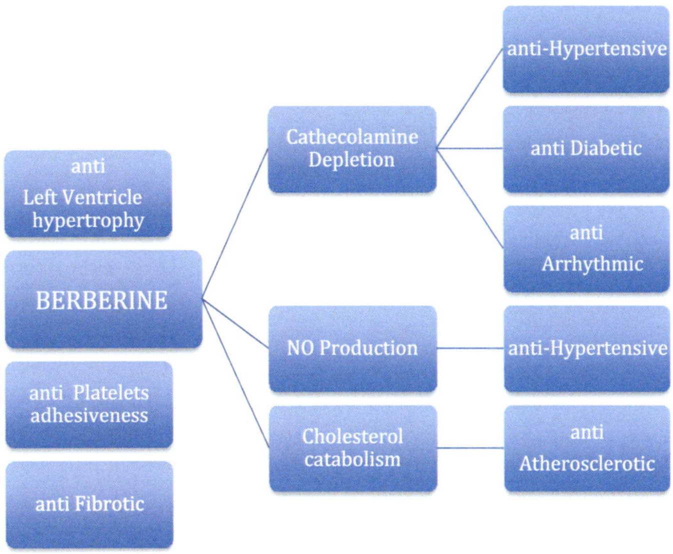

partially associated with increased nitric oxide and cAMP in left ventricular tissue. Berberine **inhibits platelet aggregation and adhesiveness** and levels of thromboxane B2, and these could be the important factors behind the **anti-ischemic activity** of berberine.

Recent research focused on the **cholesterol-lowering activity** of berberine mediated by the upregulation of hepatic LDL receptor expression and inhibition of cholesterol and triglyceride synthesis. Oral administration of berberine to hyperlipidemic hamsters for 10 days resulted in 26 and 42% decreases in total cholesterol and LDL cholesterol respectively. Human studies seem to demonstrate that berberine might **benefit the integrity and function of vascular endothelial cells** by improving protective mechanisms: increasing the **production of NO** and enhancing resistance to hyperglycemia-induced injury [7, 8, 19].

1.8 *Camelia sinensis* (Green Tea)

Green tea is produced from leaves of *Camellia sinensis*, an evergreen shrub native to Eastern Asia from Teaceae family. Green tea is the dried leaf component, whereas black tea is produced by a complex wilting and fermentation process. Tea leaves contain varying amounts of polyphenols (most of which are catechins) in addition to smaller quantities of caffeine, theanine, theobromine, theophylline, and phenolic acids. Evidence from clinical trials suggests that green tea might play a role in **metabolic syndrome** because it may have an impact on body weight, glucose homeostasis, and other cardiovascular risk factors. Green tea helps to reduce the oxidation of low-density lipoproteins, **improving cholesterol profiles**, **reducing**

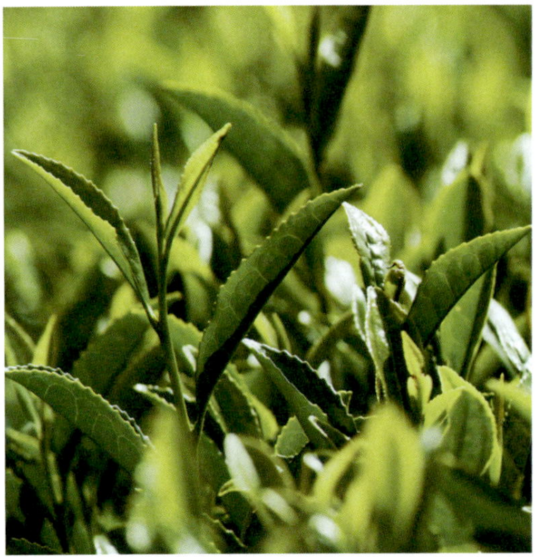

Fig. 1.4 *Camelia sinensis*

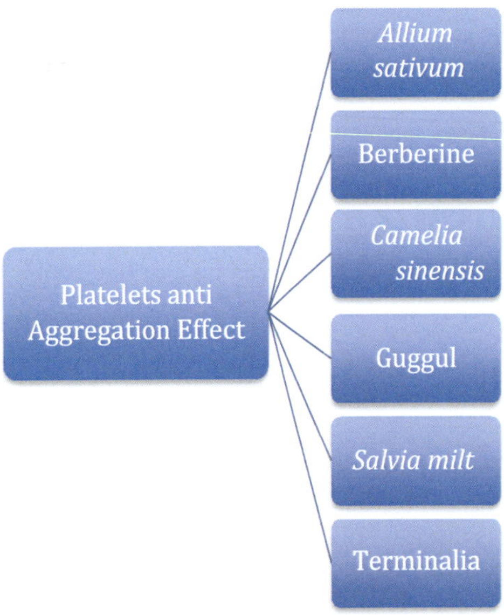

platelet aggregation, and finally antagonizing atherosclerosis [7, 8, 19–22] (Fig. 1.4).

1.9 *Commiphora mukul* (Guggul)

Guggul is a small shrub that is widely distributed in India and adjacent dry regions from the Burseraceae family. The gum has been used in Indian medicine for centuries as a cardiac tonic, and as a weight-reducing and anti-inflammatory agent.

The dry gum resin obtained from the bark of the tree **downregulates the expression of all inflammatory mediators**. Research shows that the resin of the guggul tree contains ketonic steroid compounds called guggulsterones and these have the ability to reduce the cholesterol-containing plaque. Guggul also helps to increase the metabolic rate of the body and thus is useful for **weight loss**.

Guggul, in animal experiments, was as effective as phenylbutazone and ibuprofen in acute and chronic inflammation. A study in 200 patients with **ischemic heart disease** demonstrated an improvement on electrocardiography and a decrease in episodes of dyspnea and chest pain. Guggul increases fibrinolytic activity and **decreases platelet adhesiveness,** but the most interesting activity is the improvement of **hypothyroid conditions** and an increase in triiodothyronine levels. In most studies, the use of guggul leads to a **reduction in total cholesterol** and HDL. Globally, guggul is considered an important natural remedy for preventing coronary heart disease [23, 24].

1.10 *Convallaria majalis* (Lily of the Valley)

Lily of the valley is an herbaceous perennial plant native to the forests of Northern Hemisphere of the Asparagaceae family (previously classified in the Liliaceae family). The aerial parts contain cardenolides and glycosides whose potency is not comparable to that of *Digitalis* and is also weaker than that of *Scilla*. Hence *Convallaria* is mainly used in patients with **mild heart failure**. The main advantage of *Convallaria* is its rapid onset of effects and the only remote risk of accumulation of glycosides. Furthermore, the glycosides in *Convallaria* do not affect the nerve impulse conduction system of the heart; thus, there is no risk of arrhythmias. This plant is therefore very well suited for the treatment of heart failure associated with

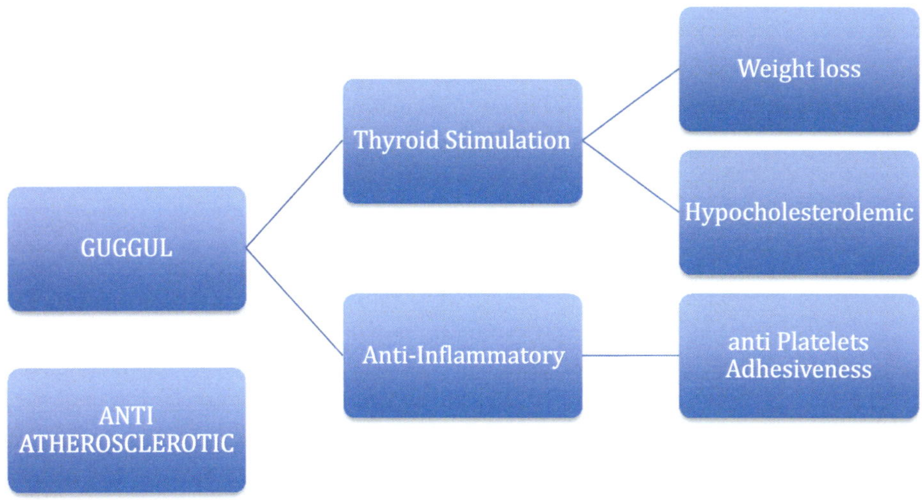

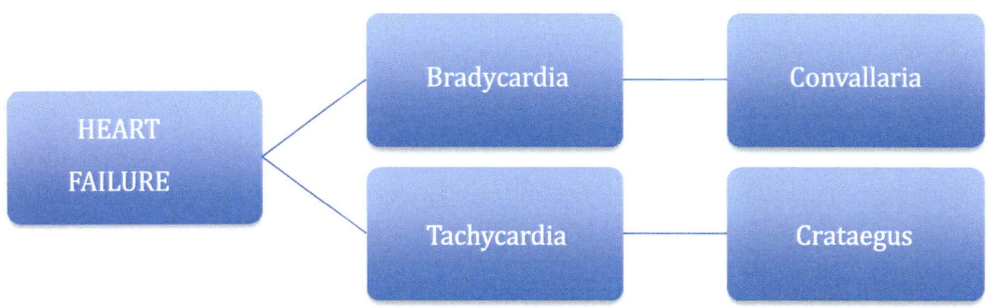

bradycardia. *Crataegus* complements *Convallaria* in the case of an "aging heart." We can classify lily of the valley as a **cardiosedative remedy**, well suited to the treatment of functional heart disorders [25].

1.11 *Crataegus oxyacantha* (Hawthorn)

Hawthorn is a spiny tree native to temperate regions in the Northern Hemisphere belonging to Rosaceae family. The use of this herb for the treatment of heart problems dates back to 1800, but the ancients probably knew already the virtues of this plant that they not casually named *Crataegus*: in the Greek language *krátos* means strength and this suggests that this plant might give the body energy through the enhancement of heart activity. Today, hawthorn is an official drug in the pharmacopoeias of Brazil, China, Czechoslovakia, France, Germany, Hungary, Russia, and Switzerland. As a measure of its incredible popularity, it is an ingredient in 213 commercial European herbal formulas, mostly for cardiovascular system.

For many years, it has been suggested that hawthorn could be used as an alternative therapy for various cardiovascular diseases, such as **angina, hypertension, hyperlipidemia, arrhythmia, and initial congestive heart failure**. Besides the **antioxidant**, **positive inotropic**, **anti-inflammatory**, and **anticardiac remodeling effects** and other **cardiovascular protective effects** of the hawthorn, active ingredients have been demonstrated in various in vivo and in vitro experiments.

The clinical efficacy of hawthorn can therefore no longer be disputed, but this plant still has

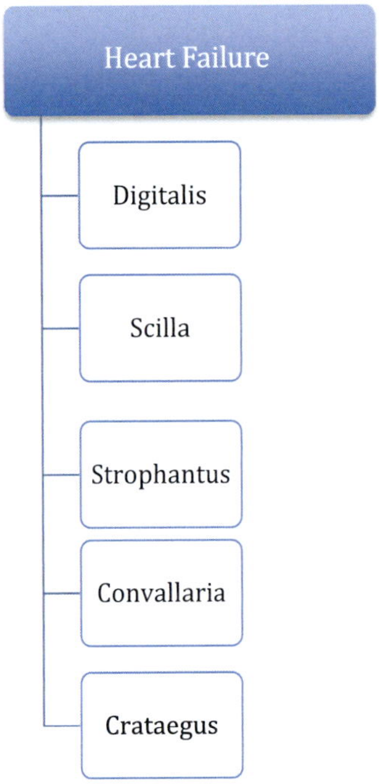

not found its rightful place in modern cardiology. Therapy shows effects after 7–8 weeks, but the pharmacologically measurable effects on the myocardium and coronary flow volume persist for several weeks, even after the administration of *Crataegus* has been discontinued.

The constituents of hawthorn are:

1. Active **dehydrocatechins** of the flavan type, also classified as oligomeric procyanidins, responsible for the **effects on coronary circulation**
2. Monomeric **flavonoids** (hyperoside, quercetin, vitexin rhamnoside), which are important for **myocardial metabolism**
3. Biogenic amines
4. Triterpene acids
5. Sterols
6. Purines
7. Catechin tannins

In any case, the research confirms that the overall effect of the extract as a whole is more significant than that of its individual constituents.

Many experimental studies in animals have confirmed that *Crataegus* increases coronary blood flow, inhibiting cAMP. Several studies also documented stimulation of myocardial contractility, through a different mechanism to that of *Digitalis*, indirectly improving myocardial energy metabolism through mitochondrial activation. This also explains why hawthorn requires a much longer period than *Digitalis* to take effect and why myocardial reactivity must exist so that the herbal drug can take effect.

It has been verified pharmacologically that *Crataegus* regulates heart rhythm and standard extracts of the plant demonstrated positive chronotropic and dromotropic effects in addition to negative bathmotropic effects. *Crataegus* increases myocardial tolerance to oxygen deficiency. An increase in cardiac volume, a reduction of peripheral vascular resistance, and an increase in cardiac performance have also been documented in various studies on animals.

Summarizing *Crataegus*:

1. Increases **coronary** and myocardial **circulation**
2. Improves myocardial contractility, mostly stimulating and **protecting mitochondria** from lipid peroxidative damage, preventing left ventricular hypertrophy and most functional and structural problems of the heart.
3. Exerts an eurythmic effect on certain types of electrical heart instabilities. *Crataegus* extract prolongs action potential duration and delays recovery. The effect is similar to the action of class III **antiarrhythmic drugs**, with a significant decrease in the total number of ventricular ectopic beats, mainly by reducing the number of beats, i.e., ventricular tachycardia.
4. Increases **myocardial tolerance to oxygen deficiency**
5. Has positive **inotropic activity**: the force of contraction of the left ventricle is clearly enhanced.
6. Has an **anti-inflammatory effect**, downregulating COX-2, TNF-α, IL-1β, and

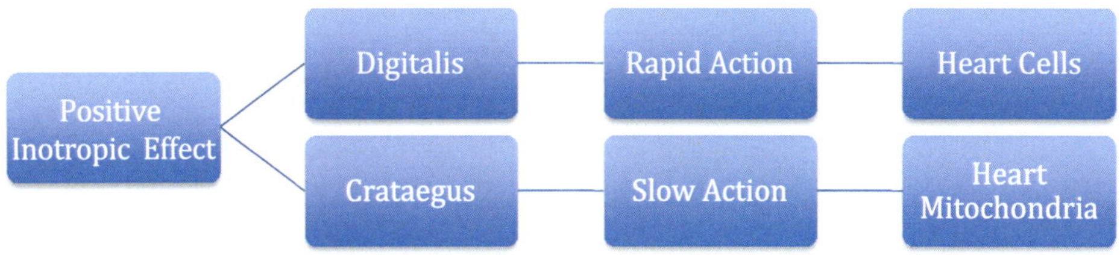

IL-6 expression, in addition to reducing nitrative stress and oxidative stress, and thus decreasing apoptosis of myocardial cells.

7. Has an **anti-platelet aggregation effect** at low doses, as indicated by the increase in bleeding time, decrease in platelet aggregation, and reduction in serum levels of thromboxane.
8. Is effective in **lowering blood lipid levels** and significantly reducing the ratio between low-density and high lipoprotein. It also increases bile acid excretion and depresses hepatic cholesterol by upregulating hepatic LDL receptors with a consequently greater influx of plasma cholesterol into the liver.
9. Significantly restores the **activity of antioxidant** enzymes such as superoxide dismutase, catalase, glutathione peroxidase, and glutathione.
10. Antagonizes **left ventricular hypertrophy** related to hypertension
11. Has a vasodilatory action on both coronary and peripheral circulation that may be mediated by the inhibition of angiotensin-converting enzyme (ACE).
12. Effectively protects against endothelial barrier dysfunction by its action on key determinants of endothelial permeability (adherens junctions, actin cytoskeleton, and contractile apparatus). Past and ongoing studies also suggest that the chronic intake of *Crataegus* might have prevented aging-related endothelial dysfunction by reducing the prostanoid-mediated contractile responses.
13. **Decreases heart rate** by sinus node suppression and progressive atrio-ventricular blockade owing to direct stimulation of the muscarinic receptor M2 and possible blockade of β-receptors
14. Significantly reduces the **deterioration of contractile function** and infarct size in rat myocardium exposed to prolonged ischemia and reperfusion. Besides, it showed an evident effect against reperfusion arrhythmias by reducing the average prevalence of malignant arrhythmias (VF + flutter) and the average prevalence of ventricular tachycardia (VT). Moreover, it prevents the isoproterenol-induced decrease in antioxidant enzyme activity .
15. Has **hypotensive action as it enhances nitric oxide** release
16. Is a support to conventional treatment because of its **positive inotropic, antiarrhythmic, and vasodilator properties**, and may provide additional benefit in symptom control (fatigue, listlessness, dyspnea under strain, pretibial edema, and rapid exhaustion), frequency of nocturnal urination, and exercise tolerance (distance walked and number of stairs ascended without fatigue).
17. Reduces **sudden cardiac death** by 39.7% and is safe for patients with heart failure. The maximal tolerated workload during bicycle exercise showed that typical heart failure symptoms as rated by the patients were reduced to a greater extent [7, 8, 13, 19, 23, 26–28].

1.12 *Cytisus scoparius* (Broom)

Cytisus is deciduous bush native to central and southern Europe and belongs to the Fabaceae family. The main alkaloid in the floral parts of the plant is sparteine, classified as an anti-arrhythmic drug. Sparteine inhibits the transport of sodium ions across the cell membrane, thereby reducing overstimulation of the nerve impulse conduction system of the heart. Pathological change in the impulse arising in the atrium is

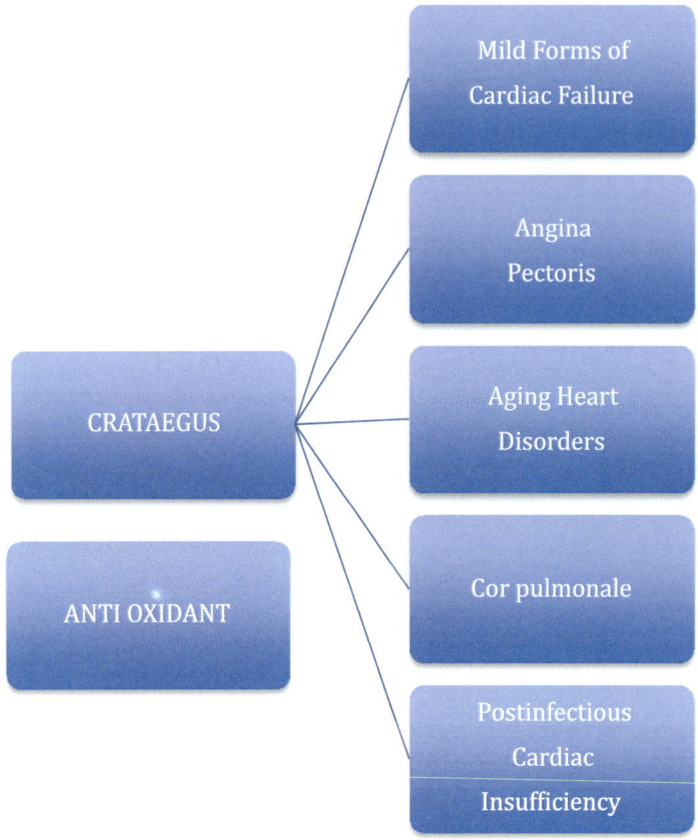

also normalized. Unlike *Digitalis* glycosides, sparteine does not have a positive inotropic effect, but still extends diastole. Broom is contraindicated in hypertension and should also be avoided in pregnancy because it increases the tonicity of the gravid uterus. The indications for *Cytisus* are **primarily functional cardiac arrhythmias mostly of the tachycardiac type, in combination with a tendency toward low blood pressure** [29].

1.13 *Digitalis purpurea*

Digitalis is a biennial plant native to Western Europe, but is found today as an ornamental plant through the world. It belongs to the Scrophulariaceae family. In Europe, its use for the treatment of heart failure has been traced back to the 10th century. In 1875, digitoxin was isolated from *Digitalis* and since then this plant has been recognized by all major pharmacopeias.

Cardiac glycosides from the leaves of *Digitalis* possess **positive inotropic effects** owing to inhibition of sodium–potassium adenosine triphosphatase; this allows calcium to accumulate in myocytes leading to the enhancement of cardiac contractility. *Digitalis* causes some **antiarrhythmic activity**, but the therapeutic index is quite narrow and it can only induce arrhythmias at higher dosages [7, 8, 19, 30].

1.14 *Gelsemium sempervirens* (Yellow Jasmine)

Gelsemium is a climbing plant native to Mexico and Guatemala and belongs to Loganiaceae family. The rootstock is used to make a tincture containing indole alkaloids. *Gelsemium* reduces

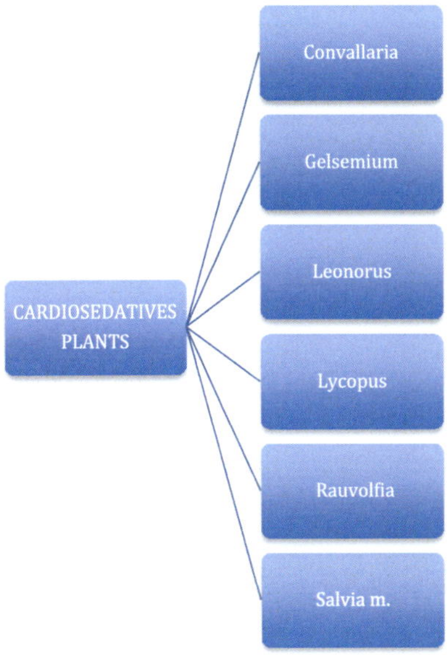

the overstimulation of the sympathetic nervous system and calms the overtonicized vascular system. This plant can be classified as **cardiosedative**. Unlike broom, it does not have a specific effect on the nerve impulse conduction system; nevertheless, it does have a calming effect on the heart in patients with **extrasystoles** and **functional heart disorders** [31, 32].

1.15 *Ginkgo biloba*

Ginkgo can be traced back more than 200 million years to fossils of the Permian geological period and is the sole survivor of the Ginkgoaceae family. Individual trees may live as long as 1,000 years and grow to a height of approximately 40 m. The main medicinal constituents are found in the leaves and include flavonoids and several terpene trilactones unique to the family. There is a seasonal variation in the content of active compounds in leaves, with the highest amounts in autumn. *Ginkgo* is traditionally used to treat **peripheral arterial occlusion** and has been demonstrated to be useful for **improving walking distances** for patients with **intermittent claudication**. *Ginkgo* extracts are used in China to treat **short-term ischemic stroke** and may be useful to shorten general and neurological recovery [7, 8, 19, 33–36].

1.16 *Hibiscus sabdariffa* (Roselle)

Hibiscus is an annual herb native to Central and West Africa and belongs to the Malvaceae family. It has a long history of traditional use for many conditions, including hypertension, liver disease, cancer, constipation, and fever. Its flowers contain various polyphenols, including anthocyanins, proanthocyanidins, flavonoids, and other pigments. Aqueous preparations of *Hibiscus* showed a dose-dependent **decreased effect on systolic** and **diastolic pressure** comparable with that of captopril and lisinopril. A **natriuretic effect** was also observed in various studies [37].

1.17 *Leonorus cardiaca* (Motherwort)

Leonorus cardiaca is an herbaceous perennial plant native to Central Asia and South East Europe and belongs to the Lamiaceae (mint) family. It contains alkaloids, bitter glycosides, and bufenolides. In particular, the alkaloid leonurine is a mild vasodilator with a relaxant effect on smooth muscles. *Leonorus* is indicated in patients with vegetative and functional heart complaints, and like valerian seems to have a primarily **sedative effect**. It must usually be used for several months to achieve adequate treatment results [38].

1.18 *Lycopus virginicus/europeus*

Lycopus virginicus/europeus is a herbaceous perennial plant growing in the wet habitats of North America and Europe. It belongs to the Lamiaceae (mint) family. Phenolic compounds, lithospermic, rosarinic, chlorogenic, and caffeic acid have been identified in both European and American plants. This herb is mainly used for hyperthyroidism and related symptoms. Extracts of the plant **reduce prolactin levels** and may be related to the suppression of TSH. Its thyrostatic activity, due to the inhibition of iodine transport and the release of preformed thyroid hormones, can be useful for tachycardia in patients with even slight hyperfunction of the thyroid gland [13, 39].

1.19 Nattokinase (Fermented Soybeans)

Nattokinase is an **enzyme** produced when the bacterium *Bacillus subtilis* natto is added to boiled soybeans of the Fabaceae family. The fermentation of soybeans is common in traditional Asian culinary practice and natto is a traditional Japanese food that has been consumed for at least 1,000 years as breakfast with rice, on toast, or as sushi. It has traditionally been used to treat heart conditions.

This enzyme catalyzes the cleavage of protein to polypeptides and is inactivated in acid conditions, and tablets of nattokinase must be have an enteric coating. It increases the activity of tissue plasminogen activator and promotes the conversion of plasminogen to plasmin, with a resultant increase in clot and thrombolysis. This enzyme has also been reported to degrade amyloid fibrils. Dietary supplements with nattokinase **suppress intimal thickening**, **modulate the lysis of mural thrombi,** and **improve arterial blood flow**. In dogs, its oral administration completely dissolves induced clots from major leg veins within 5 h. Nattokinase, in combination with pycnogenol, taken 2 h before a long flight, and every 2 h during the flight can reduce thrombotic events and edema [40–42].

1.20 *Plectranthus barbatus* (Forskolin)

This plant, also named forskolin or Indian coleus, is a perennial herb native to East Africa and the tropical regions of India and belongs to the Lamiaceae (mints) family. The main constituents are essential oils (mono and sesquiterpenes) and diterpenoids (at least 70), the most active compounds. The principal mechanism by which this plant exerts its activity is by stimulating adenylate cyclase (AC), thereby increasing cellular cAMP, which is involved in glycogen and lipid metabolism and in the relaxation of smooth muscles.

Positive inotropic action (related to the activation of AC), **augments coronary blood flow**, **increases the heart rate, decreases blood pressure**, and has been demonstrated in animal and human tests [43]. A concentration-dependent **inhibition of vascular contractility** and a **vasodilatory action** was shown in rats and rabbits. Owing to poor water solubility and low oral bioavailability, the clinical use of this plant is limited. A derived water-soluble molecule (colforsin) has been developed and is currently used in Japan (Adehl).

In addition to **smooth muscle relaxation,** forskolin exerts **strong activity on inflammatory mediators** and is often used to treat asthma due to histamine, inflammatory interleukins, and leukotrienes.

1.21 *Rauvolfia serpentina* (Indian Snakeroot)

Rauvolfia is a flowering plant native to the Indian Subcontinent and East Asia of the Apocynaceae family. It was mentioned in Sanskrit writings from around 200 B.C. There are reports of its use in a wide variety of diseases, but it was primarily used as a universal sedative. The drug is derived from the root containing more than 50 different alkaloids belonging to the monoterpenoid indole family. It exerts **sympatholytic action** via **depletion of norepinephrine** uptake into the vesicles of the noradrenergic nerve endings. As a result, reserpine has **antihypertensive and sedative properties**. Ajmaline, another constituent of the root, is known to have **anti-arrhythmic action** for membrane stabilization. *Rauvolfia* also has antimicrobial, antifungal, anti-inflammatory, anticholinergic, and antiproliferative actions. It is one of the 50 fundamental herbs of traditional Chinese medicine. Contraindications are related to vagotonic stimulation, which can result in depression, ulcers, and impotence [7, 8, 13, 44, 45].

1.22 *Ruscus aculeatus* (Butcher's Broom)

Ruscus is a low-growing common evergreen shrub that is widely distributed in Mediterranean regions and belongs to the Liliaceae family. It has a long history of use as a laxative, **diuretic,** and phlebotherapeutic agent. Early investigations during the 1950s indicated that extracts of the rhizomes of butcher's broom could induce **vasoconstriction** and therefore may be of use in the treatment of circulatory diseases. *Ruscus* is used to treat **orthostatic hypotension** and does not cause supine hypertension like other related drug therapies [46–48].

1.23 *Salvia miltiorrhiza* (Danshen)

Danshen is a perennial herb native to China's hills and belongs to the Lamiaceae (mints) family. It is considered one of the most important traditional Chinese medicines and has widespread use in Asian countries. It was the first traditional Chinese medicine to pass phase 2 clinical trials for cardiovascular indications in the USA. More than 50 compounds have been identified in danshen, mainly of two classes:

1. Lipophilic diterpenes, named tanshinones, with antibacterial, antioxidant, and antineoplastic effects.

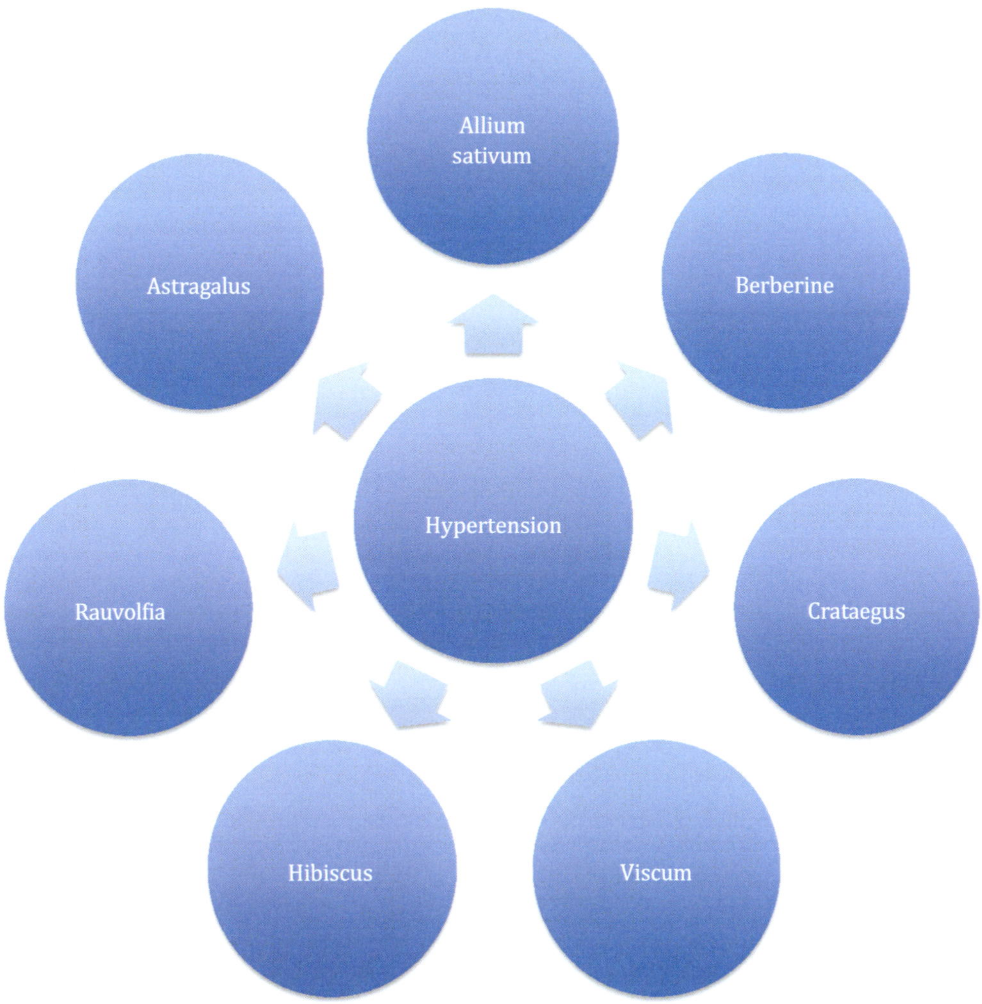

2. Polar phenolic compounds, mostly caffeic acid derivates with antioxidant and anticoagulant effects.

Many studies report the extensive use of this plant as a standard treatment for **acute ischemic stroke** in China. The injury to the vasculature following ischemia and reperfusion may be ameliorated by treatment with this plant. In vitro data suggest that this type of *Salvia* inhibits vascular smooth muscle cell proliferation and reduces intimal hyperplasia. Animal experiments demonstrated **increased cerebral microcirculation**. After ischemic stroke, the use of danshen improved neurological deficits. Animal data showed the cardioprotective activity of danshen with regard to infarct size and mortality. A meta-analysis of trials among patients with angina demonstrated an improvement in symptoms and electrocardiogram parameters compared with nitrates. Efficacy in the treatment of myocardial infarction may be due to **sedative, antioxidant, and antiplatelet effects** in addition to **improved coronary microcirculation**. Various studies demonstrated a reduction in cholesterol, triglycerides, and LDL levels with the use of the plant. Danshen is used for the management of hypertension in China, Korea, and Japan, and is thought to act via inhibition of angiotensin converting enzymes (ACE inhibitors) [39, 49, 50].

1.24 *Scilla maritima*

Scilla or *Urginea maritima* is a perennial herb native to the Mediterranean region of Liliaceae family. The bulbs of this plant contain a large number of cardioactive glycosides and *Scilla* is a cardiotonic similar to *Digitalis*. Herbalists used to claim that *Scilla* had a specific effect on right-sided heart failure. This bulb is indicated in all types of **mild to moderate heart failure**, especially when **diuretic action** is desired. Cor pulmonale associated with emphysema is a special indication for the use of the plant. Like *Digitalis, Scilla* causes dose-dependent effects such as nausea, vomiting, and cardiac arrhythmias, which are quickly reversible.

1.25 *Strophantus kombe*

This is a climbing plant found in the jungles of tropical Africa from the Apocynaceae family. The drug is made from the seeds and the tincture has a mild **cardiotonic** effect in patients with mild myocardial or coronary impairment of a primarily functional nature. It combines very well with other **antispasmodic** tinctures of herbs, such as *Convallaria*, *Valeriana*, and *Belladonna*. Administration should last for several months. In vagotonic patients, it can determine meteorism, which can be avoided by adding carminative herbs and belladonna [7, 8].

1.26 *Terminalia arjuna*

Terminalia is an evergreen tree that reaches 30 m in height and is native to northern India and Tibet. It belongs to the Combretaceae family. The bark has been used in Indian medicine for at least 3,000 years as a remedy, mostly for heart ailments. Experiments with rats demonstrated **antiplatelet** and **anticoagulant** actions similar to those of acetylsalicylic acid. Clinical studies have revealed that the use of this bark significantly reduces episodes of angina and improves diastolic function in patients with **ischemic mitral regurgitation**.

Terminalia also exerts **antioxidant**, **hypocholesterolemic,** and **hepatoprotective** actions, activities very useful in cardiac patients [51].

1.27 *Viscum album* (Mistletoe)

Viscum is a spherical evergreen shrub, which is hemiparasitic, growing on a wide variety of host trees (pine, oak, birch, and apple). It belongs to the Loranthaceae family. *Viscum* preparations have been used medicinally in Europe for centuries to treat epilepsy, infertility, hypertension, and arthritis. The most distinctive

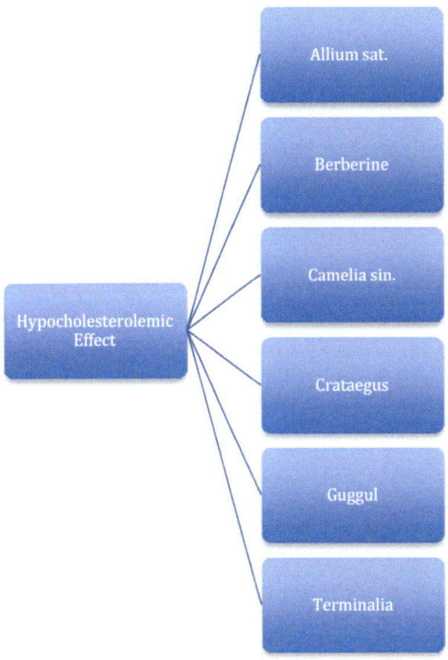

constituents are viscotoxins, lectins, flavonoids, biogenic amines, phenylpropane derivates, and lignans. None of these compounds is specifically responsible for the **antihypertensive properties** of the plant. Its effect on blood pressure is mild compared with *Rauvolfia*, but the patients report beneficial effects on **subjective symptoms of hypertension** such as **headache, dizziness, and irritability**. *Viscum* does not have any unpleasant side effects and is the long-term therapy of choice for hypertensive patients [9, 19, 52, 53].

References

1. McLean AJ et al (2004) Aging biology and geriatric clinical pharmacology. Pharmacol Rev 56 (2):163–184
2. Miller AL (1998) Botanical influences on cardiovascular disease. Altern Med Rev 3(6):422–431
3. Navarro E, Alonso PJ, Alonso SJ et al (2000) Cardiovascular activity of a methanolic extract of Digitalis purpurea spp. Heywoodii. J Ethnopharmacol 71 (3):437–442
4. Schulz R, Hänsel R (1996) Rationale Phytotherapie. Springer, Heidelberg
5. Chidsey AC, Braunwald E, Morrow AG, Mason DT (1963) Myocardial norepinephrine concentration in man—effects of reserpine and of congestive heart failure. N Engl J Med 269:653–658
6. Bianchi I (2015) Aglio (Allium sativum). Scienza Natura, Equilibrio immunitario 2(10):92–93
7. Bisset NG (1994) Herbal drugs and phytopharmaceuticals: a handbook for practice on a scientific basis. Medpharm/CRC, Boca Raton, FL, pp 83–87
8. Bone K, Mills S (2013) Principles and practice of phytotherapy. Churchill Livingstone Elsevier, Edinburgh
9. Campanili E (2004) Dizionario di fitoterapia e piante medicinali. Ed. Tecniche nuove, Milano, pp 69–72
10. Lodi G (1957) Piante Officinali Italiane. Ed. Agricole, Bologna, p 791
11. Ried K, Fakler P (2014) Potential of garlic (Allium sativum) in lowering high blood pressure: mechanisms of action and clinical relevance. Integr Blood Press Control 7:71–82
12. Yadav RK, Verma NS (1993) Effects of garlic (Allium sativum) extract on the heart rate, rhythm and force of contraction in frog: a dose-dependent study. Arzneimittelforschung 43(2):94–98
13. Bianchi I (2011) Stress conoscerlo per prevenirlo e curarlo. Mos maiorum, Milano
14. Strasburger E (1982) Trattato di Botanica, 7th edn. Antonio Delfino Editore, Roma
15. Bianchi I (2015) Astralago. Scienza Natura, Sistema immunitario 2(12):32–34
16. Toda S, Shirataki Y (1998) Inhibitory effects of isoflavones in roots of Astragalus membranaceus Bunge on lipid peroxidation by reactive oxygen species. Phytother Res 12:59–61
17. Li X-T, Zhang Y-K, Kuang H-X et al (2012) Mitochondrial protection and anti-aging activity of Astragalus polysaccharides and their potential mechanism. Int J Mol Sci 13(2):1747–1761
18. Zhu XL, Zhu BD (2007) Mechanisms by which Astragalus membranaceus injection regulates hematopoiesis in myelosuppressed mice. Phytother Res 21 (7):663–667
19. Bruneton J (1995) Pharmacognosy, phytochemistry, medicinal plants. Lavoisier, Paris, Hatton CK, trans
20. Babu A, Liu D (2008) Green tea catechins and cardiovascular health: an update. Curr Med Chem 15 (18):1840–1850
21. Oyama J, Maeda T, Sasaki M et al (2010) Green tea catechins improve human forearm vascular function and have potent anti-inflammatory and anti-apoptotic effects in smokers. Intern Med 49(23):2553–2559
22. Thielecke F, Boschmann M (2009) The potential role of green tea catechins in the prevention of the metabolic syndrome—a review. Phytochemistry 70 (1):11–24
23. Bianchi I, Bianchi V (2014) La tiroide. Mos Maiorum, Milano
24. Ojha SK, Nandave M, Arora S et al (2008) Effect of Commiphora mukul extract on cardiac dysfunction and ventricular function in isoproterenol-induced myocardial infarction. Indian J Exp Biol 46 (9):646–652
25. Schrutka-Rechtenstamm R, Kopp B, Löffelhardt W (1986) Bioconversions leading to minor cardiac glycosides in Convallaria majalis. Phytochemistry 25 (5):1107–1109

26. Holubarsch CJ et al (2000) Survival and prognosis: investigation of Crataegus extract WS 1442 in congestive heart failure (SPICE)-rationale, study design and study protocol. Eur J Heart Fail 2:431–437
27. Tauchert M et al (1999) High-dose Crataegus extract WS 1442 in the treatment of NYHA stage II heart failure. Herz 24:465–474
28. Zou QZ, Bi RG, Li JM, Feng JB, Yu AM, Chan HP, Zhen MX (1989) Effect of motherwort on blood hyperviscosity. Am J Chin Med 17:65–70
29. Jusiak L et al (1967) Analysis of alkaloid extract from the herb of Cytisus scoparius by chromatography on moist buffered paper and countercurrent distribution. Acta Pol Pharm 24(6):618
30. Warren B (2005) Digitalis purpurea. Am J Cardiol 95 (4):544
31. Chirumbolo S (2011) Gelsemine and Gelsemium sempervirens L. extracts in animal behavioral tests: comments and related biases. Front Neurol 2:31
32. Venard C, Boujedaini N, Mensah-Nyagan AG, Patte-Mensah C (2011) Comparative analysis of Gelsemine and Gelsemium sempervirens activity on neurosteroid allopregnanolone formation in the spinal cord and limbic system. Evid Based Complement Alternat Med 2011:407617
33. Bianchi I, Bianchi V (2014) Manuale di Terapia Vegetale. Mos Maiorum, Milano
34. Brinkley TE, Lovato JF, Arnold AM, Ginkgo Evaluation of Memory (GEM) Study Investigators et al (2010) Effect of Ginkgo biloba on blood pressure and incidence of hypertension in elderly men and women. Am J Hypertens 23(5):528–533
35. McKenna DJ, Jones K, Hughes K (2001) Efficacy, safety and use of Ginkgo biloba in clinical and pre-clinical applications. Altern Ther Health Med 7:70–86, 88–90
36. Zeng X, Liu M, Yang Y, Li Y, Asplund K (2005) Ginkgo biloba for acute ischaemic stroke. Cochrane Database Syst Rev (4):CD003691
37. Herrera-Arellano A, Miranda-Sanchez J, Avila-Castro P et al (2007) Clinical effects produced by a standardized herbal medicinal product of Hibiscus sabdariffa on patients with hypertension. Planta Med 73:6–12
38. Yin J, Shi GG, Wang HL (2003) Effects of Leonurus heterophyllus sweet on hemorheology and thrombosis on rat with myocardial ischaemia. Eur Heart J 24:79
39. Bianchi I (2012) Le Labiate. La Medicina Biologica, n 1–2
40. Kim JY, Gum SN, Paik JK et al (2008) Effects of nattokinase on blood pressure: a randomized, controlled trial. Hypertens Res 31(8):1583–1588
41. Pais E, Alexy T, Holsworth RE Jr, Meiselman HJ (2006) Effects of nattokinase, a pro-fibrinolytic enzyme, on red blood cell aggregation and whole blood viscosity. Clin Hemorheol Microcirc 35(1–2):139–142
42. Tal MW, Sweet BV (2006) Nattokinase for prevention of thrombosis. Am J Health Syst Pharm 63 (12):1121–1123
43. Bristow MR, Ginsburg R, Strosberg A, Montgomery W, Minobe W (1984) Pharmacology and inotropic potential of forskolin in the human heart. J Clin Invest 74(1):212–223
44. Belz GG, Butzer R, Gaus W, Loew D (2002) Camphor-Crataegus berry extract combination dose-dependently reduces tilt induced fall in blood pressure in orthostatic hypotension. Phytomedicine 9(7):581–588
45. Schlittler E (1965) Rauwolfia alkaloids with special reference to the chemistry of reserpine. Alkaloids Chem Physiol 8:287–334
46. Bouskela E, Cyrino FZ, Marcelon G (1993) Inhibitory effect of Ruscus extract and of the flavonoid hesperidine methylchalcone on increased microvascular permeability induced by various agents in the hamster cheek pouch. J Cardiovasc Pharmacol 22:225– 230
47. Cappelli R, Nicora M, Di Perri T (1988) Use of extract of Ruscus aculeatus in venous disease in the lower limbs. Drugs Exp Clin Res 14(4):277–283
48. (2001) Ruscus aculeatus (butcher's broom). Altern Med Rev 6:608–612
49. Tam WY, Chook P, Qiao M et al (2009) The efficacy and tolerability of adjunctive alternative herbal medicine (Salvia miltiorrhiza and Pueraria lobata) on vascular function and structure in coronary patients. J Altern Complement Med 15(4):415–421
50. Wang G, Wang L, Xiong ZY, Mao B, Li TQ (2006) Compound salvia pellet, a traditional Chinese medicine, for the treatment of chronic stable angina pectoris compared with nitrates: a meta analysis. Med Sci Monit 12(1):SR1–7
51. Pawar RS, Bhutani KK (2005) Effect of oleanane triterpenoids from Terminalia arjuna—a cardioprotective drug on the process of respiratory oxyburst. Phytomedicine 12:391–393
52. Andersson KE, Johannsson M (1973) Effects of viscotoxin on rabbit heart and aorta, and on frog skeletal muscle. Eur J Pharmacol 23(3):223–231
53. Rosell S, Samuelsson G (1966) Effect of mistletoe viscotoxin and phoratoxin on blood circulation. Toxicon 4(2):107–110

2 Homeopathy and Cardiovascular Disease

Ivo Bianchi

2.1 Historical Background and Basic Concepts

Homoeopathy is the name given by Samuel Hahnemann in the first years of the eighteenth century to a new therapeutic approach that was indeed as ancient as medicine. Hahnemann was not a revolutionary, but a restorer of traditional values related to a comprehensive view of medicine originating from Hippocrates, the founder of Western medicine, who recognized two different and somewhat opposing approaches to the problem of illness that were both useful for healing suffering people. The still current dichotomy of medicine is descended from these concepts:

- *Official rationalist Galenic medicine*, based on the immediacy of its conclusions and on the linearity of its concepts. This approach gave rise to the tendency to face illnesses directly, with poison to kill the germ and the bistoury to remove it. This tendency is directly connected with the modern, official form of medicine, which is quick, safe, and technically perfect.
- *Alternative empiristic Celsus medicine*, based on a global concept of man and nature, giving much importance to spiritual and psychic factors and giving rise to the tendency to face illness by far, trying to stimulate an organic reaction against the disease and often ignoring the ultimate cause of the disease itself. This approach is very important because it is directed toward the comprehension of natural laws, with an effort to find a therapy strictly related to them. This tendency, which also gave rise to alchemical research, was not and is still not immediately comprehensible. Homeopathy is within this range: it can be slow and empirical, based mostly on the intuition of the doctor, but is often successful, providing long-lasting results without side effects and at a low cost.

Homoeopathy proposes to use a wide variety of substances, both to fight the disease directly and to stimulate the physiological reactivity of the organism. This was possible by studying very carefully the toxicological reports of various activities from the plant, mineral, and animal kingdoms. There is experimental evidence that even very diluted substances are still effective if they are well prescribed. The basic principle is that the symptom or the damage caused by a toxic substance in the healthy body can be healed if present in the illness, using this same very diluted and activated substance. The skill of the doctor is to look for the specific symptoms and signs in the patient, not focussing his attention only on the pathognomonic known expressions

I. Bianchi (✉)
University Guglielmo Marconi, Rome, Italy
e-mail: dr.ivobianchi@gmail.com

M. Fioranelli (ed.), *Integrative Cardiology*, DOI 10.1007/978-3-319-40010-5_2

of the disease. Of course, the doctor must know a large number of substances and their specific effects, also using reference books or even aided by computer. The more diluted the remedy used, the more specific and precise must be the symptoms found on which to prescribe. The most active homeopathic remedies, in cardiological practice as well, are derived from the most poisonous substances and their activity is best when used with accuracy in a very diluted form. Their clinical effect is indeed bound to the precision of the prescription; if given without solid homeopathic knowledge they have no activity and can even be dangerous, inducing a disequilibrium in body reactivity. *Aconitum napellus* is a practical example of this type of remedy. Even 1 g of the root of this plant can be fatal within 2–6 h. It causes hypotension, sinus bradycardia, and fatal ventricular arrhythmias. Diluted a thousand times, this substance has been proven to be therapeutic for ventricular arrhythmias [1–3].

Some other homeopathic remedies are nevertheless not coming from toxicological studies, but from speculations on experiences of traditional herbal therapy. A great number of plants that are clinically effective, but not fully safe when used concentrated, are valid remedies when employed at low doses, though not infinitesimal, even according to traditional indications. Homeopathy gave to pharmacology many active principles used before the recent development of biochemistry that are still very interesting. *Adonis vernalis* is a practical example of this. Traditionally, this plant was used for heart conditions, including mild heart failure, irregular heartbeat, and nervous heart complaints. The use of this interesting plant was stopped same decades ago because of its toxicity. When the extract of Adonis is slightly diluted, the toxicity is no longer present, and it can be used for many cardiac indications; the best results can be seen in old, obese people with low vitality.

The author's opinion is that today, homoeopathy still represents an extraordinary therapeutic method. There is no contradiction between homeopathy and conventional remedies, and the two methods of cure could both be used by an open-minded and passionate doctor. The value of substitution therapy is undeniable (hypothyroidism, diabetes, chronic pancreatitis); nobody can deny the successes of chemotherapy and surgery and the importance to patients of the modern drugs for inflammation, acute diseases, and pain. Nevertheless, some conventional remedies are merely symptomatic, prescribed without taking into account the specific and unpredictable reactivity of the patient and the complementary homeopathic approach could help to fill this gap. As a matter of fact, there are few reasons to justify the contrast between conventional and homeopathic doctors, if both are conscious of their limitations, impartial, and always careful with regard to scientific progress. In any case, to reach the above-mentioned integration, a terminological update of homeopathy, often still using the typical language of nineteenth century medicine, is absolutely necessary. Homeopathic doctors must also know conventional medicine very well. At the same time, homeopathic remedies cannot be used in the same way as the conventional ones. The official doctor that wants to prescribe homeopathy must study homeopathic principles and materia medica in great depth.

For the homeopathic doctor, in particular, the physical and psychic constitution of the patient is crucial because it is implicated in the determination of the reactive modalities of the patient to toxins, viruses, and to various events. The most effective homeopathic remedies are prescribed after an accurate evaluation of the symptoms. For homeopathy, the disease always originates in the disequilibrium psychic, endocrine, immunological, and finally, organic. Every single and even intercurrent disease should be treated according to a global strategy aimed at gradually restoring the various levels of equilibrium.

2.2 Regional Homeopathic Remedies for the Heart

In the author's experience well-selected homeopathic remedies, can be very useful even in acute cardiological conditions. The following is a list of some of the most significant remedies based on 200 years of experience and hundreds of reported clinical cases.

1. *Aconitum napellus*
2. *Adonis vernalis*
3. *Apocinum cannabinum*
4. *Arnica montana*
5. *Arsenicum album*
6. *Aurum metallicum*
7. *Baryta carbonica*
8. *Cactus grandiflorus*
9. *Carbo vegetabilis*
10. *Chininum arsenicosum*
11. *Coffea cruda*
12. *Digitalis purpurea*
13. *Lachesis mutus*
14. *Latrodectus mactans*
15. *Gelsemium sempervirens*
16. *Glonoin*
17. *Grindelia robusta*
18. *Kali carbonicum*
19. *Kalmia latifolia*
20. *Iberis amara*
21. *Naja tripudians*
22. *Prunus spinosa*
23. *Spigelia marilandica*
24. Sumbul
25. Tabacum
26. *Veratrum album*

2.2.1 *Aconitum napellus*

Aconitum is a basic homeopathic heart remedy that is useful in acute conditions and not to be continued after pathological changes. It is indicated when there is a state of fear, anxiety, and anguish of mind and body. There is tachycardia, pain in the left shoulder, a stitch pain in the chest, but overall, anxiety and fainting. *Aconitum* is the emergency cardiac remedy that everybody should carry. Even in acute cases the most effective dilution is high (200CH-MK-XMK) and should be repeated according to the symptoms [4–6].

2.2.2 *Adonis vernalis*

A remedy specifically for rheumatic endocarditis with precordial pain, palpitation, and dyspnea. The pulse is rapid and irregular. Mitral and aortic valves are mostly affected. *Adonis vernalis* is a remedy for chronic cases and should be used for long periods at a low dilution (5–7CH, three granules morning and evening) [7–12].

2.2.3 *Apocinum cannabinum* Injeel

Remedies for the treatment of bradycardia and decompensation at an advanced stage with congestion, widespread edemas, ascites, oliguria, and anasarca. It should be used at a low dilution (5–7CH, three granules morning and evening) [7, 8, 10, 11, 13–15].

2.2.4 *Arnica montana*

A good remedy for angina pectoris with severe pain in the elbow of the left arm and stiches in the heart area. The pulse is feeble and irregular. *Arnica* is the remedy for heart insufficiency with distressing dyspnea, dropsy, and cardiac hypertrophy. This remedy can be used both in acute (high dilutions, 200CH-MK, every 12 h until amelioration) or in chronic conditions (low dilution, 5–7CH, three granules morning and evening for long periods [8, 10–22].

2.2.5 *Arsenicum album*

A remedy that acts deeply for every organ and tissue. *Arsenicum* is indicated when the patient is exhausted, restlessness, irritable, aggravated during the first part of the night, with burning pains. The heart is suffering because of smoke or alcohol and the symptoms could include: palpitations, pain, dyspnea, faintness, tachycardia, and cyanosis. The remedy is indicated in hypertension and angina pectoris with pains in the neck and occiput, especially when the left ventricle is dilated. It can be used in acute situations, but also as a basic constitutional remedy to prevent heart problems. Patients taking *Arsenicum album* are cold and they feel the cold, although they may complain of some burning pains in the chest. They look extremely anxious. Their lips are pale and sometime cyanotic. The best dilution to employ is 200CH, normally as a weekly dose, but in acute conditions, it could be administered every 3–4 h [7–11, 13, 17, 19, 21].

2.2.6 *Aurum metallicum*

The specific homeopathic remedy for arterial hypertension and for its consequences for the left ventricle. Normally, a 200CH dose is used weekly in hypertensive patients until pressure normalization. The patient feels palpitations and a variable pulse beat. The author never prescribes a remedy without a global evaluation of the patient; thus, in the case of *Aurum*, the psychological enquiry is fundamental. This remedy, especially at a high dilution, is indicated in depressed patients. They show utter worthless, profound despondency, disgust for life with thoughts of suicide. Hypertension in these patients worsens when there is cold weather and after overindulgence, loss of money, and loss of social position [7, 8, 10–13, 15, 17, 18, 20, 21].

2.2.7 *Baryta carbonica*

The remedy for cardiocirculatory problems of the elderly: the blood pressure is increased, arteries indurated, there are palpitations, and aneurysm of the aorta. This remedy for a chronic condition should be used at low dilutions (5–7CH, three granules morning and evening) for very long periods [7–11, 15, 17, 20, 21].

2.2.8 *Cactus grandiflorus*

Cactus is one of the most important homeopathic heart remedies, especially indicated in angina pectoris with suffocation, cold sweat, palpitations, vertigo, and dyspnea. The key symptom is the sense of constriction in the chest and left arm. The sensation is of an iron band around the chest. It is indicated in endocarditis with mitral insufficiency and rapid and violent pulse action. The patient may have endocardial murmurs, precordial dullness, enlarged ventricle, and low blood pressure. This remedy originates directly from phytotherapic experience and should be used at low dilutions (6-6D, 5–7CH) with frequent administration during acute phases and only morning and night when treating a chronic coronary condition [7–9, 11, 14, 17, 21].

2.2.9 *Carbo vegetabilis* Injeel

The remedy for obese patients with cardiac insufficiency, edemas, and peripheral cyanosis with cold limbs and a tendency toward heart failure. It could be used in acute cases of decompensation and in the most severe chronic cases. This is a remedy for chronic conditions to be used at low dilution (5–7CH, three granules three times a day) [7, 8, 10, 11, 13, 15, 18, 20, 21].

2.2.10 *Chininum arsenicosum*

A specific remedy for paroxysmal tachycardia with suffocative symptoms to improve air. Heart problems can occur after an acute infection and is associated with *Astragalus* (ponderal dose) when viral myocarditis is suspected or for prevention. Even in acute conditions, this remedy is better used at low dilutions (5–7CH, three granules three times a day) [7, 8, 20].

2.2.11 *Coffea cruda*

A very specific remedy, similar to aconite, that is useful for acute high pressure, violent irregular palpitations, and urinary suppression after excessive joy or surprise. High dilutions work the best

(200CH–MK), administered in relation to the symptoms [7, 8, 10, 17, 20].

2.2.12 *Digitalis purpurea*

The homeopathic and therefore harmless form of digitalis, which often causes direct or accumulated toxicity. It is homeopathically indicated in the case of weak, slow or irregular pulse with a tendency toward signs of cardiac decompensation and disorders of the electrocardiogram. This remedy can be used for long periods at low dilutions (5–7CH, three granules 2–3 times a day) [7, 8, 10, 13, 14, 17, 18, 21].

2.2.13 *Gelsemium sempervirens*

The centre of action of this remedy, a plant belonging to the Loganiaceae family, is the nervous system. There is a tendency toward motor paralysis, dizziness, drowsiness, dullness, trembling, and fear. The pulse is slow, soft, and weak and the patient feels that it is necessary to keep in motion or else the heart would stop working. *Gelsemium* at 200CH dilution is indicated in patients with anticipatory anxiety, once a week. The heart symptoms are not organic, but neurovegetative [7, 8, 10, 11, 13, 14, 17, 18, 21, 23, 24].

2.2.14 Glonoine

Glonoine is the homeopathic term for nitroglycerine, an explosive substance; therefore, its action is fast and violent, expressing upon the circulation where it causes violent pulsations, irregular congestions, and the blood rushes upward. It is indicated in vascular climacteric disturbances, suspected apoplexy, and eclampsia. Palpitations are violent, there is a throbbing of the carotids, the heart seems to be full, and cardiac pains radiate to all parts. The most frequently indicated dilutions are high (200CH-MK) and the dosage must be adapted to the specific situation [7, 8, 10, 11, 17, 18, 20].

2.2.15 *Grindelia robusta*

The remedy for the treatment of cardiac decompensation in patients suffering from chronic bronchitis. It should be used for long periods at a low dilution (5–7CH, three granules, 2–3 times a day) [7, 8, 14, 22].

2.2.16 *Kali carbonicum*

An important tissue remedy for the heart that is better indicated for elderly people with heart insufficiency, conditioning difficult breathing, and awaking from 2 to 4 a.m. Palpitations are common, with a small, soft, variable or dicrotic pulse. This is a typical chronic remedy to be used at a very low dilution (4–6D, four tablets morning and evening) [7–11, 17, 20, 21].

2.2.17 *Kalmia latifolia*

Rheumatic remedy of homeopathic materia medica that should be used as a precaution during bacterial tonsillitis. It is useful in tachycardia caused by tobacco or coffee abuse and by hyperthyroidism. Sharp pains in the epigastrium take the breath away. The action of the heart can be tumultuous with cardiac anguish. The best acting dilutions are low (5–7CH) and should be used twice a day periodically or on demand when there are symptoms [7, 8, 11, 14].

2.2.18 *Iberis amara*

A remedy with a marked action on the heart, very useful in cardiac problems such as heart hypertrophy, dyspnea, dropsy, and cardiac debility after influenza. The patient feels palpitations with vertigo and choking in the throat in addition to stitch-like pains and a sensation of weight in the cardiac region. The pulse is full, tachycardic, irregular, and violent palpitation are induced by the slightest exertion, by laughing or coughing. The best acting dilutions are low (5–7CH) and should be used 3–4 times a day when this clinical picture occurs [7, 10, 11, 14, 18].

2.2.19 *Lachesis mutus*

Lachesis is a remedy for emerging cardiovascular symptoms related to climacteric years and the menopause. Patients are very loquacious, but jealous and suspicious. They are restless and uneasy, generally aggravated on waking in the morning and when wearing anything tight. The remedy is often used in climacteric hypertension, is especially indicated when the patient has palpitations, anxiety, a feeling of constriction, and irregular beats. *Lachesis* cannot be prescribed without the typical cohort of mental symptoms; in that case, the dilution most often used is the 200CH, once a week [7–12, 17, 18, 20, 21].

2.2.20 *Latrodectus mactans*

This is the specific homeopathic remedy for severe attacks of angina pectoris. The patient has violent precordial pains radiating to the shoulders and back. The pulse is feeble and rapid, there may be cramping pains from the chest to the abdomen, and numbness of extremities. This is not a constitutional remedy like *Lachesis* or *Aurum*; thus, the best dilutions to use are low (7CH–9CH), and it is often administered until amelioration of the symptoms, and of course together with allopathic remedies and intensive care unit intervention [7, 8, 10, 17, 18, 20].

2.2.21 *Naja tripudians*

Naja is one of the most interesting homeopathic remedies for heart valve troubles. The patient manifests dragging and heaviness in the precordia with angina pains extending to the nape and neck, the left shoulder, and arm, with great anxiety and fear of death. There is marked hypotension and evidence of a damaged heart, often after an infectious disease. The heart's auscultation will reveal a condition of acute or chronic endocarditis. In acute crisis, if symptoms are typical, a high dilution of 200CH is indicated. For repairing damaged heart tissue, often when waiting for specific surgery or when surgery is not possible, a low dilution twice a day (8D, 5–7CH) is indicated [7, 8, 17–20].

2.2.22 *Prunus spinosa* Injeel

A remedy that is indicated in the treatment of congestive cardiac insufficiency with edemas in the limbs and a tendency toward anasarca and scarce urine. Almost a herbal remedy, it should be used at very low dilutions (4–6D), 3–4 times a day [7, 8].

2.2.23 *Spigelia marilandica*

Spigelia is a specific remedy for pericarditis with stitch-like pains, palpitations, dyspnea, and neuralgic pain extending from the precordia to both arms. Patients are the symptoms of the patient is aggravated by movement and need to lie on right side with head high. The hearts is often rheumatically affected by *Spigelia*, with episodes of angina pectoris and violent palpitations relieved by hot water. This remedy is works better at low dilutions (4–6D, 5–7CH), frequently administered according to the specific symptoms. In chronic pericarditis or endocarditis, it makes sense to prescribe *Spigelia* (7CH or D8), morning and evening for long periods [7–11, 17, 18, 20, 21].

2.2.24 Sumbul

Musk root, or sumbul, is the remedy for hysterical and nervous conditions. The patient is nervous, irritable, and sleepless, and has a tendency to faint for the slightest reason. It is an important remedy for nervous palpitations, high blood pressure, and cardiac asthma related to climaxis, but also to arteriosclerosis [7, 11].

2.2.25 Tabacum

Tabacum is a leading remedy for angina pectoris with coronary sclerosis and hypertension. The patient has violent palpitations, which are worsened by lying on the left side. The pulse is hard and intermittent and angina symptoms are often accompanied with nausea, cold sweat and collapse [7, 12–14, 18, 19].

2.2.26 *Veratrum album*

Perfect collapse, fainting remedy. This patient faints with strong emotions, at the least exertion, slight injury or surgery, at injections, after stools, and after vomiting. The patient has palpitations with anxiety and rapid respiration; the pulse is irregular and feeble. *Veratrum album* is a remedy for acute conditions with hypotension and is best used in a single MK dose (Tables 2.1 and 2.2) [7–9, 12, 14, 17, 18, 20].

Table 2.1 Tissue specificity of cardiological homeopathic remedies

Remedy	Tissue
Spigelia	Heart valves, endocardium
Arnica	Coronary arteries
Kali carbonicum	Right ventricle
Aurum metallicum	Left ventricle
Aconitum	Nerve tissue of the heart

Table 2.2 Functional classification of homeopathic remedies

Anti-arhythmics
– *Aconitum* – Sulfur
Anti-atheriosclerotics
– *Aurum jodatum* – *Carbo vegetalis* – *Plumbum jodatum*
Anti-degeneratives
– *Acidum formicicum* – *Arnica* – *Arsenicum album* – Phosphorus
Anti-neuralgics
– *Asclepias tuberosa* – *Ranunculus bulbosus*
Anti-hypertensives
– *Arnica* – *Aurum metallicum* – Glonoine – *Iberis* – *Lachesis* – *Melilotus* – *Plumbum jodatum* – *Spartium* – *Spigelia* – Stigmata – Sulfur – *Veratrum viride*
Anti-spasmodics
– *Aethusa* – *Asa foetida* – *Cactus*
Sympathicomimetics
– *Scilla* – Tabacum
Vagotonics
– *Spigelia*
Cardiokinetics
– *Adonis* – *Convallaria maialis* – *Crataegus* – *Digitalis* – *Kali carbonicum* – *Laurocerasus* – *Scilla* – *Spartium* – Stigmata – *Strophantus*

(continued)

Table 2.2 (continued)

Sedatives
– *Aconitum*
– *Argentum nitricum*
– *Arsenicum album*
– *Asa foetida*
– *Cactus*
– *Castoreum*
– *Crataegus*
– *Gelsemium*

References

1. Bianchi I (1992) Materia medica omotossicologica in ambito cardiocircolatorio, Rivista Italiana di Omotossicologia. Guna Editore, Milan, n 3, pp 55–62
2. Bianchi I (1989) Geriatria ed Omotossicologia, La Medicina Biologica. Guna Editore, Milan, n 1, pp 15–22
3. Bianchi I (2005) Le Basi Biologiche di Omeopatia e Omotossicologia. Guna editore, Milan
4. Bianchi I (1983) Aconitum Napellus, Rivista Italiana di Omotossicologia. Guna Editore, Milan, n 1, pp 7–8
5. Bianchi I (1983) *Aconitum napellus*—Homeopathicum, La Medicina Biologica. Guna Editore, Milan, n 1, pp 7–8
6. Bianchi I (2006) Le Ranuncolaceae Homeopathicum, La Medicina Biologica. Guna Editore, Milan, n 2, pp 43–47
7. Bianchi I, Bianchi V (2012) Bianchi's repertory of homeopathy and homotoxicology. Edizioni Mos Maiorum, Verona
8. Boericke W (1974) Pocket manual of homeopathic materia medica. Jain, New Delhi
9. Demarque D (1993) Pharmacologie et Matiere Medicale Homeopathique. Ed. CEDH, Lyon
10. Guermonprez M (1985) Matiere Medicale Homeopathique. Ed. Doin, Paris
11. Reckeweg HH (1991) Materia Medica: homeopathia antihomotoxica a selective pharmacology. Aurelia, Baden Baden
12. Stauffer K (1978) Klinische Homopathische Arzneimittellehere. Sonntag, Regensburg
13. Lippe A (1977) Materia Medica, B. Jain, New Delhi
14. Madaus G (1979) Lehrbuch der biologischen. Heilmittel, Heidelberg
15. Zissu R, Guillaume M (1988) Materia Medica Omeopatica. Ed. Marrapese, Rome
16. Bianchi I (2009) Le Asteraceae Homeopathicum, La Medicina Biologica, Milan, Guna Editore, n 2, pp 45–49
17. Clarke JH (1998) Dizionario di farmacologia omeopatica clinica. Ed. IPSA, Palermo
18. Demarque D, Jouanny J, Poitevin B (1999), Milan
19. Jayasuriya A (1988) Clinical homeopathy. Jain, New Delhi
20. Mathur KN (1979) Systematica Materia Medica, B. Jain, New Delhi
21. Nash E (1987) Leaders in homeopathic therapeutics. Jain, New Delhi
22. Voegeli A (1984) Leit und wahlanzeigende Symptome der Hoopathie. Haug, Heidelberg
23. Bianchi I (2003) Le Loganiacee (parte prima), Homeopathicum. In: La Medicina Biologica. Guna Editore, Milan, n 3, pp 43–48
24. Bianchi I (2003) Le Loganiaceae Homeopathicum, La Medicina Biologica. Guna Editore, Milan, n 3, pp 43–48

3 Low-Dose Therapy for the Treatment of Low-Grade Chronic Inflammation

Massimo Fioranelli, Marco Del Prete, Jahaira Carolina Aracena, Maria Grazia Roccia, Carlo Dal Lin, and Claudio Tomella

3.1 Introduction

From a macroscopic point of view, the inflammatory process is considered to be an event for which it is possible to identify a beginning and an end, typically represented by the appearance and subsequent disappearance of the classical signs and symptoms (*rubor, tumor, calor, dolor*, and *functio laesa*) respectively [1, 2].

However, there is a subacute form of inflammation not characterized by the classic symptoms; it may be secondary to an acute inflammatory event or exist per se as a result of a slow and progressive alteration of physiological homeostasis.

It should never be forgotten that inflammation is a defense mechanism of the physiological organism, and is activated whenever it proves necessary, to eliminate a pathogen, for example, or in a psycho-neuro-endocrine-immunology (PNEI) vision, the elimination of homotoxins not expelled through the excretory organs.

Dr HH Reckeweg, in the 1940s, pictured the inflammatory phenomena as "the sacred fire by which the body burns toxins"; the impossibility of the resolution of the physiological inflammatory process inevitably leads the body to search for a new homeostatic (but pathological) balance characterized by the activation of a low-intensity chronic inflammatory response: low-grade chronic inflammation (LGCI).

From the point of view of inflammatory and immune homeostasis, LGCI can be described as the gradual and slow move toward a state of equilibrium in a pro-inflammatory one, marked by an increase in plasma levels of Th1/Th17-derived cytokines such as interleukins (ILs)-6; -1β; -17 (autoimmunity), and tumor necrosis factor-alpha (TNF-α). The increasing concentration of these factors leads to the progressive reduction of organ function, to the reduction of the efficiency of the clearing systems (difficulty in maintaining PNEI homeostasis), and to a higher incidence of inflammation-related pathological conditions [3, 4].

One physiological process is closely reminiscent of LGCI: the aging phenomenon [5, 6]. The parameters cited are also typical markers of aging; in particular, the time course

M. Fioranelli (✉)
Department of Nuclear Physics, Sub-nuclear and Radiation, Guglielmo Marconi University, Rome, Italy
e-mail: massimo.fioranelli@gmail.com

M. Del Prete
Comitato Scientifico Amiot, Guglielmo Marconi University, Rome, Italy

J.C. Aracena • C. Tomella
Guglielmo Marconi University, Rome, Italy

M.G. Roccia
University B.I.S. Group of Institutions, Punjab Technical University, Punjab, India

C. Dal Lin
Department of Cardiological, Thoracic and Vascular Sciences, Padua University Medical School, Padova, Italy

M. Fioranelli (ed.), *Integrative Cardiology*, DOI 10.1007/978-3-319-40010-5_3

of the IL-6 plasma level is a key factor for following the performance of both the physiological aging is of LGCI, as further proof of the close connection between the two biological events.

Under conditions of healthy aging, IL-6 increases, following a nonlinear fashion, starting a slow climb near 50 years of age and reaching, in an exponential fashion, high values in centenarians; the maintenance of this physiological progression curve depicts "physiological aging" [7].

The main effect of LGCI is to anticipate the exponential phase of IL-6 growth. This results in premature aging, which accelerates the progressive impairment of organ function.

3.2 Gastrointestinal Homeostasis, Microbiota Composition and Low-Grade Chronic Inflammation

Looking at the impressive list of stressors responsible for LGCI [8–15] onset, it is clear that any organ, system, or apparatus is "immune" from the effects of chronic inflammation; however, the gastrointestinal tract is the most "sensitive" to alterations of homeostasis induced by proinflammatory triggers.

Diet, lifestyle, stress, and drugs have significant effects on the gastrointestinal tract.

At the level of the intestinal mucosa, eukaryotic and prokaryotic cells (microbiota) live closely and interact. Today, it is no longer possible to think of the human body without neglecting the relationship between it and the microbiota; thus, it is a superorganism [16, 17]. This microcosm, a real ecosystem, is able to maintain a homeostatic physiological condition through cellular and molecular interactions, finely regulated by the nervous and endocrine systems and in the maintenance of an adequate immune response, rapid, efficient, and intense so as to lead to the resolution of perturbing events without affecting the morphological and functional integrity of the structure in which it takes place. The gastrointestinal tract is characterized as a PNEI system and plays the role of homeostatic controller, not only of its own relevant compartment, but of the whole organism [18, 19].

The intestinal mucosa is able to secrete neuropeptides, neurohormones, hormones, and cytokines, carrying out nervous, endocrine, and immune functions and it is closely connected to other organs, systems, and apparatuses [20, 21]. As a result of these interactions, it is evident that the presence of a state of physiological inflammation is a normal phenomenon in the intestine, a real "function" inserted inside the mechanisms of PNEI homeostasis. The intestinal mucosa is constantly exposed to a massive antigen load represented by the commensal bacterial flora, also named microbiota. The tolerance of the microbiota is central to the maintenance of physiological inflammation in the intestine [20].

Quantitative and qualitative alterations of the microbiota may be a trigger for the onset of diseases characterized by local changes in permeability of the mucosa, such as inflammatory bowel disease (IBD), irritable bowel syndrome (IBS), gluten sensitivity, and leaky gut syndrome, but also extraintestinal diseases, such as autism spectrum disorders, the anxious–depressive syndromes, Alzheimer's disease, type II diabetes, obesity, psoriasis, rheumatoid arthritis, chronic obstructive pulmonary diseases (COPDs), or recurrent respiratory infections (IRRs).

The least common denominator of all the diseases cited is the presence of inflammation, and in particular, low-grade chronic inflammation [22–31].

3.3 Cardiovascular Risk Factors and Low-Grade Chronic Inflammation

High levels of circulating lipids (specifically, high low-density lipoprotein (LDL) and low high-density lipoprotein levels) and triglycerides, obesity, hypertension, and hyperglycemia/diabetes are generally considered the best predictive parameters for the calculation of cardiovascular risk [32–34].

The combination of the above-mentioned risk factors with some anthropometric parameters (gender, age, etc.) is mathematically interpreted and creates a numerical score used to determine the position of the subject being analyzed on the risk scale. But what are the biological mechanisms underlying the events mechanically interpreted by mathematical functions? The mechanism of LGCI is the joining link between all the cardiovascular risk factors representing the biological response to the perturbation of continuous homeostasis triggered by multiple stressors.

There are many pro-inflammatory triggers involved in LGCI onset, affecting virtually every aspect of an individual's life: Western diet; chronic stress; overweight and obesity; genetically modified organisms; environmental pollutants; drug abuse or misuse; and an inappropriate lifestyle [8–15].

The cardiovascular system, like every other tissue, organ, or system, is subject to alterations of its physiological functions due to the loss of the conditions needed for homeostasis.

Acute and especially chronic inflammatory (LGCI) conditions are potent triggers of homeostatic alterations and have an effect on cardiovascular function; every cell population, from myocardiocytes to the endothelial cells of the vessels, is therefore influenced by inflammatory mediators [35, 36].

Heart failure, heart attacks, atherosclerosis, and other cardiovascular diseases have an inflammatory component of considerable importance. In fact, among the etiological factors that cause the onset is inflammation of the myocardium.

Myocardial inflammation is secondary to a large number of triggers including infections (bacterial myocarditis), trauma mechanics, hemodynamic stress, hypertension, and not least, high levels of pro-inflammatory cytokines.

A deeper understanding of the inflammatory mechanism and the role of the specific markers C-reactive protein (CRP), IL-1, IL-6, and TNF-α [37–39] underlying the pathogenesis of chronic cardiac diseases is fundamental to the correct management of cardiovascular disease (CVD).

C-reactive protein is a key element of the inflammatory response; it is indispensable for the activation of the complement and as a phagocytosis-stimulating factor.

However, it is also one of the main events triggering inflammation that affects the blood vessel wall; CRP levels $\geq$2.4 mg/L are at high risk of CVD.

C-reactive protein is a typical acute phase reactant. It reaches a peak concentration at 48 h after inflammation onset (50,000 times higher than baseline). Its presence at a vascular level is indicative of great endothelial chronic inflammation, a fundamental factor for the triggering of atherogenic phenomena.

The importance of CRP as a marker of the individual risk of CVD has recently been highlighted by evidence that statins are able to reduce fatality rates in individuals who have a normal LDL cholesterol concentration, but increased CRP concentration, as statins directly decrease the CRP concentration.

Under IL-6 stimulation CRP is produced in the liver; macrophages are supposed to produce more IL-6 after different types of injury (infection, injury, etc.), but, interestingly, elevated levels of CRP are also detected in depressive individuals. CRP levels are completely independent of other factors linked to CRP concentration, leading to the hypothesis that a depressive mood is independent of an increase in inflammatory mediators, and, consequently, it is probably the key reason for the increased risk of CVD in depressive individuals. This interaction between a psychological disease and an increased inflammatory status clearly proves that both physiological and pathological inflammation constitute PNEI events, highlighting that alteration of the homeostatic balance (independently of the nature of the perturbing agent) has profound effects on the whole body.

Patients with chronic inflammatory diseases (e.g., rheumatoid arthritis or IBDs) are at a higher risk of CVD and related mortality. Cardiovascular risk factors are obviously a key trigger for CVD onset, but LGCI, which is also independently involved, accelerates atherosclerosis, myocardial infarction, cerebrovascular disease, and heart failure (HF). TNF-α and IL-1 could be major actors in this pathophysiology [40].

The inflammatory cytokines, IL-1α and IL-1β, are the master mediators of both local and systemic inflammatory responses underlying a broad spectrum of diseases that clearly includes CVD.

Atherosclerosis and the other CVDs have a significant inflammatory component in their etiology, and hyperlipidemia is also one of the main risk factors for hypertension and diabetes. Macrophages generate pro-inflammatory cytokines such as IL-1 and TNF-α and are deeply involved in atherosclerosis, in addition to mast cells, which generate several other cytokines (IL-6 and IFN-γ) and chemokines (MCP-1 and RANTES) [41] involved in monocyte recruitment and differentiation in the arterial endothelium.

3.4 The Prognostic Role of IL-6 in LGCI and Related Cardiovascular and Kidney Diseases

As mentioned above, IL-6 levels correlate with some of the traditional CVD risk factors [42]. Normally, IL-6 increases with age and its levels are directly associated with high blood pressure, smoking, and insulin resistance [43].

The synthesis of IL-6 increases in parallel with increasing levels of adiposity in healthy men and women. Indeed, about one-third of the total IL-6 circulating level originates from adipose tissue and this is a clear example of the direct correlation between obesity and LGCI.

Anticipating the onset of age-related diseases, IL-6 is a trigger for cardiovascular disease per se [44], but, consistent with its role in inflammatory diseases, it is also one of the best markers for risk assessment by virtue of its dependence on or independence from classic risk factors.

High levels of IL-6, independent of the source, are predictive of increased CVD risk [44–46].

Analysis of variance between the normal increasing rate of IL-6 and an altered rate can be predictive of LGCI status, even in apparently healthy subjects, intensifying the screening for CVD risk and unlinking it from classical risk factors.

Inflammation also represents the link between CVDs and chronic kidney diseases (CKD). CVDs are common in patients affected by CKD and also end-stage renal disease (ESRD) [47]. Cardiovascular mortality and total mortality are 10- to 100-fold higher in ESRD patients than in age-matched controls [48, 49]. Indeed, the risk of death after a cardiovascular fatal event in a 30-year-old ESRD subject is comparable to that of a healthy 80-year-old subject. IL-6 is one of the best inflammation markers because of its high predictive value for outcome evaluation in ESRD [49].

3.5 LGCI, Gut–Liver Axis and PNEI Homeostasis Breakdown

The LGCI constitutes the point of contact between all the pathological manifestations of the loss of PNEI homeostasis. The gastrointestinal system participates in a decisive way in the establishment and the functioning of the PNEI network; it is the key in two axes to the maintenance of the gut–brain axis and the gut–liver axis [50, 51].

Any disturbance in the intestine (alterations of the structure, function, and microbiota) affects P.N.E.I. homeostasis with alterations of immune, endocrine, neuroendocrine, and hormone responses.

As already mentioned, the loss of intestinal functional balance has as the primary result the alteration of immunological tolerance against both the microbiota and the food antigens. This results in the shift from physiological to pathological inflammation. Continuous exposure to proinflammatory triggers reduces intestinal homeostasis recovery and the continuation of this condition leads to the appearance of LGCI.

There is ample evidence for the close correlation between the alteration of the microbiota and the intestinal function and chronic liver, kidney, and cardiovascular diseases [52, 53].

Actually, the metabolic syndrome (MS) is increasingly seen as a fundamental causative agent for liver function abnormalities [54]; in particular, there is a direct link between MS and that set of liver diseases (not related to viral infections or alcohol consumption) that are referred to as non-alcoholic fatty liver disease (NFLD) [55]. Faced with this evidence, numerous studies have shown that NFLD and CVD are closely linked by common pathophysiological aspects [56]: high oxidative stress, LGCI, and atherogenic dyslipidemia [57, 58]. A further etiogenetic component of NFLD is apparently not related to those cited: the alteration of the intestinal microbiota [59, 60]. In fact, we have already seen how quantitative changes in the intestinal bacterial population constitute a powerful pro-inflammatory trigger; the resulting LGCI returns this factor into the set of common factors in NFLD and CVD.

In summary, all phenomena of altered intestinal homeostasis are potential triggers able to change the whole endocrinological, immunological, and hormonal organism. The LGCI is the unsuccessful attempt by the body to recover a homeostatic balance, and its major mediators IL-1, TNF-α, IL-6, and CRP are involved, in various ways, in the development and maintenance of all the inflammation-based diseases.

3.6 The Cellular Target of LGCI: Impaired Mitochondrial Activity and Reflexes in Cardiovascular Dysfunction

The mitochondria are a natural source of reactive oxygen species (ROS) [61], which are physiologically generated during the processes of mitochondrial respiration. Low levels of ROS are therefore physiological and fundamental for the correct operation of the electron transport chain [62, 63]; redox homeostasis is achieved through protection mechanisms managed by suitable radical scavengers, such as superoxide dismutase (SOD) and coenzyme Q10 (ubiquinone), which operates both as a carrier of electrons and as an antioxidant by exploiting the possibility of passing through partially reduced and reduced forms by accepting electrons.

An excessive presence of free radical species is universally known to be a major cause of CVD. Induced changes in the environment at a cardiovascular level by free radicals have long been studied; in particular, it has become apparent that the cytotoxic properties and atherogenic LDL cholesterol, in both native and oxidized form, are mediated by events of oxidative stress [64–67].

Low-grade chronic inflammation is a considerable source of oxidative stress caused by the subclinical elevation of proinflammatory mediators and consequent generalized alteration of cellular metabolic homeostasis. As is well known, oxidative stress, in its most typical expression is represented by an excess of ROS, and attacks the membranous structures of the cell and its genetic material. Mitochondria appear to be most sensitive to ROS subcellular organelles and numerous studies have shown that mitochondria are also particularly sensitive to the reactive nitrogen species (RNS) [68].

Mitochondrial oxidative phosphorylation is impaired by an excess of free radicals that act as inhibitors of electron transport at a mitochondrial inner membrane level. In particular, NO radicals block the reduction of molecular oxygen (O_2) to form H_2O at complex IV level [69] (a part of the electron transport chain formed by a series of multisubunit protein complexes). Physiologically, 2–4 % of electrons escape the oxidative chain forming ROS; the presence of free radicals increases this percentage, inducing excessive oxidative stress and the biological result consists in increased levels of cellular damage, dysfunction, and consequently apoptosis. Hence, fluctuations of ROS/RNS levels heavily influence organelle functions, targeting membranes and mitochondrial DNA (mtDNA) [70]. Mitochondrial damage primarily impairs the ability of cells to produce energy and also alters many cellular functions based on redox signaling pathways.

At the cardiovascular level, oxidative stress-induced mitochondrial damage is a crucial event in the onset of CVD [71, 72]. CVD patients show a high level of mtDNA degradation [73] (both deletions and sequence abnormalities) in both the heart and aorta compared with healthy subjects. It is clear that myocardiocytes and vascular endothelial cells are key targets for oxidative stress and the impaired mitochondrial functions in these cells take part in disease onset [66, 74].

Redox balance is fundamental to the maintenance of cardiovascular homeostasis. Impaired ROS scavenger synthesis at the cardiac level is linked to reduced resistance to ischemia/reperfusion damage; decreased expression of the specific superoxide dismutase 2 (SOD2) in vascular endothelium is directly linked to an increased risk of CVD [75, 76].

All main CVD risk factors share one feature: increased oxidative stress, which is the concomitant result and trigger for LGCI present in atherosclerosis, hypercholesterolemia, and diabetes; tobacco smoke-related cardiomyopathy is related to mitochondrial dysfunction and mtDNA damage at the aortic endothelium level.

The connection among oxidative stress, inflammation, and CVD risk is increasingly evident and the example of diabetes is typical. Hyperglycemia is a powerful trigger for ROS generation and, on the contrary, mitochondrial SOD2 is able to prevent hyperglycemia-associated ROS production and block NF-kB activation.

Loss of glucose homeostasis in diabetes results in increased ROS and reduced SOD2 production; loss of NF-kB translocation control results in a 2-/3-fold increase in its activation and consequently in the overexpression of pro-inflammatory mediators such as IL-1β, TNF-α, and IFN-γ. A vicious circle is established among altered homeostasis, inflammation, and oxidative stress; this results in LGCI and a progressively increasing risk of CVD.

At the mitochondrial level, a chronic inflammatory state and high oxidative stress reduce the production of energy. Coenzymatic systems are particularly susceptible to damage from ROS and inflammation. Mitochondrial coenzyme Q10 is essential for the management of the phases of aerobic ATP production [77, 78] (95% of the ATP product comes from the aerobic phase) as a basic component of the electron transport chain. The high transport capacity of electrons makes Q10 of one of the main scavengers of radical species, thus performing a fundamental antioxidant action capable of maintaining the redox equilibrium at the mitochondrial level [79].

The increased levels of oxidative stress by LGCI eventually lead to the exhaustion of buffering antioxidant systems [64]. It is significant to note that in the presence of metabolic syndrome levels of Q10, higher than the average values of a healthy subject are detected. This phenomenon describes the attempt by the body to increase its capacity to buffer the redox imbalance, but also highlights the failure of this protective mechanism: at a cardiovascular level, the loss of the ability of redox regulation results in a decline in mitochondrial function, which translates into progressive congestive heart failure (CHF).

Low-grade chronic inflammation also affects vascular endothelial functions [64, 80]. Physiological aging and pathological LGCI exert a detrimental action on endothelial cells, increasing mitochondrial oxidative stress and mitochondrial DNA damage [81]. LGCI generates an overproduction of ROS, which impairs the vasodilatory activity of nitric oxide (NO) and increases the formation of the peroxynitrite $ONOO^-$, a dangerous free radical [64].

In addition, a reduced antioxidant response mediated by erythroid-2-related factor-2 (Nrf2) and downregulation of SOD2 contribute to the induction of a chronic pro-oxidative microenvironment in chronically inflamed vessels [64].

NF-kB is sensitive to redox imbalance and it is upregulated in endothelial cells from LGCI-affected subjects. NF-kB drives a proinflammatory shift that positively feedbacks oxidative stress and its chronic activation is due to upregulated angiotensin-II signaling and impaired sirtuin expression; these events reduce the cellular protective response against acute ROS generation. A major source of damage comes from the imbalanced production of ROS. Mitochondrial ROS (mtROS) prejudice both mitochondrial structures and biogenesis through redox alteration of macromolecules, such as mitochondrial DNA (mtDNA). Structural and functional deterioration of mitochondria plays a fundamental role in cardiovascular diseases, driving both cardiac failure and vascular atherosclerotic events.

MtROS homeostasis is fundamental for the maintenance of the physiological function of mitochondria and an optimal level of oxidative stress is required [82, 83]. ROS exert a biphasic action on mitochondria metabolism: excessive production of ROS (as previously stated) impairs mitochondrial activity, but extremely low levels of oxidative stress also have negative effects on mitochondrial homeostasis.

Pharmacological or nutritional (supplementation) intervention with massive doses of antioxidant agents may impair mitochondrial functionality by blocking the respiratory electron chain and, consequently, energy production.

In the presence of cardiovascular risk with reduced cardiac and vascular functions and impaired hemodynamic homeostasis, the sustenance and/or recovery of mitochondrial redox homeostasis is important within a correct anti-inflammatory strategy.

The redox imbalance could lead to increased lipid peroxidation (including oxLDL), boosting LGCI-induced atherosclerosis; the approach to reducing this imbalance is based on the administration of antioxidants such as vitamins C and E and beta-carotene and coenzyme Q; the latter is considered the more active against lipid peroxidation [84, 85].

It is important to note that high-dose treatment with statins, one of the most important classes of anti-hyperlipidemic drugs used for primary and secondary CVD prevention, decreases plasma coenzyme Q10 concentrations with deleterious effects on cardiac function owing to muscular damage induced by the impaired mitochondrial activity.

3.7 Low-Dose Therapy for the Treatment of LGCI

Actually, there are no protocols for the treatment of chronic inflammation (including LGCI) based on the use of specific synthetic drugs, but the chronic use of anti-inflammatory drugs designed for use in acute (e.g., NSAIDs) is frequent, with dramatic consequences in terms of side effects, especially on the cardiovascular [86, 87] (increased risk of nonfatal and fatal cardiovascular events, both in heart patients and in healthy individuals) and immune systems [88] (risk of immune deficiency and the consequent high susceptibility to bacterial/viral infections).

Recently, a new pharmacology has developed and contributed to the understanding of the mechanisms of inflammation, clarifying how to act on them in respect of the biology of the inflammatory process.

It is a new paradigm that refers to pharmacological low-dose medicine: the therapeutic use of low dosages, particularly natural principles and biological molecules, such as cytokines, neuropeptides, hormones, and growth factors [89, 90].

In recent years, basic research has helped to clarify the mechanism of biological action of low doses and, at the same time, clinical research, through controlled studies, has highlighted the efficacy and safety of this innovative pharmacological approach [91–101].

Of fundamental importance in understanding the mechanisms regulating inflammation is the immune balance model; namely, the relationship of reciprocity between some lymphocyte subsets, particularly Th1/Th17 and Treg/Th2 and, as noted above, the chronobiology of cytokines involved in the inflammatory process.

Chronobiology of the inflammatory phenomenon is essential to fully appreciate the completeness of action of the milestone of low-dose anti-inflammatory drugs: Arnica comp.-Heel® (Biologische Heilmittel Heel GmbH, Baden Baden, Germany), whose formulation contains remedies with anti-inflammatory properties [102, 103].

In summary, Arnica comp.-Heel® induces the resolution of inflammation by acting on its first phase, modulating and normalizing the action of pro-inflammatory cytokines IL-1, TNF-α, and IL-6, with a mechanism of downregulation. It also acts on the second phase of inflammation by increasing the synthesis of IL-10, which, in the chronobiology of inflammation, drives the resolution phase of the inflammatory phenomenon.

Also, the possibility of acting through the use of "opponent" low-dose cytokines (that counteract the upregulation of pathological pro-inflammatory cytokines) and the use of "enhancer" low-dose cytokines (that stimulate pathologically downregulated cellular pathways) is an extraordinary opportunity for therapeutic action targeting homeostatic imbalances typical of the inflammatory phenomenon (both acute and chronic, even in the presence of an auto-immune component) and in particular LGCI.

This therapeutic hypothesis is realized by the availability of medicines containing cytokines and the anti-IL-1 antibodies low-dose activated technology sequential kinetic activation (SKA – a pharmaceutical production technique codified and standardized by GUNA Spa Milan, Italy) such as:

- Anti IL-1: suitable for the modulation of the acute inflammatory response by restoring the correct levels of circulating IL-1.
- Interleukin-10: fundamental for the management of chronic inflammatory phenomena as boosters of the resolution phase.
- Interleukin-4: suitable for the control of the triggers of autoimmune diseases; in fact, IL-4 is the main mediator of the Th2 lymphocyte response, which is depressed in the presence of auto-immune disease.

The combination of Arnica comp.-Heel® with specific antibodies anti IL-1 and interleukins allows the physician to set a strategy for the management of specific inflammatory conditions:

- Acute inflammation (Arnica comp.-Heel® + anti-IL-1)
- Chronic inflammation (Arnica comp.-Heel® + interleukin 10)
- Inflammation-based diseases with auto-immune component (Arnica comp.-Heel® + interleukin-4)

The use of the combination of Arnica comp. -Heel® + interleukin-10 is essential, especially for the specific management of LGCI within a more complex and comprehensive strategy of prevention and treatment of cardiovascular diseases.

3.8 Low-Dose Therapy for the Enhancement of Mitochondrial Functions

Pharmacological interventions, to recover mitochondrial endogenous antioxidant capacity rather than exogenous antioxidant administration, could reverse the vicious cycle of oxidative stress–inflammation, which triggers cardiovascular risk.

The so-called mitochondrial medicine represents a fundamental complement to LGCI management therapies and shows effective ways to improve antioxidant response, lowering vascular endothelial stress and myocardial functional decline, and consequently, decreasing the risk for cardiovascular disease.

Low-dose mitochondrial medicine is based on the stimulation and reactivation of the mitochondrial respiratory chain and *citric acid cycle* (Krebs's cycle) respectively, by the administration of Ubichinon compositum and Coenzyme compositum (Biologische Heilmittel Heel GmbH, Baden-Baden, Germany) as intermediate catalysts to stimulate/modulate disturbed metabolic processes.

The aim of intermediate catalyst administration is to support energy processes that are necessary for cell turnover (antidegenerative and antioxidant effects).

The Krebs' cycle and mitochondrial oxidative phosphorylation are the major cellular energy supply mechanisms. The rate of reaction in biochemistry is determined by the concentration of substrate and by the maximum saturation of the enzyme that catalyzes the reaction, according to the Michaelis–Menten law. According to this law, by administering low doses of the substrate of the various intermediates of the Krebs cycle, it is possible to obtain optimization of the reaction rate, preventing the enzymatic saturation of the reagent, namely favoring its transformation into the reaction's product.

Coenzyme compositum and Ubichinon compositum offer a simple and effective adjuvant therapy to stimulate blocked enzyme systems (the mitochondrial respiratory chain and citric acid cycle) and to restore redox homeostasis (detoxification mechanisms).

References

1. Freire MO, Van Dyke TE (2013) Natural resolution of inflammation. Periodontology 2000 63(1): 149–164
2. Alessandri AL, Sousa LP, Lucas CD, Rossi AG, Pinho V et al (2013) Resolution of inflammation: mechanisms and opportunity for drug development. Pharmacol Ther 139(2):189–212
3. Madhumitha H, Mohan V, Deepa M, Babu S, Aravindhan V (2014) Increased Th1 and suppressed Th2 serum cytokine levels in subjects with diabetic coronary artery disease. Cardiovasc Diabetol 13:1
4. Eljaafari A, Robert M, Chehimi M, Chanon S, Durand C et al (2015) Adipose tissue-derived stem cells from obese subjects contribute to inflammation and reduced insulin response in adipocytes through differential regulation of the Th1/Th17 balance and monocyte activation. Diabetes 64(7):2477–2488
5. Franceschi C, Campisi J (2014) Chronic inflammation (inflammaging) and its potential contribution to age-associated diseases. J Gerontol A Biol Sci Med Sci 69 [Suppl 1]:S4–S9
6. Pinti M, Cevenini E, Nasi M, De Biasi S, Salvioli S et al (2014) Circulating mitochondrial DNA increases with age and is a familiar trait: implications for "inflamm-aging". Eur J Immunol 44(5): 1552–1562
7. Franceschi C, Bonafè M, Valensin S, Olivieri F, De Luca M et al (2000) Inflamm-aging. An evolutionary perspective on immunosenescence. Ann N Y Acad Sci 908:244–254
8. Barbaresko J, Koch M, Schulze MB, Nöthlings U (2013) Dietary pattern analysis and biomarkers of low-grade inflammation: a systematic literature review. Nutr Rev 71(8):511–527
9. Hueston CM, Deak T (2014) The inflamed axis: the interaction between stress, hormones, and the expression of inflammatory-related genes within key structures comprising the hypothalamic-pituitary-adrenal axis. Physiol Behav 124:77–91
10. Lee H, Lee IS, Choue R (2013) Obesity, inflammation and diet. Pediatr Gastroenterol Hepatol Nutr 16(3):143–152
11. Carman JA, Vlieger HR, Ver Steeg LJ et al (2013) A long-term toxicology study on pigs fed a combined genetically modified (GM) soy and GM maize diet. J Org Syst 8(1):38–54
12. Samsel A, Seneff S (2013) Glyphosate's suppression of cytochrome P450 enzymes and amino acid biosynthesis by the gut microbiome: pathways to modern diseases. Entropy 15(4):1416–1463
13. Adler UC (2011) Low-grade inflammation in chronic diseases: an integrative pathophysiology anticipated by homeopathy? Med Hypotheses 76 (5):622–626
14. Lee BJ, Bak YT (2011) Irritable bowel syndrome, gut microbiota and probiotics. J Neurogastroenterol Motil 17(3):252–266
15. Henson J, Yates T, Edwardson CL, Khunti K, Talbot D et al (2013) Sedentary time and markers of chronic low-grade inflammation in a high risk population. PLoS One 8(10):e78350
16. Festi D, Schiumerini R, Eusebi LH, Marasco G, Taddia M et al (2014) Gut microbiota and metabolic syndrome. World J Gastroenterol 20(43): 16079–16094
17. Fujimura KE, Slusher NA, Cabana MD, Lynch SV (2010) Role of the gut microbiota in defining human health. Expert Rev Anti Infect Ther 8(4): 435–454
18. Bauer PV, Hamr SC, Duca FA (2016) Regulation of energy balance by a gut-brain axis and involvement of the gut microbiota. Cell Mol Life Sci 73(4): 737–755
19. Bercik P, Collins SM (2014) The effects of inflammation, infection and antibiotics on the microbiota-gut-brain axis. Adv Exp Med Biol 817: 279–289
20. Collins SM, Bercik P (2009) The relationship between intestinal microbiota and the central nervous system in normal gastrointestinal function and disease. Gastroenterology 136(6):2003–2014
21. Forsythe P, Kunze WA, Bienenstock J (2012) On communication between gut microbes and the brain. Curr Opin Gastroenterol 28(6):557–562
22. Kovatcheva-Datchary P, Arora T (2013) Nutrition, the gut microbiome and the metabolic syndrome. Best Pract Res Clin Gastroenterol 27(1):59–72
23. Olivares M, Laparra JM, Sanz Y (2013) Host genotype, intestinal microbiota and inflammatory disorders. Br J Nutr 109 [Suppl 2]:S76–S80
24. Hughes PA, Zola H, Penttila IA, Blackshaw LA, Andrews JM et al (2013) Immune activation in irritable bowel syndrome: can neuroimmune interactions explain symptoms? Am J Gastroenterol 108 (7):1066–1074
25. Kelly JR, Kennedy PJ, Cryan JF, Dinan TG, Clarke G et al (2015) Breaking down the barriers: the gut microbiome, intestinal permeability and stress-related psychiatric disorders. Front Cell Neurosci 9:392
26. De Punder K, Pruimboom L (2015) Stress induces endotoxemia and low-grade inflammation by increasing barrier permeability. Front Immunol 6: 223
27. Pietrzyk L, Torres A, Maciejewski R, Torres K (2015) Obesity and obese-related chronic low-grade inflammation in promotion of colorectal cancer development. Asian Pac J Cancer Prev 16(10): 4161–4168
28. Esser N, Paquot N, Scheen AJ (2015) Anti-inflammatory agents to treat or prevent type 2 diabetes, metabolic syndrome and cardiovascular disease. Expert Opin Investig Drugs 24(3):283–307

29. Wojdasiewicz P, Poniatowski ŁA, Szukiewicz D (2014) The role of inflammatory and anti-inflammatory cytokines in the pathogenesis of osteoarthritis. Mediators Inflamm 2014:561459
30. Bleau C, Karelis AD, St-Pierre DH, Lamontagne L (2015) Crosstalk between intestinal microbiota, adipose tissue and skeletal muscle as an early event in systemic low-grade inflammation and the development of obesity and diabetes. Diabetes Metab Res Rev 31(6):545–561
31. Jin C, Flavell RA (2013) Innate sensors of pathogen and stress: linking inflammation to obesity. J Allergy Clin Immunol 132(2):287–294
32. Berger S, Raman G, Vishwanathan R, Jacques PF, Johnson EJ (2015) Dietary cholesterol and cardiovascular disease: a systematic review and meta-analysis. Am J Clin Nutr 102(2):276–294
33. Stojanović S, Ilić MD, Ilić S, Petrović D, Djukić S (2015) The significance of adiponectin as a biomarker in metabolic syndrome and/or coronary artery disease. Vojnosanit Pregl 72(9):779–784
34. Turker Y, Baltaci D, Turker Y, Ozturk S, Sonmez CI et al (2015) Investigation of relationship of visceral body fat and inflammatory markers with metabolic syndrome and its components among apparently healthy individuals. Int J Clin Exp Med 8(8): 13067–13077
35. Larsen SB, Grove EL, Würtz M, Neergaard-Petersen S, Hvas AM et al (2015) The influence of low-grade inflammation on platelets in patients with stable coronary artery disease. Thromb Haemost 114 (3):519–529
36. Guarner V, Rubio-Ruiz ME (2015) Low-grade systemic inflammation connects aging, metabolic syndrome and cardiovascular disease. Interdiscip Top Gerontol 40:99–106
37. Corrado E, Rizzo M, Coppola G, Fattouch K, Novo G et al (2010) An update on the role of markers of inflammation in atherosclerosis. J Atheroscler Thromb 17(1):1–11
38. Bustamante A, Sobrino T, Giralt D, García-Berrocoso T, Llombart V et al (2014) Prognostic value of blood interleukin-6 in the prediction of functional outcome after stroke: a systematic review and meta-analysis. J Neuroimmunol 274(1-2): 215–224
39. Kaptoge S, Seshasai SR, Gao P, Freitag DF, Butterworth AS et al (2014) Inflammatory cytokines and risk of coronary heart disease: new prospective study and updated meta-analysis. Eur Heart J 35 (9):578–589
40. Dinarello CA, van der Meer JW (2013) Treating inflammation by blocking interleukin-1 in humans. Semin Immunol 25(6):469–484
41. Spinas E, Kritas SK, Saggini A, Mobili A, Caraffa A et al (2014) Role of mast cells in atherosclerosis: a classical inflammatory disease. Int J Immunopathol Pharmacol 27(4):517–521
42. Wollert KC, Drexler H (2001) The role of interleukin-6 in the failing heart. Heart Fail Rev 6 (2):95–103
43. Nicklas BJ, Penninx BW, Cesari M, Kritchevsky SB, Newman AB et al (2004) Association of visceral adipose tissue with incident myocardial infarction in older men and women: the Health, Aging and Body Composition Study. Am J Epidemiol 160(8): 741–749
44. Dessein PH, Solomon A, Woodiwiss AJ, Norton GR, Tsang L et al (2013) Marked independent relationship between circulating interleukin-6 concentrations and endothelial activation in rheumatoid arthritis. Mediators Inflamm 2013:510243
45. Nishida H, Horio T, Suzuki Y, Iwashima Y, Tokudome T et al (2011) Interleukin-6 as an independent predictor of future cardiovascular events in high-risk Japanese patients: comparison with C-reactive protein. Cytokine 53(3):342–346
46. Su D, Li Z, Li X, Chen Y, Zhang Y et al (2013) Association between serum interleukin-6 concentration and mortality in patients with coronary artery disease. Mediators Inflamm 2013:726178
47. Kon V, Yang H, Fazio S (2015) Residual cardiovascular risk in chronic kidney disease: role of high-density lipoprotein. Arch Med Res 46(5): 379–391
48. Wang AY, Lam CW, Chan IH, Wang M, Lui SF et al (2010) Sudden cardiac death in end-stage renal disease patients: a 5-year prospective analysis. Hypertension 56(2):210–216
49. Elewa U, Sanchez-Niño MD, Martin-Cleary C, Fernandez-Fernandez B, Egido J et al (2012) Cardiovascular risk biomarkers in CKD: the inflammation link and the road less traveled. Int Urol Nephrol 44 (6):1731–1744
50. Dai X, Wang B (2015) Role of gut barrier function in the pathogenesis of nonalcoholic Fatty liver disease. Gastroenterol Res Pract 2015:287348
51. Vajro P, Paolella G, Fasano A (2013) Microbiota and gut-liver axis: their influences on obesity and obesity-related liver disease. J Pediatr Gastroenterol Nutr 56(5):461–468
52. Compare D, Coccoli P, Rocco A, Nardone OM, De Maria S et al (2012) Gut–liver axis: the impact of gut microbiota on non alcoholic fatty liver disease. Nutr Metab Cardiovasc Dis 22(6):471–476
53. Minemura M, Shimizu Y (2015) Gut microbiota and liver diseases. World J Gastroenterol 21(6): 1691–1702
54. Saito T, Mochizuki T, Uchida K, Tsuchiya K, Nitta K (2013) Metabolic syndrome and risk of progression of chronic kidney disease: a single-center cohort study in Japan. Heart Vessels 28(3):323–329
55. Ferolla SM, Silva LC, de Lourdes Abreu Ferrari M, da Cunha AS, dos Santos Martins F et al (2015) Dietary approach in the treatment of nonalcoholic fatty liver disease. World J Hepatol 7(24): 2522–2534

56. Lim S, Oh TJ, Koh KK (2015) Mechanistic link between nonalcoholic fatty liver disease and cardiometabolic disorders. Int J Cardiol 201:408–414
57. Lonardo A, Sookoian S, Pirola CJ, Targher G (2015) Non-alcoholic fatty liver disease and risk of cardiovascular disease. Metabolism 65(8):1136–1150
58. Than NN, Newsome PN (2015) A concise review of non-alcoholic fatty liver disease. Atherosclerosis 239(1):192–202
59. Giannelli V, Di Gregorio V, Iebba V, Giusto M, Schippa S et al (2014) Microbiota and the gut-liver axis: bacterial translocation, inflammation and infection in cirrhosis. World J Gastroenterol 20(45): 16795–16810
60. Barrios C, Beaumont M, Pallister T, Villar J, Goodrich JK et al (2015) Gut-microbiota-metabolite axis in early renal function decline. PLoS One 10(8): e0134311
61. Dan Dunn J, Alvarez LA, Zhang X, Soldati T (2015) Reactive oxygen species and mitochondria: a nexus of cellular homeostasis. Redox Biol 6:472–485
62. Brady NR, Hamacher-Brady A, Westerhoff HV, Gottlieb RA (2006) A wave of reactive oxygen species (ROS)-induced ROS release in a sea of excitable mitochondria. Antioxid Redox Signal 8(9–10): 1651–1665
63. Gusdon AM, Fernandez-Bueno GA, Wohlgemuth S, Fernandez J, Chen J et al (2015) Respiration and substrate transport rates as well as reactive oxygen species production distinguish mitochondria from brain and liver. BMC Biochem 16:22
64. El Assar M, Angulo J, Rodríguez-Mañas L (2013) Oxidative stress and vascular inflammation in aging. Free Radic Biol Med 65:380–401
65. Ballinger SW (2005) Mitochondrial dysfunction in cardiovascular disease. Free Radic Biol Med 38(10): 1278–1295
66. Mikhed Y, Daiber A, Steven S (2015) Mitochondrial oxidative stress, mitochondrial DNA damage and their role in age-related vascular dysfunction. Int J Mol Sci 16(7):15918–15953
67. Yao X, Carlson D, Sun Y, Ma L, Wolf SE et al (2015) Mitochondrial ROS induces cardiac inflammation via a pathway through mtDNA damage in a pneumonia-related sepsis model. PLoS One 10(10):e0139416
68. Willems PH, Rossignol R, Dieteren CE, Murphy MP, Koopman WJ (2015) Redox homeostasis and mitochondrial dynamics. Cell Metab 22(2): 207–218
69. Singh S, Zhuo M, Gorgun FM, Englander EW (2013) Overexpressed neuroglobin raises threshold for nitric oxide-induced impairment of mitochondrial respiratory activities and stress signaling in primary cortical neurons. Nitric Oxide 32:21–28
70. Bogeski I, Niemeyer BA (2014) Redox regulation of ion channels. Antioxid Redox Signal 21(6):859–862
71. Tocchi A, Quarles EK, Basisty N, Gitari L, Rabinovitch PS (2015) Mitochondrial dysfunction in cardiac aging. Biochim Biophys Acta 1847(11): 1424–1433
72. Herrera A, Garcia I, Gaytan N, Jones E, Maldonado A et al (2015) Endangered species: mitochondrial DNA loss as a mechanism of human disease. Front Biosci (Schol Ed) 7:109–124
73. Sobenin IA, Zhelankin AV, Mitrofanov KY, Sinyov VV, Sazonova MA et al (2015) Mutations of mitochondrial DNA in atherosclerosis and atherosclerosis-related diseases. Curr Pharm Des 21 (9):1158–1163
74. Koene S, Smeitink J (2011) Mitochondrial medicine. J Inherit Metab Dis 34(2):247–248
75. Fukai T, Ushio-Fukai M (2011) Superoxide dismutases: role in redox signaling, vascular function, and diseases. Antioxid Redox Signal 15(6):1583–1606
76. Harrison CM, Pompilius M, Pinkerton KE, Ballinger SW (2011) Mitochondrial oxidative stress significantly influences atherogenic risk and cytokine-induced oxidant production. Environ Health Perspect 119(5):676–681
77. Yang YK, Wang LP, Chen L, Yao XP, Yang KQ et al (2015) Coenzyme Q10 treatment of cardiovascular disorders of ageing including heart failure, hypertension and endothelial dysfunction. Clin Chim Acta 450:83–89
78. Forsberg E, Xu C, Grünler J, Frostegård J, Tekle M et al (2015) Coenzyme Q10 and oxidative stress, the association with peripheral sensory neuropathy and cardiovascular disease in type 2 diabetes mellitus. J Diabetes Complications 29(8):1152–1158
79. Linnane AW, Kios M, Vitetta L (2007) Coenzyme Q (10) – its role as a prooxidant in the formation of superoxide anion/hydrogen peroxide and the regulation of the metabolome. Mitochondrion 7(Suppl): S51–S61
80. Smith BJ, Lightfoot SA, Lerner MR, Denson KD, Morgan DL et al (2009) Induction of cardiovascular pathology in a novel model of low-grade chronic inflammation. Cardiovasc Pathol 18(1):1–10
81. Ungvari Z, Kaley G, de Cabo R, Sonntag WE, Csiszar A (2010) Mechanisms of vascular aging: new perspectives. J Gerontol A Biol Sci Med Sci 65(10): 1028–1041
82. Ristow M (2014) Unraveling the truth about antioxidants: mitohormesis explains ROS-induced health benefits. Nat Med 20(7):709–711
83. Ristow M, Schmeisser K (2014) Mitohormesis: promoting health and lifespan by increased levels of reactive oxygen species (ROS). Dose Response 12 (2):288–341
84. Poljsak B, Šuput D, Milisav I (2013) Achieving the balance between ROS and antioxidants: when to use the synthetic antioxidants. Oxid Med Cell Longev 2013:956792
85. Tikhaze AK, Konovalova GG, Lankin VZ, Kaminnyi AI, Kaminnaja VI et al (2005) Effect of ubiquinone Q(10) and antioxidant vitamins on free radical oxidation of phospholipids in biological

membranes of rat liver. Bull Exp Biol Med 140(2): 181–183

86. Ghosh R, Alajbegovic A, Gomes AV (2015) NSAIDs and cardiovascular diseases: role of reactive oxygen species. Oxid Med Cell Longev 2015: 536962
87. Taubert KA (2008) Cardiology patient pages. Can patients with cardiovascular disease take nonsteroidal antiinflammatory drugs? Circulation 117 (17):e322–e324
88. Habib I, Mazulis A, Roginsky G, Ehrenpreis ED (2014) Nonsteroidal anti-inflammatory drugs and inflammatory bowel disease: pathophysiology and clinical associations. Inflamm Bowel Dis 20(12): 2493–2502
89. Lotti T, Perra A (2014) Bases and principles of low dose medicine and P.N.E.I. foundations of low dose pharmacology. Pigm Disord 1:e101
90. Fioranelli M, Roccia MG (2014) Twenty-five years of studies and trials for the therapeutic application of IL-10 immunomodulating properties. From high doses administration to low dose medicine new paradigm. J Integr Cardiol 1(1):2–6
91. Gariboldi S, Palazzo M, Zanobbio L, Dusio GF, Mauro V et al (2009) Low dose oral administration of cytokines for treatment of allergic asthma. Pulm Pharmacol Ther 22:497–510
92. D'Amico L, Ruffini E, Ferracini R, Roato I (2012) Low dose of IL-12 stimulates T cell response in cultures of PBMCs derived from non-small cell lung cancer patients. J Cancer Ther 3:337–342
93. Cardani D, Dusio GF, Luchini P, Sciarabba M, Solimene U et al (2013) Oral administration of interleukin-10 and anti-IL-1 antibody ameliorates experimental intestinal inflammation. Gastroenterol Res 6:124–133
94. Radice E, Miranda V, Bellone G (2014) Low-doses of sequential-kinetic-activated interferon-gamma enhance the ex vivo cytotoxicity of peripheral blood natural killer cells from patients with early-stage colorectal cancer. A preliminary study. Int Immunopharmacol 19:66–73
95. Roberti ML, Ricottini L, Capponi A, Sclauzero E, Vicenti P et al (2014) Immunomodulating treatment with low dose Interleukin-4, Interleukin-10 and Interleukin-11 in psoriasis vulgaris. J Biol Regul Homeost Agents 28:133–139
96. Luchetti P (2014) Increasing of visual function in patients with retinal atrophy treated with drugs of Low Dose Medicine. Monocentric retrospective observational study. Minerva Oftalmol 56(3-4):53–61
97. Barygina V, Becatti M, Lotti T, Moretti S, Taddei N et al (2015) Treatment with low-dose cytokines reduces oxidative-mediated injury in perilesional keratinocytes from vitiligo skin. J Dermatol Sci 79 (2):163–170
98. Lotti T, Hercogova J, Wollina U, Chokoeva AA, Zarrab Z et al (2015) Vitiligo: successful combination treatment based on oral low dose cytokines and different topical treatments. J Biol Regul Homeost Agents 29 [1 Suppl]:53–58
99. Radice E, Bellone G, Miranda V (2015) Enhancement of the immunostimulatory functions of ex vivo-generated dendritic cells from early-stage colon cancer patients by consecutive exposure to low doses of sequential-kinetic-activated IL-4 and IL-12. A preliminary study. Transl Oncol 8(4):327–338
100. Lotti T (2015) Successful combination treatment for psoriasis with phototherapy and low-dose cytokines: a spontaneous, retrospective observational clinical study. Hautarzt 66(11):849–854
101. Tessaro I, Modina SC, Franciosi F, Sivelli G, Terzaghi L, Lodde V et al (2015) Effect of oral administration of low-dose follicle stimulating hormone on hyperandrogenized mice as a model of polycystic ovary syndrome. J Ovarian Res 8(1): 64
102. Porozov S, Cahlon L, Weiser M, Branski D, Lider O et al (2004) Inhibition of IL-1β and TNF-α secretion from resting and activated human immunocytes by the homeopathic medication Traumeel®S. Clin Dev Immunol 11(2):143
103. González de Vega C, Speed C, Wolfarth B, González J (2013) Traumeel vs. diclofenac for reducing pain and improving ankle mobility after acute ankle sprain: a multicentre, randomised, blinded, controlled and non-inferiority trial. Int J Clin Pract 67(10):979–989

Acupuncture in Cardiovascular Diseases

4

Giuseppe Lupi and Manuela Cormio

4.1 Historical Background, the Beginning and the Diffusion

Acupuncture is one of the traditional Chinese medicine (TCM) techniques, with at least a 3,000-years history. It originated in China and the Chinese name is *Zhenjiu*, meaning needle and moxa, the two methods used to stimulate the acupoint. The occidental word "acupuncture" comes from the Latin words *acu* (needle) and *punctura*. Acupuncture is the treatment of illness by sticking needles in the skin at particular points on the body's surface, called acupoints. These points, described for the first time in a book in the second century BC, the *Huang-di Nei-jing* (the Emperor Huangdi's Canon of Medicine), are the same as those used today for medical treatments [1].

The West had already encountered acupuncture and TCM in ancient times, since the third century AD, even if, in the Middle Ages, the exchange of knowledge was limited because of the impossibility of meeting and comparing ideas. Only with the discovery of the Indies did direct trade with China favor closer relations, bringing to Europe the echoes of some of the TCM doctrines, such as the theory of the canals/meridians and the acupuncture points, along with other TCM techniques such as phytotherapy, diet therapy, and gymnastics. There were two reasons for this limited initial knowledge: first, the difficulties in translating a doctrine that was widely different from ours and in addition written in Chinese ideographs; the second reason was the scarce scientific and medical preparation of the diplomats and priests, above all Jesuits, who carried out these first translations. Later, during the seventeenth century, European doctors, particularly Dutch and German, who had had direct contact with China through the Dutch East Indies Company, translated Chinese medical texts. In the eighteenth century, more information reached Europe, mostly from French doctors and diplomats who had lived in the Far East. In the USA, news of this medicine arrived later: the first English translation of a French text on acupuncture was only published in 1826. All these contacts, although fascinating from a cultural point of view, did not, however, lead to a real comparison between the Western medical and academic world and the cultural and scientific heritage of acupuncture and TCM, which, in fact, tended to create ethnographical and anthropological rather than medical and scientific interest.

G. Lupi (✉)
Zhejiang Chinese Medical University, Hangzhou, China

Centro Medico di Agopuntura, Corso Dante 126, 10126 Torino, Italy
e-mail: info@centromedicoagopuntura.it

M. Cormio
Centro Medico di Agopuntura, Corso Dante 126, 10126 Torino, Italy

M. Fioranelli (ed.), *Integrative Cardiology*, DOI 10.1007/978-3-319-40010-5_4

It was only in the twentieth century, after the First World War, that western countries began to show a serious interest in acupuncture: the first real treatise on acupuncture in the West was the *Précis de la Vrai Acupuncture Chinoise* by George Soulié de Morant, the first volume of which was published in 1939. Interest grew after World War II and increased in the 1970s, at the end of the Cultural Revolution and the renewal of closer relations between China and the West.

In the USA, the beginning of greater awareness is usually considered to date from 1973, the year of Richard Nixon's visit to China, when one of the accompanying journalists underwent acupuncture treatment. As the news spread, it aroused a good deal of interest. In Europe, this process had already begun some years earlier, although its diffusion was slower and more gradual than in North America. However, the real spread of acupuncture in the West only began in the 1970s. At first acupuncture grew in popularity, but during the 1980s, this gradually extended to all the disciplines of TCM: massage and physiokinesiotherapy, dietetics and pharmacology, and psycho-corporal and medical gymnastics. In Italy, acupuncture was introduced slightly later than in other western countries; it began to spread from the 1960s/1970s, consolidating its expansion in the 1980s and becoming a deep-rooted medical practice by the 1990s. This diffusion began within small restricted groups of pioneers and interested persons linked mainly to the French Schools of Acupuncture. France, as we have already seen, thanks to its colonies, had scientific and cultural channels open with Vietnam and was certainly a leading nation in the early spread of acupuncture in continental Western Europe [2].

4.2 Acupuncture in Cardiovascular Diseases

4.2.1 Introduction

In the TCM, the heart is the most important organ and is described as the "Emperor" of all the internal organs. It is the seat of the mind, the ruler of blood circulation, and the source of the vascular system. Covered by the pericardium for protection, it is regarded as the "monarch organ" and the "supreme ruler of the *Zang-Fu* organs," which in TCM is the collective name for all internal organs. There are five *Zang* organs (heart, lung, spleen, liver, and kidney) and six *Fu* organs (gallbladder, stomach, small intestine, large intestine, bladder, and triple energizer). The *Zang* organs are mostly solid organs, characterized functionally as transforming, producing, and storing essential substances, but not discharging them; the *Fu* organs are characterized functionally by transforming and digesting food and drink and discharging metabolites.

The five *Zang* organs are regarded as the core structure and functions of the human body. Each organ is related to certain sense organs and tissues and is named based on the anatomy, but is not confined to anatomical entities; in fact, each can be regarded as a functional system.

The heart is described in *The Canon of Medicine and the Classic of Difficulties* (first or second century B.C.) as an organ "situated in the thorax" with its "apex contacting the diaphragm and the lung and its beat can be seen or felt under the left nipple, serving as the source of the pulse beat." In the *Yi Xue Ru Men* or *The ABC of Medicine* (1575), the authors wrote: "the Heart looks like a lotus in bud, below the Lungs and above the Liver." From this description, made many years ago, the heart in Chinese Medicine apparently refers to the same organ as in Western medicine [3, 4].

4.2.2 Physiology and Pathology

In TCM, the main physiological functions of the heart are to rule the blood and vessels and house the mind (Shen). The heartbeats drive blood to circulate through vessels to nourish the body, and this concept is similar to that of Western Medicine. To make this physiological function possible, two basic factors are necessary: a normal quantity of blood in the heart and vessels and a dynamic force that drives blood to circulate (Heart Qi). This is a very important aspect because normal heartbeats depend on adequate Heart Qi; only when Heart Qi is abundant can the Heart beat at a normal rate, rhythm, and strength, maintaining a normal blood circulation. On the other hand, a normal blood circulation also depends on the appropriate volume of heart blood. Thus, in the TCM, heart pathology, if Heart Qi is insufficient, there will be cardiac palpitations, shortness of breath, and a weak pulse. In severe cases, the patient can show precordial pain and a rapid and irregular or hesitant pulse. All these symptoms can be treated with acupuncture in a plan of integrative medicine: when the acupuncturist is a medical doctor, he uses western drugs along with all the tools of TCM.

In TCM, the heart is the "house of the mind"; it governs mental activities including consciousness, thinking, expression, and behavior. According to this function, the "heart," in Chinese medicine, refers to a part of the central nervous system, particularly the cerebral cortex. This concept seems to be entirely different from that of modern Western medicine. As previously mentioned, in TCM, different organs are not confined to anatomical entities; thus, not only the heart but also all the *Zang* organs take charge of mental activities and emotions. This is one of the holistic views of Chinese medicine, that all mental activities are reflections of the physiological functions of the organs.

Among the *Zang-Fu* organs, the heart is the supreme ruler; thus, as it is the commander of all *Zang-Fu* organs, the heart controls all the mental activities pertaining to the other organs. It can therefore be concluded that the Heart plays the most important role in higher nervous activity. The heart is the house of "Shen"; *Shen* means the comprehensive manifestation of life activities especially the spirit, consciousness, and thinking. This explains why in TCM the correct functioning of all the *Zang-Fu* organs is so important for preventing and curing cardiovascular diseases, and why it is fundamental to control different etiological factors such as joy, sadness, anger, the correct diet, the quality of life, etc. [3].

The same is the case in Western medicine: heart diseases constitute an essential problem of contemporary, developed societies. Despite continual progress being made in pharmacotherapy and in invasive cardiology, the number of heart disease cases has been systematically increasing and heart disease remains the world's number one killer [5]. The reason could be the complex etiology of these diseases; thus, to try to reduce the incidence of pathological heart conditions we must use different treatments. This is possible with integrative medicine, such as acupuncture; conventional medical treatment including lifestyle changes (stopping smoking, modifying diet, and increasing exercise); western drugs such as statins, nitrates, angiotensin-converting-enzyme (ACE) inhibitors, angiotensin II receptor blockers, calcium channel blockers, beta blockers, and antiplatelet drugs; and surgery such as coronary artery bypass grafts [6].

4.2.3 Cardiovascular Pathological Conditions: Evidence

As one of the oldest healing practices in the world, acupuncture has been used for several thousand years to treat many illnesses. In 2003, the World Health Organization (WHO) published a list of evidence-based conditions for which acupuncture could be used [7]. Specific to cardiology, angina pectoris, hypotension, and hypertension were listed. In recent years, however, the effectiveness of acupuncture in the treatment of these and other manifestations of cardiovascular diseases, such as ischemia, arrhythmias, and heart failure, and its effect on heart rate variability (HRV), have been studied and a large number of randomized controlled trials (RCTs) have been published [8].

4.3 Hypertension

Since the 1980s, various authors have demonstrated that several types of experimental hypertension, arrhythmias, and the defense reaction-induced pressure responses can be inhibited by electroacupuncture (EA), whereas hypotension and bradycardia can be alleviated by EA. Several experimental studies have been performed on this subject, from the vast epidemiological impact, above all to clarify the mechanisms of action of acupuncture on the control of the whole cardiovascular function and the possibility of influencing the autonomous nervous system.

Since 1984, numerous works provided by the Russian school have been published and even if planned otherwise, show the effectiveness of acupuncture in the control of light and modest hypertension, underlining at the same time the immediate effect of acupuncture on the pressure values and on the normalization of other parameters inherent to the neurovegetative and psychic functions [2].

A work in which the authors used real acupuncture versus sham acupuncture in ten patients suffering from hypertension revealed, in the group treated with real acupuncture, an immediate reduction of the diastolic pressure values. The acupoints used were Taichong LR3, Zusanli ST36, Quchi LI11, and the auricular point of hypertension [9].

In a controlled study, published in 1997, the authors have documented the increase in the systolic and diastolic pressure values in 50 patients not undergoing drug treatment. The authors also reported a significant decrease in renin activity, whereas the values of vasopressin and cortisol remained unchanged [10].

Thanks to the large number of studies published, in 2002, the WHO reported that acupuncture is suitable for treating primary hypotension and early essential hypertension. It has been reported that the influence of acupuncture on hypertension may be related to its regulatory effect on the level of serum nitrogen monoxide. For primary hypotension, acupuncture seems to be more effective than general tonics. For mild and moderate essential hypertension, the hypotensive effect of acupuncture is much more potent than that of placebos and is comparable with that of certain conventional hypotensive agents [11]. The importance of the integrative treatment has been shown in a recent meta-analysis; in fact, the authors's results were consistent with the notion that acupuncture significantly lowers blood pressure in patients taking antihypertesive medications [12]. In addition, acupuncture is often effective for relieving subjective symptoms, and it has no side effects. The long history of clinical practice has proven that acupuncture has curative effects, but the physiological basis requires more scientific study. In a recent systematic review, the authors explored the clinical evidence for or against acupuncture as a treatment of various types of cardiac arrhythmias, concluding that several studies demonstrated that acupuncture may be an effective treatment [13].

We know that overactivity of the sympathetic nervous system commonly initiates and sustains blood pressure (BP) elevation in patients with essential hypertension [14], but also the overactivity of the renin–angiotensin–aldosterone system can cause BP elevation [15]. From the beginning, the pharmacological approach to hypertension has been the regulation of one or both of these systems that are responsible for regulating BP and fluid balance in the body; however, from the clinic, we know that unfortunately, many patients require two or more drugs for optimal control [16]. Another problem due to the Western medicine is the difficulty of providing a safe therapy with fewer adverse side effects [17]. Yin et al. [18] examined the use of individualized manual acupuncture (different acupoints in different patients after syndrome differentiation) versus noninvasive sham as an add-on therapy for hypertensive patients concurrently treated with various antihypertensive medications. A significant reduction in both systolic and diastolic BP was observed in the acupuncture compared with the sham group. A preliminary study examining point-specific responses such as hypertension control found that applying EA at Jianshi PC5–Neiguan PC6 and Zusanli ST36–Shangjuxu ST37 once weekly for 8 weeks reduced peak and average systolic and peak diastolic BP by 5 mmHg or more in 70% of patients, whereas EA at Pianli LI6–Wenliu LI7 and Guangming GB37–Xuanzhong GB39 did not consistently lower BP [19]. EA reinforcement treatment at Jianshi PC5–Neiguan PC6 and Zusanli ST36–Shangjuxu ST37 once a month maintained the reduction in BP over the 6-month period. In a meta-analysis published in 2014, examining RCTs using real versus sham acupuncture for the treatment of hypertension, four trials qualified for the analysis. This meta-analysis suggested that acupuncture might significantly lower systolic BP and diastolic BP in patients taking antihypertensive medications, but only lower diastolic BP in unmedicated patients. Most of these patients received individualized manual acupuncture treatment using TCM principles to guide the selection of acupoints [12].

4.3.1 Hypertension in TCM

Acupuncture generally works by harmonizing the body's energy balance: in parts of the body where there is too much energy, the needles help to remove the excess and bring the body back into balance. From the TCM perspective, hypertension is a disorder of the *yin–yang* balance, and the treatment is aimed at restoring this balance. It is usually caused by emotional factors, diet, and constitutional defects that lead to an imbalance of yin and yang in the liver, spleen, and kidneys. Since balance restoration takes a considerable period of time, from the beginning an integrative therapy is needed, but once there is a therapeutic effect, this can often last for a long period. In addition, during Chinese medical treatment, the patient's general condition improves first and the blood pressure lowers later [3, 20].

1. Hyperactivity of liver yang and up-flaming of liver fire. The liver is closely related to psychic and emotional activities: mental stress or anger may cause hyperactivity of the liver yang, resulting in irritability, headache, dizziness, flushing face and red eyes, bitterness in the mouth, tinnitus, aversion to heat, insomnia, and constipation.
2. Yin deficiency of the liver and kidneys and a deficiency of yin with exuberant yang. The kidneys use their essence to produce marrow, and the brain is the "sea of marrow." In kidney yin deficiency, nourishment of the brain is often impaired and dizziness occurs. There may be other symptoms, such as a hot sensation in the palms and pain in the heels, tinnitus, and insomnia. Kidney yin deficiency is usually accompanied by deficiency of all the body's yin, in particular, liver yin, with the consequent exuberant liver yang. In this case, the relative excessiveness of yang may still lead to irritability, headache, and aggravate dizziness.
3. Deficiency of both yin and yang. Protracted yin deficiency may involve yang; besides dizziness, there may be symptoms such as cool limbs and an aversion to coldness, palpitations, nocturia, and edema.
4. Internal retention of phlegm-damp. Improper diet, overwork, and stress may damage the transporting and transforming functions of the spleen, resulting in the production of damp and phlegm. Retained phlegm-damp gives rise not only to dizziness, but sometimes numbness of the limbs, headache with the sensation of pressure in the head, a sensation of oppression in the chest, and hypertension [3, 20].

4.3.2 Acupuncture

Common points are [3, 20]:

Baihui (GV20), Fengchi (GB20), Zusanli (ST36), Quchi (LI11), Taichong (LR3), auricular point of hypertension

Additional points are:

1. Hyperactivity of liver yang and up-flaming of liver fire: Xingjian (LR2)
2. Yin deficiency of liver and kidneys and deficiency of yin with exuberant yang: Sanyinjiao (SP6), Taixi (KI 3)
3. Deficiency of both yin and yang: Zhaohai (KI6), Qihai (CV6), Guanyuan (CV4)
4. Interior retention of phlegm-damp: Jianshi PC5, Neiguan (PC6), Shangjuxu (ST37), Fenglong (ST40)

4.4 Myocardial Infarction and Coronary Heart Disease

We know that the autonomic nervous system plays an important role in the modulation of cardiac electrophysiology and arrhythmogenesis [21]. In general, acupuncture is believed to stimulate the nervous system and cause the release of neurochemical messenger molecules; the resulting biochemical changes influence the body's homeostatic mechanisms, thus promoting physical and emotional well-being.

Acupuncture therapy has been confirmed to be effective in treating cardiovascular diseases in clinical practice, and the acupuncture-induced balance of the autonomic nervous system activities is one of its key mechanisms [22]. Several randomized controlled trials show evidence for acupuncture in the treatment of coronary heart disease, including angina pectoris and myocardial infarction.

Myocardial ischemia and the consequent cardiac damage resulting from a lack of blood flow to the heart muscle can lead to cell death or infarction [23]. The severity and duration of post-ischemic changes depend on the length and intensity of the ischemia and can ultimately lead to heart failure [24]. Norepinephrine, a neurotransmitter released by the sympathetic nervous system, can increase the extent of ischemia by increasing demand for myocardial oxygen and causing coronary vasoconstriction [25], and the increases in sympathetic activation during myocardial ischemia can also lead to arrhythmias and increase infarct size [26].

Since the 1980s, various studies have been published to evaluate the effects of acupuncture on myocardial ischemia. Chen et al. [27] showed that the stimulation of the acupoint Neiguan PC6 increases myocardial contractility in congestive cardiomyopathy; the stimulation of the acupoint Shaofu HT8 instead decreases the contractive force of the myocardium and turns out to be positive in patients with hypertrophic cardiomyopathy. Li et al. [28] described the positive effects of acupuncture on cardiovascular function in patients with acute myocardial infarction. In this study, the authors compared the clinical and instrumental data of a group of patients treated only using drug therapy with those obtained in another group subjected to acupuncture and drug therapy combined.

Liu et al. [29] studied the effects of acupuncture on 100 patients suffering from coronary heart disease in a blinded controlled study. The authors used an acupuncture group and two control groups, one composed of healthy volunteers treated as patients, the other of subjects suffering from coronary heart disease treated with sham acupuncture at non-acupuncture points. In the subjects treated with true acupuncture, a significant increase in the contractility of the rear ventricular wall and an increase in the volume of the cardiac output, in contrast to the trend of the control group. It is interesting to note that in healthy subjects, significant variations in the cardio-circulatory function have not been highlighted.

In a study performed by Ballegaard et al. [30] on 49 patients with angina (two groups: real acupuncture vs sham acupuncture), the authors showed a reduction of 50% in the angina attacks and in the use of nitro-derivative medicines in both groups, the patients who underwent the real acupuncture also showed significant changes in resistance to stress (+9%) and timing of onset of angina pain (+10%) compared with the sham group.

In human trials, Ballegaard et al. [31] demonstrated that 3 weeks of manual acupuncture (seven treatments) at Neiguan PC6, Zusanli ST36, and Jueyinshu BL14 in normotensive patients with >50% coronary stenosis, positive stress tests, and severe refractory angina significantly increased cardiac working capacity, compared with sham (points in outside meridians, same dermatome). Ballegaard et al. [32] also conducted a 2-year prospective, nonrandomized trial (on a group of 105 angina patients) to explore the cost savings potential of acupuncture followed by acupressure as part of a lifestyle program. Among the most interesting data, we note the improvement in the New York Heart Association (NYHA) index (evaluating the general conditions of the cardiac patient and their quality of life): the patients with a grade of NYHA 0–1, without any limitation in their day-to-day life, comprised only 8% at the beginning of the study; they proportion increased to 53% by the end of the first year and to 63% after 5 years. The economic benefit of $32,000 (USA) per patient was also evaluated, resulting from a reduction of 90% in the hospitalization time and 70% for surgical services [33]. An investigation by Richter et al. demonstrated that manual acupuncture (manipulated only once upon insertion) at Neiguan PC6, Tongli HT5, Xinshu BL15, Pishu BL20, and Zusanli ST36, administered three times for 30 min each week for 4 weeks reduced the number of angina attacks, the intensity of pain, and ST segment depression compared with placebo [34].

The WHO states that encouraging results have been reported for a number of controlled studies on the treatment of heart disease with acupuncture, particularly in psychosomatic heart disorders, such as cardiac neurosis [11]. In coronary heart disease, acupuncture has been shown by various authors to be effective in relieving angina pectoris [35]; its beneficial influence has been demonstrated during coronary arteriography. Cardiological, neurophysiological, and psychological observations, made in mutually independent studies, indicated that acupuncture improved the working capacity of the heart in patients with angina pectoris and activated autoregulatory cardiovascular mechanisms in healthy persons [11]. A systematic review of 16 randomized controlled trials (RCTs) found that acupuncture added to conventional drugs reduced the occurrence of acute myocardial infarction. Compared with drugs alone, both acupuncture alone and acupuncture plus conventional drugs proved more effective at relieving angina symptoms and improving electrocardiography. However, compared with conventional treatment, acupuncture alone showed a longer delay before its onset of action, probably indicating that it is not suitable for the emergency treatment of myocardial infarction [36].

A laboratory trial by Zhou et al. examined the response to EA in a model of myocardial ischemia–reperfusion (MIR) injury in six different groups of rabbits. The authors have studied the responses with EA Jianshi PC5–Neiguan PC6 (2 Hz for 30 min) at different times and with different association. The authors concluded that EA reduces ischemia–reperfusion injury through both opioid and protein kinase C-dependent mechanisms and has the potential to play an important role in the clinical treatment of cardiac ischemia [37].

From the literature, we notice that clinical improvement and cardiovascular benefits were gained with manual acupuncture using EA at Jianshi PC5–Neiguan PC6 and Zusanli ST36–Shangjuxu ST37 in non-ischemic patients. We hypothesize that we might obtain good results in ischemic patients too, but further studies are needed to confirm.

4.4.1 Coronary Heart Disease in TCM

The common feature of angina pectoris is impaired blood flow in the vessels of the heart. Coronary heart disease is usually related to aging, weakness, improper diet, and emotional factors that often lead to inactivation of chest yang, stagnation of cold and phlegm in the collaterals, in addition to Qi stagnation and blood stasis. Excessive rich food may impair the spleen and stomach, producing endogenous phlegm-damp or leading to Qi deficiency. When phlegm-damp invades the heart, it impedes the flow of Qi and blood, resulting in angina pectoris, but in angina pectoris, the heart, spleen, kidneys, and liver may be involved; deficiency of Qi, yin, and yang are the fundamental pathological changes; and blood stasis, Qi stagnation, phlegm-damp accumulation, and cold are the precipitating factors [3, 20].

4.4.2 Acupuncture

Common points are [3, 20]:

Xinshu (BL15), Juque (CV14), Tanzhong (CV17), Neiguan (PC6), Tongli (HT5), Shaofu HT8

Additional points are:

1. Obstruction by phlegm: Fenglong (ST40), Taiyuan (LU9), Jianshi PC5
2. Retention of blood stasis in the collaterals: Geshu (BL17), Xuehai (BL10)
3. Deficit of the Spleen: Pishu (BL20), Sanyinjiao (SP6), Zusanli (ST36), Shangjuxu (ST37)

4.5 Rhythm Disorders

Arrhythmia refers to the abnormal frequency and rhythm of the heart beating. We know that cardiac arrhythmias constitute one of the most significant risk factors for heart disease [38]; ischemia and increases in sympathetic activity are causal factors for both supraventricular and ventricular arrhythmias [39].

Given that acupuncture reduces ischemia and inhibits sympathetic outflow, it could also be used as a modality in the treatment of cardiac arrhythmias that are related to augmented sympathetic outflow and sympathetic/parasympathetic imbalance [40]. A study conducted by Liptak et al. in 1980 on 33 patients with extra systoles shows that both acupuncture and EA can considerably reduce the number of extra systoles during needle stimulation, whereas the heart rate remains unchanged; to explain these clinical data, the author suggests an effect at the level of the vegetative and neuroendocrine system [41]. Another survey conducted in subjects with normal sino-atrial conduction has also shown that EA stimulation of the acupoints Neiguan PC6 and Jianshi PC5 significantly shortens the sino-atrial contraction time compared with the control group not subjected to any stimulation [42].

Shi et al. in 1995 studied changes in heart rhythm components at low and high frequency in coronaropathic patients treated in acupoint Neiguan PC6. The results show a significant improvement only as far as the low frequency is concerned, also emphasizing that manual acupuncture reached maximum impact within 10 min from the beginning of the treatment; the values returned to standard 20–30 min later, without any rebound effect [43]. In experimental models, it was demonstrated that EA at Neiguan PC6 and Zusanli ST36 reduced premature ventricular contractions and ventricular tachycardia [44]. A meta-analysis by Kim et al. [13] was published, examining the effectiveness of acupuncture in the treatment of cardiac arrhythmias. This chapter evaluated the response of paroxysmal supraventricular tachycardia, premature ventricular contractions (PVCs), and atrial fibrillation to acupuncture. Given that the majority of studies were of low methodological quality and included small sample sizes, Kim et al. cautiously concluded that acupuncture may be an effective treatment for arrhythmias.

4.5.1 Arrhythmias in TCM

Arrhythmias are attributed to the yin–yang imbalance of the heart, disorders in nourishing the heart, or disturbances of the heart by phlegm-fire or blood stasis. This disease is usually caused by a weak constitution, emotional stimulation, excessive anxiety, and invasion of pathogenic factors that lead to heart malnutrition due to Qi deficiency, blood, yin and yang, or by phlegm-fire attacking the heart, and stagnation of the heart's blood [3, 20]. These causes can be summarized as follows:

1. Deficiency of Qi and blood: palpitation and shortness of breath aggravated by dizziness, insomnia, and lassitude.
2. Deficiency of yin with exuberant yang: palpitations and restlessness accompanied by dizziness, tinnitus, bitterness in the mouth, and insomnia.
3. Phlegm-fire: restlessness and oppression in the chest, palpitations, insomnia and disturbed sleep, expectoration with sticky sputum, and dry mouth.

4. Qi stagnation and blood stasis: palpitation and oppression in the chest, sometimes with pectoral pain, amnesia, and insomnia [3, 20].

4.5.2 Acupuncture

Common points are [3, 20]:

Xinshu (BL15), Jueyinshu (BL14), Neiguan (PC6), Shenzhu (GV12), Shendao (GV11), Shenmen (HT7)

Additional points are:

1. Deficiency of Qi and blood: Danzhong (CV17), Guanyuan (CV4), Zusanli (ST36), Sanyinjiao (SP6), Pishu (BL20), Geshu (BL17)
2. Deficiency of Qi and yin: Qihai (CV6), Yinlingquan (SP9), Zusanli (ST36), Taixi (KI3)
3. Phlegm-fire: Chize (LU5), Feishu (BL13), Fenglong (ST40), Jianshi PC5
4. Qi stagnation and blood stasis: Qihai (CV6), Xuehai (SP10), Danzhong (CV17), Ximen (PC4)

4.6 Conclusion

Heart diseases constitute the essential problem of contemporary developed societies. Despite the continual progress in pharmacotherapy and in invasive cardiology, the number of heart disease cases has been systematically increasing, and heart disease remains the number one killer in the world. Much effort is made to try to reduce the incidence of pathological heart conditions, but we know that to reach this goal we must use different treatments: integrative medicine, such as acupuncture and integrative conventional medical treatment including lifestyle changes such as stopping smoking, modifying diet, and increasing exercise. The number of studies to evaluate the efficacy of manual acupuncture or EA to treat symptoms of heart disease is large, and even if the quality is low, it appears that this ancient therapy may be beneficial in several cardiovascular disease conditions. EA appears to be useful in patients with mild to moderate hypertension, whether antihypertensive drugs are used or not. Acupuncture can also be used in all those patients who elect to remain unmedicated because of unwanted side effects. Certainly, it can provide a treatment alternative for patients with myocardial ischemia, it may help to treat arrhythmias, and can reduce angina and the need for nitroglycerin. The last but not least, when integrated into a holistic program, may produce cost savings. Thus, thanks to all these positive therapeutic effects, the lack of side effects [45], and the relatively low cost, the use of acupuncture and more specifically EA may be warranted, although a large number of high-quality studies is needed.

From the different studies published, it appears that the most common acupoint used in the treatment of cardiovascular diseases is Neiguan PC6. Point stimulation may be manual or electrical, but, to reduce the difference between clinicians and lead to more consistent clinical outcomes, it is better to administer EA at Jianshi PC5–Neiguan PC6 at 2 Hz for 30 min. In various published meta-analyses it appears that one of the most important biases in acupuncture research is the protocol: for the same pathologyical condition different clinicians use different numbers and acupoints, without the correct TCM differentiation. Therefore, more research is needed to determine the correct selection of acupoints and which other points may or may not provide an added benefit. At this time, it appears that employing EA at Zusanli ST36–Shangjuxu ST37 in conjunction with Jianshi PC5–Neiguan PC6 might provide optimal clinical cardiovascular responses. In conclusion, acupuncture is a save and safety therapy with no side effects that can be used as integrative medicine to treat some cardiovascular diseases.

4.7 Cardiology and Myofascial Trigger Points

During the past few decades, myofascial trigger points (MTrPs) and myofascial pain syndrome

(MPS) have received much attention in the scientific and clinical literature. Researchers worldwide are investigating various aspects of MTrPs, including their specific etiology, pathophysiology, histology, referred pain patterns, and clinical applications [46, 47].

Although Dr. Janet Travell (US President JF Kennedy's MD) (1901–1997) is generally credited for bringing MTrPs to the attention of healthcare providers, MTrPs have been described and rediscovered for several centuries by various clinicians and researchers. In the late 1930s, Travell, who at that time was a cardiologist and medical researcher, became particularly interested in muscle pain [48].

Chronic myofascial pain can mimic or accompany cardiovascular disease [49]. The reader needs to be familiar with the MTrPs.

4.7.1 Clinical Aspects of Myofascial Trigger Points

An MTrP is described as "a hyperirritable spot in skeletal muscle that is associated with a hypersensitive palpable nodule in a taut band."

The classical and most commonly used description of trigger points is that by Travell and Simons [48]. They defined trigger points as the presence of exquisite tenderness at a nodule in a palpable taut band (of muscle). Trigger points can produce referred pain, either spontaneously or on digital compression. The clinical definition came to be that trigger points are localized areas of deep tenderness within a taut band of muscle. They exhibit a local twitch response (muscle fasciculation) or jump sign (whole body movement) in response to digital pressure or dry needling. In their text, Simons et al. [48] also produced body maps of common trigger point locations and their referral zones. These locations have been noted to have significant similarities to acupuncture points used in traditional Chinese medicine for the relief of pain [50].

Myofascial trigger points are the hallmark characteristics of MPS and feature motor, sensory, and autonomic components. Motor aspects of MTrPs may include disturbed motor function, muscle weakness as a result of motor inhibition, muscle stiffness, and restricted range of motion. Sensory aspects may include local tenderness, referral of pain to a distant site, and peripheral and central sensitization. Peripheral sensitization can be described as a reduction in threshold and an increase in responsiveness of the peripheral ends of nociceptors, whereas central sensitization is an increase in the excitability of neurons within the central nervous system. Signs of peripheral and central sensitization are allodynia (pain due to a stimulus that does not normally provoke pain) and hyperalgesia (an increased response to a stimulus that is normally painful). MTrPs are painful on compression. A detailed clinical history, examination of movement patterns, and consideration of muscle referred-pain patterns assist clinicians in determining which muscles may harbor clinically relevant MTrPs. Muscle pain is perceived as aching and poorly localized. There are no laboratory or imaging tests available that can confirm the presence of MTrPs, which are identified through the palpation technique. The presence of a so-called local twitch response (LTR), referred pain, or reproduction of the person's symptomatic pain increases the certainty and specificity of the diagnosis of MTrPs.

Myofascial pain syndromes can be primary or secondary conditions. When they are secondary, they occur as a manifestation of another disorder. A regional pain referral from a visceral disorder can induce secondary MPS. Visceral disorders induce central sensitization with hypersensitivity and expansion in the number and size of receptive fields. Central sensitization is topographically organized in the spinal cord, being segmentally predominant at the level of the affected viscera. The associated MPS tend to be regional, but are related to the segmental innervation of the affected viscera. Regional MPS in turn can mimic visceral disease or be the diagnostic sign of visceral disease. Cardiac disease, gastrointestinal disorders, hepatic and biliary disorders, irritable bowel syndrome, and interstitial cystitis are some of the conditions in which MPS can occur secondarily or that they mimic.

The most common etiological mechanisms include: low-level muscle contractions, uneven intramuscular pressure distribution, direct trauma, unaccustomed eccentric contractions, eccentric contractions in unconditioned muscle, and maximal or submaximal concentric contractions [51].

4.7.2 MTrPs in Cardiology

Chest pain is a common presenting symptom in primary care. The foremost concern among most patients is that the underlying cause of the pain may be related to their heart. However, once patients have been referred to secondary care for investigations, as many as half of them are diagnosed with noncardiac chest pain. As an example, the trigger points in the pectoralis major and minor muscles can produce symptoms that are nearly identical to the pain associated with having a heart attack or angina pectoris. Referred pain from these trigger points is experienced in the chest, front of the shoulder, down the inside of the arm, and along the inside of the elbow [49].

First and foremost, everything described below assumes that a cardiac source of chest pain has been ruled out by a cardiologist. Only after being cleared by a cardiologist should this myofascial source of chest pain be investigated.

4.7.3 Which Muscles May Be Involved in Cardiology?

There may be a TrP on the right-side pectoralis major between the fifth and sixth ribs about midway between the nipple and the outer edge of the sternum that may be involved with cardiac arrhythmias. Treating the TrP may eliminate the arrhythmia. Pectoralis major MTrPs cause pain under the sternum. They also transmit pain to the front of the chest and breast, extending down to the little finger side of the arm to the fourth and fifth fingers. MTrPs on the left side often mimic heart-attack pain.

Pectoralis MTrPs can occur in any of the muscle layers, in any place, but they are most common in certain areas. At the collarbone, they cause local pain and refer pain over the front of the shoulder. In the breastbone area, MTrPs can broadcast intermittent, intense pain to the front of the chest and down the inner aspect of the arm. This can include a feeling of chest tightness, often mistaken for angina. These MTrPs can radiate pain to the inside top of the forearm, and to the little finger side of the hand, including the last two or more fingers. If there are arrhythmias and no other signs of heart problems, check for MTrPs. Chest pain that persists after a heart attack is frequently caused by these MTrPs.

Pectoralis minor MTrPs are most often located in an area about midway between the clavicle and nipple, and about midway between the edge of the breastbone and the outer edge of the upper arm. These MTrPs send pain over the front of the chest and shoulder. Pain may run down the inner side of the arm and include the last three fingers. Pain from a left side pectoralis minor MTrP can mimic angina. These MTrPs can also entrap the axillary artery and the brachial plexus nerve. The radial pulse may disappear as your patient moves the arm to different positions [48]. When you relieve the TrP, the pulse is restored.

Shortness of breath is often due to MTrPs in the serratus anterior muscle and is commonly associated with a "stitch in the side." There is referred pain to the side and to the back of the chest. This includes the lower interior border of the shoulder blade and sometimes the pain runs down the inner area of the arm, hand, and the last two fingers. There may be air hunger, with panting or mouth breathing. In severe cases, there is chest pain, even at rest. The nerve going to the serratus anterior muscle may be entrapped because of scalene muscle MTrPs. These MTrPs may also contribute substantially to the pain of a heart attack [48]. It can also cause a catch in the lower inner side of the shoulder blade. Serratus posterior inferior MTrPs produce an unusual ache radiating over and around the muscle. Iliocostalis thoracis MTrPs at mid-chest level send pain upward toward the shoulder and sideways toward the chest wall. Trigger points on the left side in this area cause pain that is often mistaken for angina.

All major scalene muscles can refer pain to the front and back of the body in a widespread pattern. At the front, they cause persistent aching pain over the chest and down the front and back of the arm to the forearm. The patient may report that the chest feels tight. On the left side, this pain may be mistaken for angina. There may be numbness, tingling, and odd sensations in the fourth and fifth fingers and in the little finger side of the hand and forearm.

Intercostal MTrPs cause primarily local aching pain. Palpate for these MTrPs around the ribs. They are most often located on the front of the body, close to the side. The patient may not be able to endure pressure on these MTrPs. The pain increases when s/he takes a deep breath, coughs, or sneezes. In the area near the breastbone, these MTrPs may cause cardiac arrhythmia [48].

Diaphragm MTrPs refer pain in two different directions, using two different neural pathways. One sends pain to the upper border of the shoulder on the same side as the MTrP, from MTrPs in the diaphragm dome. MTrPs along the edges send pain to the edges of the ribs close by. Diaphragm MTrPs can cause the "stitch in the side," chest pain, or inability to draw a full breath. The pain will be most intense on exhalation after a deep breath. These MTrPs cause restricted rotation of the spine upon twisting to look behind. Chronic cough and paradoxical breathing perpetuate these MTrPs, as will head-forward, slumped-shouldered posture. Local impact trauma, chest surgery (chest retractors are likely to leave clusters of MTrPs in their wake), herpes zoster, and rib fractures are also possible initiating and perpetuating factors, as are tumors, and some repetitive exercises.

Many cases of Raynaud's phenomenon have a TrP component. Numbness and odd sensations of the fourth and fifth fingers are common with these MTrPs. There may be peculiar sensations over some parts of the forearm and over the palmar side of the first three and a half fingers. Paradoxical breathing perpetuates this TrP, as does poor posture. Check standing and sitting movements and ask about sleep positions. Blood vessel entrapment by these MTrPs does not produce the hand puffiness associated with scalene entrapment. Connective tissue MTrPs in scar tissue of the attachment area in some rotator cuff tissues may cause referred tenderness, hot prickling pain, and lightning-like jabs to the pectoralis area.

Chest tightness may also be due to MTrPs in the sternalis muscle. Sternalis MTrPs cause a deep ache under the breastbone, extending over the entire region of the breastbone and below. This can cover the upper chest and front of the shoulder on the same side, including the underarm and upper arm on the little finger side up to the elbow, and produces an ache that feels like a heart attack or angina and is independent of body movement. Trigger points can occur anywhere within the sternalis, but they are often found in the upper two-thirds and to the left of center at mid-sternal level.

Myofascial trigger points in the jaw and neck can contribute to referred chest pain. Overburdening these muscles can cause MTrPs, which can be formed during a heart attack or other visceral disease. When a coronary artery disease occurs, if the patient has angina or has had a heart attack, s/he probably has MTrPs, as these events can be initiating factors. Treating the MTrPs may reduce the symptom level.

If these or any MTrPs keep recurring, in spite of proper treatment, the perpetuating factor must be found. There could be a visceral problem, for example. Such organic disease can cause MTrPs. Relieving the MTrPs may relieve the symptoms for a short period, but the underlying problem is still there.

4.7.4 Trigger Point Therapy

Trigger point therapy is essentially divided into invasive and non-invasive techniques. Non-invasive techniques are those that have been traditionally employed by physical and manual therapists. In recent years, there has been a marked increase in the use of invasive therapies, in particular, acupuncture (needle therapy), to manage trigger points.

Needling involves multiple advances of an acupuncture-type needle into the muscle in the region of a trigger point, aiming to reproduce the patient's symptoms, visualize local twitch responses, and achieve relief of muscle tension and pain. In an early study, dry needling was found to be equivalent to local anesthetic, corticosteroid, and coolant spray in the treatment of lower back pain.

The major drawback to the use of dry needling over local anesthetic injection is the higher incidence of post-treatment soreness. This would appear to be maximal in the 24 h after therapy and is usually manageable with heat packs and stretching, but may be intolerable to some patients, and therefore care with patient selection is important.

References

1. Stein RA, Oz MC (eds) (2004) Complementary and alternative cardiovascular medicine. Humana, Totowa, NJ
2. Vari AA (2000) Agopuntura: evidenze cliniche e sperimentali aspetti legislativi e diffusione in Italia. Casa Editrice Ambrosiana, Mila
3. Xie Z (2000) Practical traditional Chinese medicine. Foreign Language Press, Beijing
4. Cheng X (1987) Chinese acupuncture and moxibustion. Foreign Languages Press, Beijing
5. Piepoli MF, Corrà U, Adamopoulos S et al (2012) Secondary prevention in the clinical management of patients with cardiovascular diseases. Core components, standards and outcome measures for referral and delivery: a Policy Statement from the Cardiac Rehabilitation Section of the European Association for Cardiovascular Prevention & Rehabilitation. Endorsed by the Committee for Practice Guidelines of the European Society of Cardiology. Eur J Prev Cardiol 21:664–681
6. Peterssen S, Peto V, Scarborough PRM (2005) Coronary heart statistics. British Heart Foundation, London
7. Zhang X (2002) Acupuncture: teview and analysis of reports on controlled clinical trials. World Health Organization, Geneva
8. Painovich J, Longhurst J (2015) Integrating acupuncture into the cardiology clinic: can it play a role? Acta Physiol Sin 67(1):19–31
9. Williams T, Mueller K, Cornwall MW (1991) Effect of acupuncture point stimulation on diastolic blood pressure in hypertensives subjects: a preliminary study. Phys Ther 71(7):523–529
10. Chiu YJ, Chi A, Reid IA (1997) Cardiovascular and endocrine effects of acupuncture in hypertensive patients. Clin Exp Hypertens 19(7):1047–1063
11. WHO (2002) Acupuncture: review and analysis of reports on controlled clinical trials. World Health Organization, Geneva
12. Li DZ, Zhou Y, Yang YN et al (2014) Acupuncture for essential hypertension: a meta-analysis of randomized sham-controlled clinical trials. Evid Based Complement Alternat Med 2014:279478
13. Kim TH, Choi TY, Lee MS, Ernst E (2011) Acupuncture treatment for cardiac arrhythmias: a systematic review of randomized controlled trials. Int J Cardiol 149(2):263–265
14. Oparil S, Zaman MA, Calhoun DA (2003) Pathogenesis of hypertension. Ann Intern Med 139:761–776
15. Weir MR, Dzau VJ (1999) The renin-angiotensin-aldosterone system: a specific target for hypertension management. Am J Hypertens 12:205S–213S
16. Chobanian AV, Bakris GL, Black HR, Cushman WC, Green LA, Izzo JL Jr, Jones DW, Materson BJ, Oparil S, Wright JT Jr, Roccella EJ (2003) Joint National Committee on Prevention, Detection, Evaluation, and Treatment of High Blood Pressure. Hypertension 42:1206–1252
17. Claxton AJ, Cramer J, Pierce C (2001) A systematic review of the associations between dose regimens and medication compliance. Clin Ther 23:1296–1310
18. Yin C, Seo B, Park HJ et al (2007) Acupuncture, a promising adjunctive therapy for essential hypertension: a double-blind, randomized, controlled trial. Neurol Res 29 [Suppl 1]:S98–S103
19. Li P, Cheng L, Liu DM, Painovich J et al (2014) Long-lasting inhibitory effect of electroacupuncture in hypertensive patients; role of catecholamine, renin and angiotensin. FASEB J 28:1140.3
20. Zhao J (2002) Chinese acupuncture and moxibustion. Publishing House of Shanghai University of TCM, Shanghai
21. Shen MJ, Zipes DP (2014) Role of the autonomic nervous system in modulating cardiac arrhythmias. Circ Res 114(6):1004–1021
22. Wang YL, Yu Z, Xu B (2014) Progress of studies on mechanisms of acupuncture underlying regulation of cardiac function via autonomic nervous system. Zhen Ci Yan Jiu 39(1):83–86
23. Remme WJ (2000) Overview of the relationship between ischemia and congestive heart failure. Clin Cardiol 23:IV4–IV8
24. Braunwald E, Kloner RA (1982) The stunned myocardium: prolonged, postischemic ventricular dysfunction. Circulation 66:1146–1149
25. Hashimoto M, Okamoto M, Yamagata T et al (1993) Abnormal systolic blood pressure response during exercise recovery in patients with angina pectoris. J Am Coll Cardiol 22:659–664
26. Harris AS, Otero H, Bocage AJ (1971) The induction of arrhythmias by sympathetic activity before and

after occlusion of a coronary artery in canine heart. J Electrocardiol 4:434–443
27. Chen SX, Bao S, Chang P et al (1983) Preliminary investigation on the effect of acupuncture of Neiguan and Shaofu on cardiac function of idiopathic cardiomyopathy. J Tradit Chin Med 3(2):113–120
28. Li CJ, Bi LG, Zhu BJ et al (1986) Effects of acupuncture on left ventricular function, microcirculation, cAMP, and cGMP of acute myocardial infarction patients. J Tradit Chin Med 6(3):157–161
29. Liu FZ, Li JL, Liu GZ et al (1986) Clinical observation of effects of acupuncture on angina pectoris. In: Research on acupuncture, moxibustion and acupuncture anaesthesia. Science Press, Bejing, pp 861–875
30. Ballegaard S, Pedersen F, Pietersen A et al (1990) Effects of acupuncture on moderate, stable angina pectoris: a controlled study. J Intern Med 227:25–30
31. Ballegaard S, Jensen G, Pedersen F, Nissen VH (1986) Acupuncture in severe, stable angina pectoris: a randomized trial. Acta Med Scand 220:307–313
32. Ballegaard S, Norrelund S, Smith DF (1996) Cost-benefit of combined use of acupuncture, Shiatsu and lifestyle adjustment for treatment of patients with severe angina pectoris. Acupunct Electrother Res 21:187–197
33. Ballegaard S, Johannessen A, Karpatschof B et al (1999) Addition of acupuncture and self-care education in treatment of patients with severe angina pectoris may be cost beneficial: an open prospective study. J Altern Complement Med 5(5):405–413
34. Richter A, Herlitz J, Hjalmarson A (1991) Effect of acupuncture in patients with angina pectoris. Eur Heart J 12:175–178
35. Xu L, Xu H, Gao W, Wang W, Zhang H, Lu DP (2013) Treating angina pectoris by acupuncture therapy. Acupunct Electrother Res 38(1-2):17–35
36. Chen J, Ren Y, Tang Y, Li Z, Liang F (2012) Acupuncture therapy for angina pectoris: a systematic review. J Tradit Chin Med 32(4):494–501
37. Zhou W, Ko Y, Benharash P et al (2012) Cardioprotection of electroacupuncture against myocardial ischemia-reperfusion injury by modulation of cardiac norepinephrine release. Am J Physiol Heart Circ Physiol 302:H1818–H1825
38. Zheng ZJ, Croft JB, Giles WH, Mensah GA (2001) Sudden cardiac death in the United States, 1989 to 1998. Circulation 104:2158–2163
39. Kalman JM, Munawar M, Howes LG et al (1995) Atrial fibrillation after coronary artery bypass grafting is associated with sympathetic activation. Ann Thorac Surg 60:1709–1715
40. Chung JW, Yan VC, Zhang H (2014) Effect of acupuncture on heart rate variability: a systematic review. Evid Based Complement Alternat Med 2014:819871
41. Liptak V, Habeler G, Egger J (1980) Influence of acupuncture and electro-acupuncture on heart rate and extrasystoles. Wien Med Wochenschr 130 (20):668–670
42. Xi IA, Zou P, Song T (1993) Effect of electro-acupuncture at Neiguan P6 on sino-atrial conduction in patients without sick sinus syndrome. Chung Kuo Chung His I Chiech Ho Tsa Chih 13(11):663–664
43. Shi X, Wang ZP, Liu KX (1995) Effect of acupuncture on heart rate variability in coronary heart disease patients. Chung Kuo Chung His I Chiech Ho Tsa Chih 15(9):536–538
44. Guo X, Jia R, Cao Q et al (1981) Inhibitory effect of somatic nerve afferent impulses on the extrasystole induced by hypothalamic stimulation. Acta Physiol Sin 33:343–350
45. MacPherson H, Thomas K, Walters S (2001) The York acupuncture safety study: prospective survey of 34 000 treatments by traditional acupuncturists. BMJ 323:486–487
46. Shah JP, Thaker N, Heimur J, Aredo JV, Sikdar S, Gerber L (2015) Myofascial trigger points then and now: a historical and scientific perspective. PM R 7 (7):746–761
47. Dommerholt J, Grieve R, Hooks T, Layton M (2015) A critical overview of the current myofascial pain literature—October 2015. J Bodyw Mov Ther 19 (4):736–746
48. Simons DG, Travell JG, Simons LS (1999) Travell and Simons' myofascial pain and dysfunction: the trigger point manual, vol I, 2nd edn. The upper body. Williams and Wilkins, Baltimore, MD
49. Travell J, Rinzler SH (1948) Pain syndromes of the chest muscles: resemblance to effort angina and myocardial infarction, and relief by local block. Can Med Assoc J 59:333–338
50. Melzack R, Stillwell D, Fox E (1977) Trigger points and acupuncture points for pain: correlations and implications. Pain 3:3–23
51. Gerwin R (1994) Neurobiology of the myofascial trigger point. Baillieres Clin Rheumatol 8:747–762

5 Metabolic Cardiology

Massimo Fioranelli, Mara Piccoli, Maria Grazia Roccia, Veronica Di Nardo, Andrea Lozzi, Claudio Tomella, and Carlo Dal Lin

The heart consumes more energy than any other organ, pumping approximately 5 L of blood per minute at rest and up to 24 L/min during vigorous exercise. It needs about 6 kg of adenosine triphosphate (ATP) every day, which is 20–30 times its own weight. The main contributors to ATP synthesis are fatty acids (70%), through β-oxidation, and glucose (30–40%), through aerobic glycolysis. Because of this dependence on oxidative energy production, increases in cardiac activity are dependent on instantaneous parallel increases in oxygen availability and ATP production [1].

Almost all the energy (about 90% of ATP) is produced in the mitochondrial respiratory chain, through oxidative phosphorylation. Recent studies [2] showed that resting cardiac energy metabolism is inversely associated with heart rate. These data may explain the prognostic role of the heart rate as demonstrated by epidemiological studies. Therefore, maintaining adequate mitochondrial metabolism is essential to ensure adequate heart contractility.

5.1 Mitochondria Dysfunction and Heart Failure

Damage to the mitochondria in endothelial cells is the initial process of atherosclerosis [3, 4]. Traditional risk factors for cardiovascular disease, such as smoking, obesity, high blood sugar, high cholesterol, and high triglycerides, are all linked to dysfunctional mitochondria [5–14]. Nutrients that enhance mitochondrial function (such as coenzyme Q10 and L-carnitine) improve clinical and symptomatic indicators of congestive heart failure (CHF) [15–17]. The mitochondria in cells of elderly people are mostly dysfunctional, whereas young individuals have virtually no mitochondrial damage [18, 19].

Many natural compounds can be useful in the treatment of cardiovascular diseases. This chapter analyzes the molecules that we think more useful in producing energy in the heart.

M. Fioranelli, MD (✉)
Department of Nuclear Physics, Sub-nuclear and Radiation, Guglielmo Marconi University, Rome, Italy
e-mail: massimo.fioranelli@gmail.com

M. Piccoli
UO Cardiologia, Policlinico L.di Liegro, Rome, Italy

M.G. Roccia, PhD
University B.I.S. Group of Institutions, Punjab Technical University, Punjab, India

V. Di Nardo, PhD • C. Tomella, MD
Guglielmo Marconi University, Rome, Italy

A. Lozzi, MD
Comitato Scientifico Amiot, Milan, Italy

C. Dal Lin, MD
Department of Cardiological, Thoracic and Vascular Sciences, Padua University Medical School, Padova, Italy

M. Fioranelli (ed.), *Integrative Cardiology*, DOI 10.1007/978-3-319-40010-5_5

5.1.1 L-Carnitine

The amino acid L-carnitine is required to transport fatty acids into the mitochondria to be burned for energy production. It is mostly highly concentrated in organs in which there is a high energy requirement, such as the heart and skeletal muscle. Levels of L-carnitine decline in patients with heart failure. Many studies have shown that patients with heart failure who take L-carnitines show an improvement in the ejection fraction [20–22]. The recommended dose is 1–3 g/day.

5.1.2 Coenzyme Q10 (CoQ10)

Many nutrients and supplements have shown an effect on heart contraction; coenzyme Q10 is the most powerful supplement in heart failure.

Coenzyme Q10 plays a key role in cell bioenergetics both mitochondrial (respiratory chain) and at the level of ATP-producing oxidative phosphorylation chain, located in the inner mitochondrial membrane, and plays an antioxidant role in relation to low-density lipoprotein (LDL), in particular, in its reduced form, ubiquinol, which represents 80% of the total coenzyme Q10 in human plasma and protects biological membranes and lipoproteins. The normal value range of CoQ10 in human plasma is 0.8–1.2 mg/L. Being a lipophilic substance in the gastrointestinal tract, it is incorporated into chylomicrons, then passes into the lymphatic vessels, and ends in the bloodstream. The degree of absorption when ingested orally is very poor, because of its insolubility in water and the high molecular weight, and it is very important to the choice of the pharmaceutical formulation, which allows high solubility [23].

CoQ10 levels decrease with age and may be low in people with cancer, certain genetic disorders, diabetes, heart conditions, HIV/AIDS, muscular dystrophies, and Parkinson's disease. Oxidative modification of LDLs in arterial walls is thought to be an initial event for atherosclerosis development. Reduced coenzyme Q10 (CoQ10H2) inhibits LDL oxidation in vitro. Co-supplementation in α-tocopherol and coenzyme Q10 in apolipoprotein E-deficient mice is effective at inhibiting atherosclerosis [24]. (Although coenzyme Q10 supplementation promises a decrease in atherosclerosis, additional research is needed to determine whether this supplementation can inhibit the development or progression of atherosclerosis in humans.) In heart failure, too, small intervention trials of therapy with coenzyme Q10 (100–300 mg/day of coenzyme Q10 for 1–3 months) in patients with congestive heart failure, in conjunction with conventional medical therapy, have demonstrated improvements in some cardiac function measures, but previously other researchers have found that supplementing the diet with 100–200 mg/day of coenzyme Q10 did not significantly improve left ventricular ejection fraction or exercise performance in heart failure patients [25, 26]. A 2006 meta-analysis of ten randomized controlled trials found that coenzyme Q10 supplementation (99–200 mg/day for 1–6 months) in heart failure patients resulted in a significant improvement in left ventricular ejection fraction [27].

The coenzyme Q10 has been shown to reduce the remodeling mechanism that adversely modifies the heart geometry, leading to dilatation and contractility dysfunction [28, 29].

We recommend a dose 100–600 mg/day, according to the severity of heart disease.

5.1.3 Creatine

Cardiac creatine levels are reduced in chronic heart failure and supplementation should be useful in chronic heart failure. When patients with heart failure were given 20 g of creatine per day, an increase in the contractile force was observed [30]. Creatine supplements improve skeletal muscle force and restore a normal muscle metabolism in heart failure. We usually use a loading phase with 15–20 g per day, followed by a week with a dose of 2–5 g/day.

5.1.4 D-Ribose

An insufficient supply of ATP may play a role in ischemic CHF. Ribose is a pentose sugar and is the core of the ATP molecule. Ribose enhances the recovery of depressed myocardial ATP levels and provides improvement in myocardial diastolic compliance in a setting of myocardial ischemia [31, 32].

D-Ribose enhances cardiac metabolism in entering the pentose phosphate pathway to form ribose-5-phosphate counteracting the rate-limiting enzymes of glucose-6-phosphate dehydrogenase and 6-phosphogluconate dehydrogenase.

Several studies have shown that D-ribose shortens the time needed to regenerate deficient myocardial ATP levels following ischemia. Decreased availability of myocardial ATP may allow calcium to remain fixed to troponin longer in diastole, leading to diastolic dysfunction. This supplement is strategic in the treatment of heart failure. We recommend a dose between 10 and 15 g per day; after a week the dose may be reduced to 5 g twice daily [33].

5.1.5 Hawthorn

Hawthorn extract improves symptoms of heart failure. It contains flavonoids and oligomeric proanthocyanidins. Cardiovascular effects include a positive inotropic effect. Hawthorn possesses vasodilatation properties, reduces blood pressure, inhibiting the angiotensin-converting enzyme, and exerts a heart control rate in a manner similar to digoxin, reducing chronotropic properties [34, 35].

This herb should be a useful treatment in mild forms of heart failure. Hawthorn is usually well tolerated; the most common side effects are dizziness, vertigo, and nausea. This herbal remedy has the potential to cause hypotension and should be used with caution with conventional medications used in the treatment of hypertension. Gastrointestinal complaints, fatigue, sweating, rash, palpitations, headache, sleeplessness, agitation, and circulatory disturbances have been reported. Potential adverse drug–herb interactions may exist between hawthorn and some drugs, such as anticoagulants and cardiac glycosides. The dosage varies between 600 and 1,800 mg/day.

5.1.6 Lipoic Acid

Alpha-lipoic acid, a compound rich in sulfur, plays an essential role in the metabolic processes involved in energy production. It exerts an effect mainly on the mitochondria; it is a cofactor of several enzymes that participate in the glucose conversion process, the fatty acids, and other energy ATP sources. Alpha-lipoic acid is also active in the regeneration of reduced glutathione and vitamin C (ascorbic acid). Lipoic acid is a powerful antioxidant, similar to glutathione. Because oxidative stress is associated with a decrease in cardiac function, the lipoic acid may be an aid in the treatment of heart failure [36, 37].

5.1.7 Pyrroloquinoline Quinone

Pyrroloquinoline quinone (PQQ) is a quinone disodium salt that is produced through a fermentation process. It was initially classified as a vitamin B complex after being identified by Japanese researchers in 1979. Although it is distributed within the body, this molecule is particularly concentrated in specific locations, such as the heart, brain, and red blood cells. The PQQ can be obtained through certain foods (beans, potatoes, parsley, green tea, and kiwi) or dietary supplements. This molecule interferes with many metabolic processes and influences a number of enzymes and proteins, the so-called quinoprotein, which adjusts and modulates the activity. The PQQ has significant antiaging properties and has antioxidant activity 100 times more potent than vitamin

C. Although CoQ10 optimizes mitochondrial function, PQQ activates genes that govern mitochondrial reproduction, protection, and repair. Mitochondrial DNA decreases by 40% in failing hearts [38, 39]. We recommend a dosage of 10–20 mg/day. Although it has been clinically shown that 20 mg of PQQ is necessary to effectively support cognitive function, 10 mg of PQQ or even less has been clinically shown to induce mitochondrial biogenesis.

5.1.8 Taurine

Taurine is a so-called "conditional amino acid," an amino acid that can be produced by the body. Instead an "essential amino acid" should be provided by the diet because it cannot be produced by the organism. Supplementation of taurine is necessary in infants who are not breastfed because their ability to produce the amino acids is not yet fully developed and cow's milk does not provide enough taurine. Also, in enteral and parenteral feeding it is added to nutritional products. This amino acid exerts a potent antioxidant effect.

Taurine is one of the main intracellular osmolytes and therefore provides an important contribution to the regulation of cell volume. It has the effect of an ACE inhibitor. The mechanism of action appears to be that of the modulation of hyperactivity of the sympathetic nervous system, particularly activated in the case of stress [40].

Taurine is a supplement useful in the treatment of CHF, hypertension, and hypercholesterolemia.

5.1.9 Vitamin D

The deficiency of vitamin D is related to a reduction of the contractile function of the heart. Many scholars believe that the increase in plasma pro-inflammatory cytokines may contribute to heart failure. Vitamin D has a cardioprotective effect as an anti-inflammatory molecule.

The many actions attributed to vitamin D reflect the wide tissue distribution of its receptors, the vascular smooth muscle cells, endothelium, immune cells, and cardiomyocytes, tissue for which the total vitamin D modulates the immune and inflammatory conditions.

Clinical studies have reported associations between low plasma levels of vitamin D and other aspects of the cardiovascular system (CV), such as hyperactivity of the renin–angiotensin–aldosterone system, high blood pressure, coronary calcification, glucose metabolism disorders, and cardiovascular disease.

Vitamin D has a potent immunomodulatory effect: laboratory studies show that it inhibits the production of prostaglandins and cyclo-oxygenase-2, modulates the synthesis of matrix metalloproteinases and many of the pro-inflammatory cytokines, and increases the synthesis of interleukin-10, leading to the modulation of inflammation [41–44].

5.2 Low-Dose Therapy

Low-dose medicine represents an innovative medical paradigm for the treatment of cardiovascular diseases. It has emerged from the latest knowledge in the field of molecular biology, the psycho-neuro-endocrine immunology (PNEI) vision, and research into nano-concentration pharmacology.

In recent years, research in the field of low-dose medicine has had a huge impact and several studies, both preclinical and clinical, have been published with the evidence for the theoretical bases of this innovative branch of medicine [45–55].

Low-dose therapy is characterized by the administration of remedies, such as natural substances (plants, minerals, animal derivatives) at various ultralow doses and, in particular, biological molecules (neuropetides, cytokines, hormones, and growth factors) at the physiological low dose that is within the range of picomoles or femtomoles/ml concentration. All these substances only have biological activity if they have undergone a process of sequential kinetic activation (SKA). SKA is a technique patented by GUNA Laboratories (GUNA, Milan, Italy), using a standardized method. The remedies undergo to a shaking process (vertical shaking; 10 cm motion range; shaking speed corresponding to 100 oscillations over 10 s), sequentially diluted in saline solution (serial dilution 1:100), and kinetically energized by a mechanically applied force [45].

According to the physiological regulating medicine (PRM) theory, all the diseases are due to a lack of communication among the three main homeostatic control systems (central nervous system, neurovegetative system and endocrine system, immune system).

Neuro-endocrine immunological regulation is a complex system in which one can only intervene therapeutically by using delicate elements such as low-dose cytokines, neuropeptides, and hormones, at the precise concentrations mentioned above, that is, the concentration that is sufficient to restore the physiological function of the membrane receptors.

The action mechanism of activated low-dose cytokines, neuropeptides, and hormones involves sensitizing or activating some cell or plasmatic receptor units through an upregulation mechanism (a result of their extreme dilution, which is the same physiological dilution as these substances: from micrograms 10^{-6} to fentograms 10^{-15}). This sensitization of receptors enables chain reactions (complex systems) to be triggered with the subsequent recovery of the biological function of the entire neuro-immune-endocrine network.

The opportunity to use homeopathically activated cytokines, hormones, and neuropeptides for therapeutic purposes originated primarily from the discovery that their physiological concentration, both in plasma and tissues, was very close to that of the low–medium dilutions used in homeopathy. Nowadays, we use, more correctly, the term "low doses." Each cytokine and hormone has a precise range of physiological concentrations at which it has a regulatory (physiological) effect [56].

For the support of mitochondrial metabolism and the Krebs cycle, we use the following multicomponent low-dose medications:

Heel Coenzyme Compositum:

- Stimulates the enzymatic systems.
- Stimulates the energy metabolism.
- Stimulates intracellular detoxification.

Composition:
Krebs cycle intermediates:
Vitamin C D6–vitamin B1 D6, vitamin B2 D6–vitamin B6 D6, Nikotinsaureamid D6, Ac. cis-aconitum D8, A. citricum D8, Ac. fumaricum D8, Ac. alfa-chetoglut. D8, Ac. DL-malicum D8, Ac. succinicum D8, baryum oxalsuccinicum D10, natrium oxalaceticum D6, natrium pyruvicum D8.
Cystein D6, ATP D10, NAD D8-coenzyme A D8, cerium oxalicum D8, alfa-liponsaure D6, pulsatilla D6, hepar sulfuris D10, sulfur D10, beta vulgaris rubra D4, manganum phosphoricum D6, magnesium oroticum D6.

Heel Ubichinon Compositum
It is extremely useful for stimulating the functioning of mitochondrial quinone. The quinones are contained in low-dose concentrations to prevent excessive stimulation induced by overdoses that can lead to a surplus of free radicals. Their use in low doses speeds up the reaction of the quinones and the resumption of oxidative phosphorylation and energy production.
Composition:
Anthrachinon D10, naphtochinon D10, parabenzochinon D10, ubichinon D10, hydrochinon D8, trichinoyl D10, ATP D10, istamin D10, NAD D10, manganum phosphoricum D8, magnesium gluconicum D10, natrium oxalaceticum D8, coenzima A D10, Ac. lipoico D8, adicum L (+) – lacticum D6, vitamin C D6, vitamin B1 D6, vitamin B2 D6, vitamin B6 D6, myrtillus D4, colchicum D4, podophyllum D4, conium D4, hydrastis D4, galium aparine D6, sulfur D8

These remedies are useful in heart failure and in the aging heart in general.

References

1. Westerhof N, Boer C, Lamberts RR, Sipkema P (2006) Cross-talk between cardiac muscle and coronary vasculature. Physiol Rev 86:1263–1308
2. Fragassu G, De Co belli F, Spudalorc R (2011) Resting cardiac energy metabolism is inversely associated with heart rate in healthy young adult men. Am Heart J 162(1):136–141
3. Schleicher M, Shepherd BR, Suarez Y et al (2008) Prohibitin-1 maintains the angiogenic capacity of endothelial cells by regulating mitochondrial function and senescence. J Cell Biol 180(1):101–112
4. Oeseburg H, Iusuf D, van der Harst P, van Gilst WH, Henning RH, Roks AJ (2009) Bradykinin protects against oxidative stress-induced endothelial cell senescence. Hypertension 53(2):417–422
5. Yang Z, Harrison CM, Chuang GC, Ballinger SW (2007) The role of tobacco smoke induced mitochondrial damage in vascular dysfunction and atherosclerosis. Mutat Res 621(1–2):61–74
6. Knight-Lozano CA, Young CG, Burow DL et al (2002) Cigarette smoke exposure and hypercholesterolemia increase mitochondrial damage in cardiovascular tissues. Circulation 105(7):849–854
7. Jia L, Liu Z, Sun L et al (2007) Acrolein, a toxicant in cigarette smoke, causes oxidative damage and mitochondrial dysfunction in RPE cells: protection by I-alpha-lipoic acid. Invest Ophthalmol Vis Sci 48 (1):339–348
8. Yang Z, Knight CA, Mamerow M et al (2004) Prenatal environmental tobacco smoke exposure promotes adult atherogenesis and mitochondrial damage in apoE−/− mice fed a chow diet. Circulation 110 (24):3715–3720
9. Bach D, Pich S, Soriano FX et al (2003) Mitofusin-2 determines mitochondrial network architecture and mitochondrial metabolism. A novel regulatory mechanism altered in obesity. J Biol Chem 278 (19):17190–17197
10. Li M, Absher M, Liang P, Russell JC, Sobel BE, Fukagawa NK (2001) High glucose concentrations induce oxidative damage to mitochondrial DNA in explanted vascular smooth muscle cells. Exp Biol Med 226:450–457
11. Vanhorebeek I, Ellger B, De Vos R et al (2009) Tissue-specific glucose toxicity induces mitochondrial damage in a burn injury model of critical illness. Crit Care Med 37(4):1355–1364
12. Madamanchi NR, Runge MS (2007) Mitochondrial dysfunction in atherosclerosis. Circ Res 100 (4):460–473
13. Graier WF, Malli R, Kostner GM (2009) Mitochondrial protein phosphorylation: instigator or target of lipotoxicity? Trends Endocrinol Metab 20 (4):186–193
14. Maasen JA (2008) Mitochondria, body fat and type 2 diabetes: what is the connection? Minerva Med 99 (3):241
15. Mortensen SA, Vadhanavikit S, Muratsu K, Folkers K (1990) Coenzyme Q10: clinical benefits with biochemical correlates suggesting a scientific breakthrough in the management of chronic heart failure. Int J Tissue React 12(3):155–162
16. Langsjoen PH, Langsjoen AM (2008) Supplemental ubiquinol in patients with advanced congestive heart failure. Biofactors 32(1–4):119–128
17. Serati AR, Motamedi MR, Emami S, Varedi P, Movahed MR (2010) L-carnitine treatment in patients with mild diastolic heart failure is associated with improvement in diastolic function and symptoms. Cardiology 116(3):178–182
18. Short KR, Bigelow ML, Kahl J et al (2005) Decline in skeletal muscle mitochondrial function with aging in humans. Proc Natl Acad Sci USA 102(15): 5618–5623
19. Linnane AW, Kovalenko S, Gingold EB (1998) The universality of bioenergetic disease: age-associated cellular bioenergetic degradation and amelioration therapy. Ann N Y Acad Sci 854:202–213
20. Goa KL, Brogden RN (1987) L-carnitine: a preliminary review of its pharmacokinetics, and its therapeutic use in ischaemic cardiac disease and primary and secondary carnitine deficiencies in relationship to its role in fatty acid metabolism. Drugs 34:1–24
21. Mancini M, Rengo F et al (1992) Controlled study on the therapeutic efficacy of propionyl-L-carnitine in patients with congestive heart failure. Arzneimittelforschung 42:1101–1104
22. Pucciarelli G, Mastursi M et al (1992) The clinical and hemodynamic effects of propionyl-L-carnitine in the treatment of congestive heart failure. Clin Ter 141:379–384
23. Bhagavan HN, Chopra RK (2006) Coenzyme Q10: absorption, tissue uptake, metabolism and pharmacokinetics. Free Radic Res 40(5):445–453
24. Thomas SR, Leichtweis SB, Pettersson K et al (2001) Dietary cosupplementation with vitamin E and coenzyme Q(10) inhibits atherosclerosis in apolipoprotein E gene knockout mice. Arterioscler Thromb Vasc Biol 21(4):585–593
25. Belardinelli R, Mucaj A, Lacalaprice F et al (2006) Coenzyme Q10 and exercise training in chronic heart failure. Eur Heart J 27(22):2675–2681
26. Khatta M, Alexander BS, Krichten CM et al (2000) The effect of coenzyme Q10 in patients with congestive heart failure. Ann Intern Med 132 (8):636–640
27. Gao L, Mao Q, Cao J, Wang Y, Zhou X, Fan L (2011) Effects of coenzyme Q10 on vascular endothelial function in humans: A meta-analysis of randomized controlled trials. Atherosclerosis 221(2):311–316
28. Fedak PW, Verma S et al (2005) Cardiac remodeling and failure: from molecules to man (part I). Cardiovasc Pathol 14:1–11
29. Weisberg AD, Albornoz F et al (2005) Pharmacological inhibition and genetic deficiency of plasminogen activator inhibitor-1 attenuates angiotensin II/salt-induced aortic remodeling. Arterioscler Thromb Vasc Biol 25:365–371

30. Bemben MG, Lamont HS (2005) Creatine supplementation and exercise performance: recent findings. Sports Med 35(2):107–125
31. Sole MJ, Jeejeebhoy KN (2000) Conditional nutritional requirements and the pathogenesis and treatment of myocardial failure. Curr Opin Clin Nutr Metab Care 3(6):417–424
32. Tveter KJ, St. Cyr JA, Bianco RW, Einzig S, Foker JE (1988) Ribose enhanced recovery of diastolic function after global myocardial ischemia. Pediatr Res 23:226A (abstract)
33. Omran H, Illien S, MacCarter D, St CJ, Luderitz B (2003) D-Ribose improves diastolic function and quality of life in congestive heart failure patients: a prospective feasibility study. Eur J Heart Fail 5(5):615–619
34. Tauchert M (2002) Efficacy and safety of crataegus extract WS 1442 in comparison with placebo in patients with chronic stable New York Heart Association class-III heart failure. Am Heart J 143:910–915
35. Schwinger RH, Pietsch M et al (2000) Crataegus special extract WS 1442 increases force of contraction in human myocardium cAMP-independently. J Cardiovasc Pharmacol 35:700–707
36. Maxwell SR (1993) Can anti-oxidants prevent ischaemic heart disease? J Clin Pharm Ther 18:85–95
37. Carlson DA et al (2007) The plasma pharmacokinetics of R-(+)-lipoic acid administered as sodium R-(+)-lipoate to healthy human subjects. Altern Med Rev 12(4):343–351
38. Chowanadisai W, Bauerly KA, Tchaparian E, Wong A, Cortopassi GA, Rucker RB (2010) Pyrroloquinoline quinone stimulates mitochondrial biogenesis through cAMP response element-binding protein phosphorylation and increased PGC-1alpha expression. J Biol Chem 285(1):142–152
39. Karamanlidis G, Nascimben L, Couper GS, Shekar PS, del Monte F, Tian R (2010) Defective DNA replication impairs mitochondrial biogenesis in human failing hearts. Circ Res 106(9):1541–1548
40. Schaffer SW, Lombardini JB et al (2000) Interaction between the actions of taurine and angiotensin II. Amino Acids 18:305–318
41. Achinger SG, Ayus JC (2005) The role of vitamin D in left ventricular hypertrophy and cardiac function. Kidney Int Suppl 95:S37–S42
42. London GM, Guerin AP, Verbeke FH et al (2007) Mineral metabolism and arterial functions in end-stage renal disease: potential role of 25-hydroxyvitamin D deficiency. J Am Soc Nephrol 18(2):613–620
43. Zittermann A, Schleithoff SS, Tenderich G, Berthold HK, Korfer R, Stehle P (2003) Low vitamin D status: a contributing factor in the pathogenesis of congestive heart failure? J Am Coll Cardiol 41(1):105–112
44. Schleithoff SS, Zittermann A, Tenderich G et al (2006) Vitamin D supplementation improves cytokine profiles in patients with congestive heart failure: a double-blind, randomized, placebo-controlled trial. Am J Clin Nutr 83(4):754–759
45. Gariboldi S, Palazzo M, Zanobbio L, Dusio GF, Mauro V et al (2009) Low dose oral administration of cytokines for treatment of allergic asthma. Pulm Pharmacol Ther 22(6):497–510
46. D'Amico L, Ruffini E, Ferracini R, Roato I (2012) Low dose of IL-12 stimulates T cell response in cultures of PBMCs derived from non small cell lung cancer patients. J Cancer Ther 3:337–342
47. Cardani D, Dusio GF, Luchini P, Sciarabba M, Solimene U et al (2013) Oral administration of interleukin-10 and anti-IL-1 antibody ameliorates experimental intestinal inflammation. Gastroenterol Res 6(4):124–133
48. Radice E, Miranda V, Bellone G (2014) Low-doses of sequential-kinetic-activated interferon-gamma enhance the ex vivo cytotoxicity of peripheral blood natural killer cells from patients with early-stage colorectal cancer. A preliminary study. Int Immunopharmacol 19(1):66–73
49. Roberti ML, Ricottini L, Capponi A, Sclauzero E, Vicenti P et al (2014) Immunomodulating treatment with low dose interleukin-4, interleukin-10 and interleukin-11 in psoriasis vulgaris. J Biol Regul Homeost Agents 28(1):133–139
50. Luchetti P (2014) Increasing of visual function in patients with retinal atrophy treated with drugs of low dose medicine. Monocentric retrospective observational study. Minerva Oftalmol 56(3–4):53–61
51. Barygina V, Becatti M, Lotti T, Moretti S, Taddei N, Fiorillo C (2015) Treatment with low-dose cytokines reduces oxidative-mediated injury in perilesional keratinocytes from vitiligo skin. J Dermatol Sci 79 (2):163–170
52. Lotti T, Hercogova J, Wollina U, Chokoeva AA, Zarrab Z, Gianfaldoni S et al (2015) Vitiligo: successful combination treatment based on oral low dose cytokines and different topical treatments. J Biol Regul Homeost Agents 29[Suppl 1]:53–58
53. Radice E, Bellone G, Miranda V (2015) Enhancement of the immunostimulatory functions of ex vivo-generated dendritic cells from early-stage colon cancer patients by consecutive exposure to low doses of sequential-kinetic-activated IL-4 and IL-12. A preliminary study. Transl Oncol 8(4):327–338
54. Lotti T (2015) Successful combination treatment for psoriasis with phototherapy and low-dose cytokines: a spontaneous, retrospective observational clinical study. Hautarzt 66(11):849–854
55. Tessaro I et al (2015) Effect of oral administration of low dose follicle stimulating hormone on hyperandrogenized mice as model of polycystic ovary syndrome. J Ovarian Res 8:64
56. Fioranelli M, Roccia MG (2014) The history of low dose medicine research. Review of preclinical and clinical studies with low dose SKA cytokines since 2009. Interdiscip J Microinflammation 1:115. doi:10.4172/ijm.1000115

6 Medicinal Mushrooms

Ivo Bianchi

The use of mushrooms in medicine dates back to the ancient Egyptians and Chinese cultures that used them to promote general health and longevity.

Overall, there are 100,000 types of mushrooms and of these, at least 270 species are considered to possess therapeutic properties, including anticancer activity. The terms "medicinal mushrooms" or "mycotherapy" are now gaining worldwide recognition. Many mushrooms suitable for feeding used in traditional folk medicine, including *Lentinus edodes*, *Grifola frondosa*, *Hericium erinaceus*, *Flammulina velutipes*, *Pleurotus ostreatus*, and *Tremella mesenterica*; these are also a source of relatively pure bioactive compounds for medical usage, whereas other, non-edible species, such as *Ganoderma lucidum*, *Schizophyllum commune*, and *Trametes versicolor*, are used only for their medicinal properties. *Ganoderma* species have the longest history of medicinal usage, dating back at least four millennia. In Japan, this mushroom is known as *Reishi* or *manetake* (10,000-year mushroom), and in China, as *ling zhi* (mushroom of immortality). It is the mushroom that is most frequently depicted in ancient Japanese, Korean, and Chinese art, and has been extensively utilized in Chinese royal tapestries. *Reishi* is also the most interesting mushroom with regard to cardiology [1].

Recent advances in biochemical techniques have allowed the partial isolation and purification of compounds from medicinal mushrooms, especially polysaccharides, exhibiting anticancer activities. Several mushroom polysaccharides have proceeded into clinical trials in cancer patients almost exclusively in the Far East, although some have begun in the United States. Lentinan, *Schizophyllum*, and *Coriolus* have been the most intensively studied of the medicinal mushroom. In animal models, lentinan has been shown to possess anti-neoplastic activity, to prevent metastasis, and to inhibit cancer growth. Most medicinal mushrooms seem to act as non-specific immuno-stimulants, though some have direct cytotoxic effects. They activate many kinds of immune cells that are important for the maintenance of immune homeostasis [2]. Some medicinal mushroom polysaccharides have been shown to be multi-cytokine inducers, capable of modulating gene expression of various cytokines via cell membrane receptors [3]. These studies will be given specific importance with regard to the effects of medicinal mushrooms on cytokines, because some of the most important heart problems are related to inflammatory cytokine activation [3–5].

Apart from their immune-activating properties related to their content of β-glucans

I. Bianchi (✉)
University Guglielmo Marconi, Rome, Italy
e-mail: dr.ivobianchi@gmail.com

M. Fioranelli (ed.), *Integrative Cardiology*, DOI 10.1007/978-3-319-40010-5_6

Fig. 6.1 General chemical composition of mushrooms

- **Proteins 10-40%**
- Carbohydrates 3-21%
- Lipids (free fatty acids) 2-8%
- **Insoluble fibers 3-35%**
- Minerals specifics and of substrate
- Vitamins
  - **B1, B2, Niacin, Biotin**
  - **Vit.C**
  - **Vit D2** (Ergosterols)
- Low caloric content

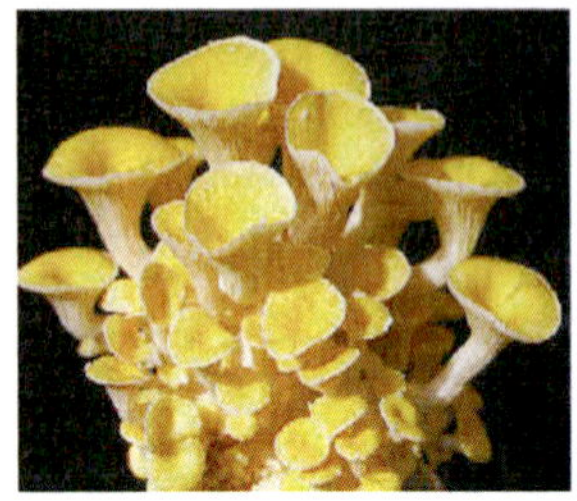

and other polysaccharides, almost all medical mushrooms exert a favorable effect on cardiovascular pathological conditions working on metabolic syndrome, often the basic underlying factor [6]. Medical mushrooms and their extracts, polysaccharide fractions, and isolated compounds possess hypoglycemic, cholesterol- and triglyceride-lowering ability, hypotensive effects, and weight-managing activity by influencing satiety [7]. In particular, the mushroom mycelium, made by an indigestible fiber called "chitin," is very active in inhibiting absorption of fats and sugars from the bowel. The most important medicinal mushrooms for cardiovascular problems are reviewed (Fig. 6.1).

6.1 *Auricularia auricula* (Jew's Ear)

This is a jelly-type fungus that grows mostly on wood (either alive or dead) with a semi-translucent fruiting body. It is an immune tonic because it stimulates DNA and RNA synthesis by human lymphocytes in vitro. It is anticoagulant and antidiabetic with a cytoprotective effect on pancreatic islets demonstrated in mice. *Auricularia* lowers total cholesterol, triglyceride, and lipid levels in general [8]. It decreases lipofuscin content of the heart muscle and consequently has an anti-aging effect [9–15].

6.2 *Cordyceps sinsensis* (Caterpillar Fungus)

It is a fungus of the genus *Ascomycetes* found in the high altitude of the Tibetan plateau that parasitizes mostly caterpillars. The wild form of the fungus is rare and expensive, but a strain isolated from the wild form is cultivated industrially and extensively used worldwide for its properties. Its activity is similar to ginseng and is said to be more potent. The first documented use was in 620 AD, during the Tang Dynasty. It is currently used for strengthening of the body after exhaustion or a long-term illness, impotence, backaches and is an antidote for opium poisoning. In traditional Chinese medicine, *Cordyceps* has also been used to treat respiratory and cardiovascular diseases. It is also useful in immune disorder and has been employed in association with cancer chemotherapy treatments and surgery. It is also believed to be a remedy for weakness and fatigue and is often prescribed as a "rejuvenator" to increase energy. This fungus is very rich in nucleosides: adenine, adenosine, uracil, uridine, guanidine, guanosine, hypoxanthine, inosine, thymine, thymidine and deoxyuridine. It also contains: all essential amino acids, immunoglycans, polyamine, sterols, fatty acids, vitamins (B1, B2, B12, E, and K). Some specific compounds are: cordycepin and other adenosine derivates such as ergosterol (provitamin D), mannitol, cordyheptapeptide A. *Cordyceps* has a long history of traditional medical use in heart disease. Adenosine and other contained nucleosides are thought to be responsible for the effect seen in animal studies. A vasodilatory action has also been reported in the hypotensive and vasorelaxant effects. Reduced heart rate and restoration from arrhythmias have also been shown in animals. Long-term studies in cardiac failure have described the effect of *Cordyceps* in improving cardiac function, arrhythmias, and overall quality of life. Fibrinolytic action of a *Cordyceps* extract has been shown in vitro on bovine and human serum. Platelet aggregation has been inhibited in rabbits and in human platelets in vitro. Extracts of the fungus showed a positive effect on hyperlipidemias.

Cordyceps mushrooms improve aerobic capacity, endurance, and post-workout recovery. It works at a mitochondrial level, increasing ATP synthesis. It also stimulates antioxidant synthesis, explaining the benefits in athletes who can train more effectively for longer periods of time, and can recover more quickly [16, 17].

The effect of *Cordyceps sinensis* on the Th1/Th 2 cytokines was investigated and after treatment with this mushroom, the serum levels of IL-2 and IL-10 significantly increased and decreased respectively. Thus, this mushroom has no anti-inflammatory effect at a cardiovascular level, but stimulates heart strength, and is thus useful in cardiac insufficiency, complementary to CoQ10 [1, 3].

6.3 *Gandoderma lucidum* (Reishi)

Ganoderma lucidum, also named Reishi, is a purplish brown fungus with a long stalk, brown spores, and a fan-shaped cap with a shiny, varnish-coated appearance. It grows on decaying wood, especially on oak or Japanese plum. Reishi has been used in traditional medicine for more than 4000 years for treating fatigue, asthma, cough and liver ailments. It has the reputation of promoting longevity. The Chinese name, *ling zhi,* means "herb of spiritual potency." The Japanese name for this fungus is *mannentake*, meaning "10,000-year-old mushroom [3]."

Ganoderma lucidum is high in polysaccharide content, with at least 36 different compounds identified, including immunostimulating β-D-glucans and triterpene antioxidants. Minerals such as calcium, magnesium, potassium, and germanium have been reported from Reishi. Lanostane, coumarins, ergosterol, and cholesterol are also components of this fungus.

Ganoderic acids triterpene constituents of Reishi decrease high blood pressure through inhibition of angiotensin-converting enzyme. Decreased biosynthesis of cholesterol, enhanced anti-oxidase activity, decreased platelet aggregation, and reduced lipid peroxidation have been demonstrated in animal and in vitro experiments. The polysaccharide content of Ganoderma is responsible for possible anticancer and immunostimulatory effects. Contraindications have not been identified [18–23].

The well-known immunomodulatory effect of *Ganoderma lucidum* is mediated through increased levels of IL-1β, IL-12 expression, and is thus also useful in heart conditions [24].

6.4 *Lentinus edodes* (Shiitake)

This is a light amber fungus found on fallen broadleaf trees, especially oak, maple, walnut, beech, and chestnut, and is indigenous to Japan and China. Eritadenine, an active compound isolated from Shiitake, has been shown to lower blood levels of cholesterol and lipids [25]. The fungus also stimulates tyrosinase activity, which lowers blood pressure. The administration of *Lentinus edodes*, increases, in experimental animal and human peripheral blood mononuclear cells, the expression levels of IL-2 and TNF α. Laboratory and clinical results suggest that Lentinus edodes might induce Th1 immune responses, which are extremely useful for preventing and treating infectious diseases, often also affecting the heart [7, 26].

Decrease	Total Cholesterol	LDL Cholesterol	Triglycerides	Platelets Aggregation	Hypertension	Blood Sugar
Auricularia	+++	++	+	++	+	+
Cordyceps	+	+	++		++	++
Lentinus	++		++			+
Ganoderma	+			+	++	+
Grifola	++		++		++	++
Pleurotus	+++					+
Tremella	++	++				++
Coriolus	+			+		
Coprinus						++

Fig. 6.2 Medicinal mushrooms and metabolic syndrome. *LDL* low-density lipoprotein

6.5 *Pleurotus ostreatus* (Oyster Mushroom)

It lowers serum low-density lipoprotein, cholesterol, and triglyceride levels. *Pleurotus* is useful, even in hereditary hypercholesterolemia and cures hepatic steatosis derived from chronic alcohol ingestion. These activities are useful in most cardiac problems (Fig. 6.2) [27, 28].

References

1. Hobbs C (1986) Medicinal mushrooms – an exploration of tradition, healing and culture. Botanica Press, Williams
2. Bianchi I (2008) I Funghi Medicinalinella Pratica Clinica. Nuova Ipsa Ed
3. Bianchi I, Bianchi V (2013) Guarire con i 12 Funghi Medicinali Mos Maiorum Ed
4. Dudhgaonkar S, Thyagarajan A, Sliva D (2009) Suppression of the inflammatory response by triterpenes isolated from the mushroom Ganoderma lucidum. Int Immunopharmacol 9(11):1272–1280
5. Lindequist U, Niedermeyer TH, Jülich WD (2005) The pharmacological potential of mushrooms. Evid Based Complement Alternat Med 2(3):285–299
6. Bianchi I Micoterapia, Integrazione salutare con I Funghi Medicinali. Sci Nat 2(2):24–29
7. Bianchi I (2007) I Funghi Homeopathicum, La Medicina Biologica, Guna Editore, Milan, vol 2–3, pp 57–61/41–45
8. Chen G, Luo YC, Li BP, Li B, Guo Y, Li Y, Su W, Xiao ZL (2008) Effect of polysaccharide from Auricularia auricula on blood lipid metabolism and lipoprotein lipase activity of ICR mice fed a cholesterol-enriched diet. J Food Sci 73(6):H103–H108
9. Kaneda T, Tokuda S (1996) The hypocholesterolemic effect of two edible mushrooms: *Auricularia auricula* (tree-ear) and *Tremella fuciformis* (white jelly-leaf) in hypercholesterolemic rats. Nutr Res 1699 (10):1721–1725
10. Quél Kho YS, Vikineswary S, Abdullah N, Kuppusamy UR, Oh HI (2009) Antioxidant and nitric oxide synthase activation properties of *Auricularia auricula*. J Med Food 12(1):167–174
11. Ukai S, Kiho T, Hara C, Kuruma I, Tanaka Y (1983) Antioxidant capacity of fresh and processed fruit bodies and mycelium of *Auricularia auricula*-judae. J Pharmacobiodyn 6(12):983–990
12. Wu Q, Tan Z, Liu H, Gao L, Wu S, Luo J, Zhang W, Zhao T, Yu J, Xu X (2010) Chemical characterization of Auricularia auricula polysaccharides and its pharmacological effect on heart antioxidant enzyme activities and left ventricular function in aged mice. Int J Biol Macromol 46(3):284–288
13. Ye TM, Qian LB, Cui J, Wang HP, Ye ZG, Xia Q et al (2010) Auricularia auricular polysaccharide protects myocardium against ischemia/reperfusion injury. Zhongguo Ying Yong Sheng Li Xue Za Zhi 26 (2):154–158
14. Yi MA, Tang J, Han C (2005) Isolation and purification of polysaccharides from wood ear (Auricularia auricular) and their hypoglycemic, hypolipidemic and antioxidant activities. IFT Annual Meeting. ift.confex.com 18B-13
15. Yoon SJ, Yu MA, Pyun YR, Hwang JK, Chu DC, Juneja LR, Mourão PA (2003) The nontoxic mushroom Auricularia auricula contains a polysaccharide with anticoagulant activity mediated by antithrombin. Thromb Res 112(3):151–158
16. Colson SN et al (2005) Cordyceps sinensis- and Rhodiola rosea-based supplementation in male cyclists and its effect on muscle tissue oxygen saturation. J Strength Cond Res 19(2):358–363

17. Koh JH et al (2003) Antifatigue and antistress effect of the hot-water fraction from mycelia of *Cordyceps sinensis*. Biol Pharm Bull 26(5):691–694
18. Berger A et al (2004) Cholesterol-lowering properties of *Ganoderma lucidum* in vitro, ex vivo, and in hamsters and minipigs. Lipids Health Dis 3:2
19. Boh B et al (2007) Ganoderma lucidum and its pharmaceutically active compounds. Biotechnol Annu Rev 13:265–301
20. Hikino H et al (1985) Isolation and hypoglycemic activity of ganoderans A and B, glycans of *Ganoderma lucidum* fruit bodies. Planta Med 4:339–340
21. Komoda Y et al (1989) Ganoderic acid and its derivatives as cholesterol synthesis inhibitors. Chem Pharm Bull (Tokyo) 37(2):531–533
22. Liu J, Kurashiki K, Shimizu K, Kondo R (2006) Structure-activity relationship for inhibition of 5alpha-reductase by triterpenoids isolated from *Ganoderma lucidum*. Bioorg Med Chem 14 (24):8654–8660
23. Patocka J (1999) Anti inflammatory triterpenoids from mysterious mushroom Ganoderma lucidum and their potential possibility in modern medicine. Acta Med 42(4):123–125. Department of Toxicology; Purkyne Military Medical Academy, Hradec Kralove
24. Yu Q et al (2012) Macrophage immunomodulatory activity of a purified polysaccharide isolated from *Ganoderma atrum*. Phytother Res 27(2):186
25. Delaš I, Beganović J, Bogdanović T, Delaš F (2008) Effects of dietary supplementation of Shiitake mushroom on fatty acid composition and cholesterol content of hen egg yolks, 4th World Congress of Food Science and Technology, Shanghai: Chinese Institute of Food Science and Technology, p 153
26. Bisen PS, Baghel RK, Sanodiya BS, Thakur GS, Prasad GB (2010) Lentinus edodes: a macrofungus with pharmacological activities. Curr Med Chem 17 (22):2419–2430
27. Liu X et al (2010) Extraction and antioxidant activities of intracellular polysaccharide from Pleurotus sp. mycelium. Int J Biol Macromol 47 (2):116–119
28. Mizutani T et al (2010) Hypolipidemic effect of *Pleurotus eryngii* extract in fat-loaded mice. J Nutr Sci Vitaminol (Tokyo) 56(1):48–53

Microbiome and Cardiac Health

7

Enrico Biffi

7.1 Gut Microbiota and Microbiome

7.1.1 The "Complexity" in the Relationship Between the Human Host and Its Microbiome: The Superorganism

"*All diseases begin in the gut.*" This is a statement from Hippocrates, who lived in Greece from 460 to 370 B.C. His statement became reality, secondary to innovative relevant studies. Indeed, there is a close relationship between gut microbiota and the host in that they share the same environment during the phylogenetic development of humans [1]. This intimate coevolution resulted in an interlocking symbiotic relationship in which the microbiota plays a regulatory role at various levels: immune, metabolic, neuroendocrine, and even behavioral; thus today a microbiota–gut–brain axis can be defined [2].

Studies using 16S ribosomal RNA surveys and direct sequencing of genetic material showed that the human gut microbiota is a complex community of 100 trillion archaeal and bacterial cells, including more than one thousand species. Each compartment of the gastrointestinal tract (mouth, esophagus, stomach, small and large intestines, rectum, and anus) represents a different chemical environment, and consequently habitable microorganisms (the quantity and quality of the species) differ notably in each compartment. The microbial genome (microbiome) of the human intestine was recently studied by important projects such as the European MetaHIT Consortium [3] and the Human Microbiota Project [4]. These allow more than 3.3 million genes in the gut of 124 Europeans subjects to be sequenced, an number 150 times larger than that of the human host.

This huge number of genes includes those encoding for regulatory functions of the host organism. For example, the microbiome provides very important biosynthetic pathways that extend the host's metabolic capacity.

To understand the importance of the relationship between microflora and the host, the human body should be considered a "dynamic system," or thermodynamically, as an "open system" that exchanges information with the environment to increase its level of organization. Some of this information is exchanged with the microbiota, which is, in turn, another dynamic system. In this type of system, the responses are sensitive to the current conditions. This means that a certain factor may have an effect on the dynamics of the organism based on the overall conditions of the system at that time. Therefore, the answer is based on the input mode: "if . . . then . . ."

E. Biffi (✉)
Brescia, Italy
e-mail: biffienrico@alice.it

M. Fioranelli (ed.), *Integrative Cardiology*, DOI 10.1007/978-3-319-40010-5_7

The effects of the relationships among the elements constituting a dynamic system go beyond the mere addition of the interactions leading to the emergence of new system configurations that can result in the evolution or involution of parts or of the whole system. Furthermore, the coexistence of stable and unstable parts of the system does not allow the true response to each input to be predicted. Today, everything leads us to consider the bodies of mammals as "superorganisms," considering the complexity of the interactions among all their subcomponents and the environment, finally defining it as a "functional field." This research on the relationship existing between microbiota and host gives variable and nonrepeatable results, differing according to standard and acquired scientific criteria [5]. The environment is very important for the composition of gut microbiota and it can be preponderant to the genetic predisposition. The composition of bacterial flora of the gut is highly sensitive to changes in the environment secondary to food and drugs, especially antibiotics. Several research works showed that this correlates with major alterations in the gut microbiota [6], resulting in the dysregulation of host immune homeostasis and an increased susceptibility to diseases [7].

New culture-independent techniques based on polymerase chain reaction (PCR) amplification, cloning, and sequencing of the 16S ribosomal RNA gene [8] and microbial DNA sequencing revolutionized the characterization of microbial communities and demonstrated that the mammalian gut microbiota is dominated by four bacterial phyla: Bacteroidetes and Proteobacteria, which are gram-negative, and the gram-positive Actinobacteria and Firmicutes, with relatively lower numbers, and one Archaea (Euryarchaeota) belonging to Verrucomicrobia, Fusobacteria, Cyanobacteria, Lentisphaerae, Spirochaetes, and TM7. Firmicutes is the largest bacterial phylum and includes 200 genera: *Ruminococcus, Bacillus, Lactobacillus, Mycoplasma*, *Clostridium*, and the butyrate producers *Eubacterium, Faecalibacterium, Roseburia*. Bacteroidetes includes *Bacteroides*, *Prevotella*, and *Xylanibacter*. Actinobacteria phylum includes *Collinsella* and *Bifidobacterium; Escherichia* and *Desulfovibrio* are Proteobacteria. Verrucomicrobia include *Akkermansia*, and Euryarchaeota includes *Methanobrevibacter* which is involved in intestinal methanogenesis.

Firmicutes and Bacteroidetes are the most important components of microbiota in metabolism regulation of the host.

Different studies and statistical analysis [9] recently identified three human "enterotypes" characterized by an enrichment of members of the *Bacteroides* (enterotype 1), *Prevotella* (enterotype 2), and *Ruminococcus* (enterotype 3) clades, not dictated by age, gender, body weight, or ethnicity. Arumugam et al. [9] hypothesize the potential diagnostic use of microbial markers. Indeed, although individual biological characteristics of the host, such as gender, age, and body mass index (BMI), cannot explain the listed enterotypes, data-driven marker genes or functional modules can be identified for each of these host properties.

In contrast, Arumugam et al. [9], in a follow-up study, concluded that only the first two enterotypes (*Bacteroides* and *Prevotella*) were supported by new data, whereas evidence for the enterotype 3 (*Ruminococcus*) was lacking. According to Wu et al., the first two enterotypes in particular are strongly influenced by diet. This means that one enterotype will dominate over the other depending on the diet: *Prevotella* prevails in the gut microbiota of people who prefer eating vegetables typical of agrarian societies; *Bacteroides* predominate in people who eat animal proteins and saturated fats, components characteristic of a Western diet. According to the study by Wu et al., microbiome composition modifies detectably within 24 h after a high-fat/low-fiber or low-fat/high-fiber diet starts, but enterotype identity changes after 10 days. Therefore, alternative enterotype states are associated with a long-term diet.

The identification of three enterotypes is currently an issue under discussion. Several research works do not seem to support the main concept of independence by location, gender, age, BMI, and health status argued by Arumugam et al. [9], leaving the debate still open.

7.2 The Role of Gut Microbiome in the Metabolism of the Host and Cardiac Health

An increasing number of studies demonstrate the role of the microbiome in health and cardiovascular diseases (CVDs). The pathogenetic mechanisms by which the microbiota of mammals influence the onset of cardiovascular diseases are multiple and complex, but all seem to result in a fundamental mechanism: low-grade inflammation. This can occur due to the bacteria themselves [11] or bacterial endotoxins [12] or to metabolic products of bacterial lipids. An alternative pathogenetic mechanism is the bacteria's ability to modify the host metabolism, causing metabolic diseases such as metabolic syndrome (MS), which is strictly correlated with CVDs. The gut microbiome can play an important pathogenetic role in vascular disease through two modes: direct and indirect interference with the host metabolism can cause vascular system inflammation.

7.2.1 Functional Relationship Between the Gut Microbiome and the Host Metabolism in Health and Disease

Development of MS is secondary to a complex process involving genetic and environmental factors. Several findings demonstrate microbial influences on lipid and glucose metabolism, sense of satiety, and chronic low-grade inflammation, which are known to be involved in MS.

Therefore, microflora and diet play a key role in the pathogenesis of MS; these elements are mutually connected. The gut microbiome interacts with the host metabolism to indirectly influence and control energy expenditure and fat storage [1, 13, 14]. This seems to be influenced by the composition of the bacterial flora, which depends on the type of diet. Therefore, all the factors modifying microbial composition and intestinal microbiota function (diet, antibiotics and other drugs, stress, infections, etc.) cause bacterial variability decrease [6], which leads to altered guest metabolism. The alteration of the intestinal barrier, caused by many factors (dysbiosis, local low-grade inflammation, drugs, stress, diet, alcohol, etc.), thus increasing continuous passage in the portal and systemic circulation of endotoxins in low doses, induces a low-grade systemic chronic inflammation (LGSCI) via translocation of TLR ligands (Fig. 7.1) [15–17].

7.2.2 Gut Microbiota Composition, Metabolic Phenotype, and Disease Risk

Several studies on animals (rats and mice) and humans demonstrate that obese and lean phenotypes are associated with different gut microbial compositions with a different Firmicutes–Bacteroidetes ratio and low levels of *Methanobrevibacter smithii*, the leading representative of the gut microbiota archaea [18]. Many studies showed an increase in Firmicutes and Actinobacteria in obese phenotype in animals [19] and humans [14]. These data support the Firmicutes–Bacteroidetes ratio as one of the important key factors in obesity that seems to be modulated by a weight-reduction diet.

Moreover, several research works emphasize the correlation between the concentration of certain *Lactobacillus* species and obesity in both humans [20] and animals [21]. Million et al. [21] observed increasing levels of *Lactobacillus reuteri* and depletion of *Bifidobacterium animalis* species in microbiota of obese test animals. Genetically, obese ob/ob mice encoding the hormone leptin promoting satiety have higher levels of Firmicutes and lower levels of Bacteroidetes at their cecal microbiota than their wild-type littermates. This condition remains unchanged when they are fed with a low-fat, polysaccharide-rich diet.

Various bacterial species were associated with obesity: *Staphylococcus aureus*, *Escherichia coli*, *Faecalibacterium prausnitzii*. However, other research works did not confirm the "typical

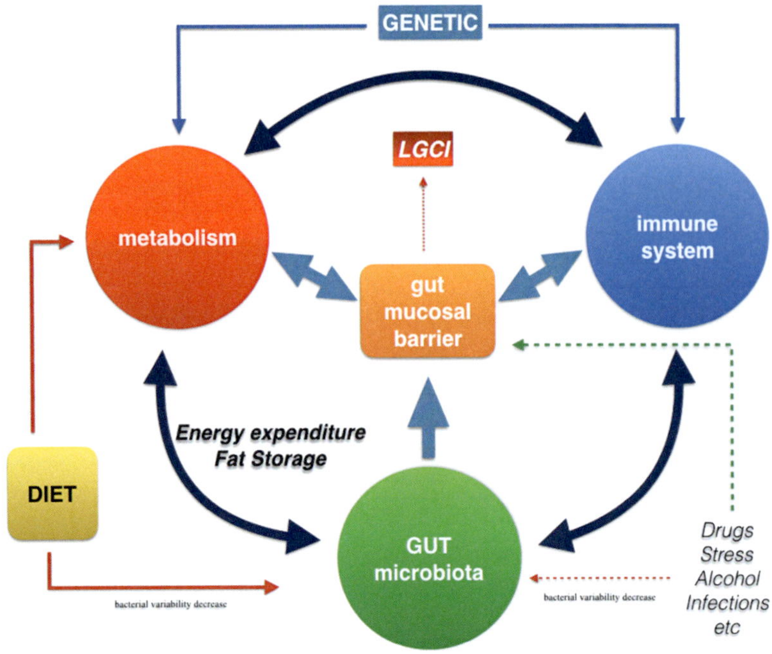

Fig. 7.1 Genetic and environmental factors in the pathogenesis of metabolic syndrome (MS)

change" detected by the above mentioned investigators. For example, Schwiertz et al. [18] showed an even lower Firmicutes–Bacteroidetes ratio in obese human adults compared with lean controls. They observed no differences between obese and lean subjects in the numbers of Bacteroidetes dosed in the fecal sample.

These different findings would suggest that the connection among diet, microbiota composition, and host metabolic regulation is a complex process in obesogenesis. The behavior of the microbiota–host metabolic regulation interactive axis varies in any individual according to development stages and environmental conditions such as diet, use of antibiotics and other drugs, and other factors that substantially reduce bacterial diversity [6], the contribution of the genetic background of the host being understood. Indeed, within an individual the same microbial products may achieve either a beneficial or an adverse effect. The "metacommunity theory" [22] could be used to explain the dynamics of the human microbiome, and in particular, compositional variability within and between the hosts. The "metacommunity" concept is an important way of thinking about linkages between different spatial scales in ecology. According to this theory, the diversity of the microbiome changes at different body sites, between people, with age and with diet. This leads to the realization of different environments within and between different individuals who are exposed to temporal variation and between populations. Most likely, the metagenomic-based functional aspects are more important than the difference at the phylum level of the microbiota.

7.2.3 Diet, Microbiota, and Host Metabolism

The impact of diet on microbiota composition appears to be more relevant than obesity [23]. Gut microbiota composition depends on different eating habits. In Burkina Faso children with a predominantly vegetarian diet, microbiota showed specific abundance in Bacteroidetes than Firmicutes, and bacterial augmentation of bacteria with enzymes enables hydrolysis of cellulose and xylan, and also of members of the genera *Prevotella* and *Xylanibacter*. However, Enterobacteriaceae (*Shigella* and *Escherichia*) were significantly under-represented. Otherwise, Firmicutes and Proteobacteria were more abundant in European children with a Western diet [24]. We can speculate that gut microbiota might have co-evolved with the polysaccharide-rich diet of African children, allowing them to maximize energy intake from fibers and protecting them from inflammation and non-infectious colonic diseases by modulating gut-associated lymphatic tissue (GALT). This study on microbiota composition of European and African children seems to confirm the evidence of Arumugam et al. [9] concerning three enterotypes dominated by a different genus—*Bacteroides*, *Prevotella*, or *Ruminococcus*.

A dietary intervention for a few days is not sufficient to change individual enterotype. A controlled feeding study of ten subjects showed that microbiome composition changed within 24 h of initiating a high-fat/low-fiber or low-fat/high-fiber diet, but that enterotype identity remained stable during the 10-day study [25].

Cani et al. [26] demonstrated in mice that a very high-fat (HF) diet induced change in gut microbiota composition associated with an increase in weight gain, adiposity, insulin resistance, and other symptoms of MS. The same authors only detected a reduction of *Bifidobacterium* spp. [27, 28] and *Bacteroides*-related bacteria, *Eubacterium rectale-Blautia coccoides* group, *Lactobacillus* spp., and *Roseburia* spp. content [26]. Several other studies confirmed the altered Firmicutes–Bacteroidetes ratio in mice fed with an HF diet [19, 23].

The increase in circulating bacterial endotoxins such as lipopolysaccharides (LPS) emphasizes the relationship among diet, microbiota, host metabolism, and low-grade inflammation. An HF diet induces changes in the microbiota composition accompanied by an increase in circulating Gram-negative *Proteobacteria* responsible, to avoid the induction of inflammatory local response and an increase in the passage of LPS from the gut lumen to the gut interstitium, where it can activate TLR4 on afferent nerve terminals [29].

Intestinal microflora change could precede the establishment of the obese phenotype and could contribute to its development. Several findings in obesity mouse models demonstrated that at a higher fat diet increases the production of Resistin-like molecule beta (RELMβ) in the stools and in the serum [30]. Furthermore, the same mechanism plays a role in humans too [30]. RELMβ is one of three isoforms of the *RELM* gene family [31] and it is produced by goblet cells secondary to microbial intestinal colonization [30]. The genetic activation of RELMβ is started via interleukin 4 by antigenic stimulation of the Th2 immunity response [32]. On the contrary it is inhibited by interferon γ through a Th1-mediated immunity response. RELMβ regulates the gut microbiota composition both by stimulating production of defensins, and regulating functions of the intestinal barrier at innate mucosal immunity [33], which results in macrophages activation. Moreover, a recent study proved the metabolic effects of RELMβ on intestinal homeostasis of glucose and induction of insulin resistance. RELMβ regulates intracellular transport mechanism of glucose by an increase in glucose transporter (GLUT2) expression, a passive low affinity transporter. This allows the output of glucose through the basal membranes of the enterocytes.

RELMβ expression is augmented both in genetic (ob/db mice) and nongenetic obesity murine models [34] induced by an HF diet. Indeed, an in vitro study showed how saturated fatty acids directly induce the expression of RELMβ [34].

A direct relationship has been demonstrated between expression levels of RELMβ and microbiota composition in RELMβ knockout mice; those showed an increase in Firmicutes rather than Bacteroidetes [23]. In cohort study, Hildebrandt et al. [23] demonstrated that RELMβ knockout mice remained comparatively lean when subjected to the HF diet. They found that consistent changes in microbial communities could be seen upon switching to the HF diet for both wild-type and RELMβ knockout mice. It was established that the HF diet itself, and not the obese state, was responsible for the altered microbiota. The action carried out by RELMβ on both the intestinal microbiota and the glucose homeostasis may explain the link between diet and modification of the intestinal microbiota. This could be related to the direct action carried out by RELMβ on the secretion of intestinal antimicrobial peptides. The reduced secretion of β-defensin I (and/or other members of the defensin family), induced by RELMβ, could be responsible for impaired composition of the microbiota induced by HF diets (Fig. 7.2).

7.3 From Leaky Gut Syndrome and Chronic Low-Grade Inflammation to Cardiometabolic Syndrome

7.3.1 The Gut Microbiota and Innate Immunity Regulation of the Host

The mammalian immune system uses two lines of defense. Innate immunity is the first line and responds to numerous nonspecific numerous exogenous and endogenous pathogenetic factors; adaptive immunity is the second line, which

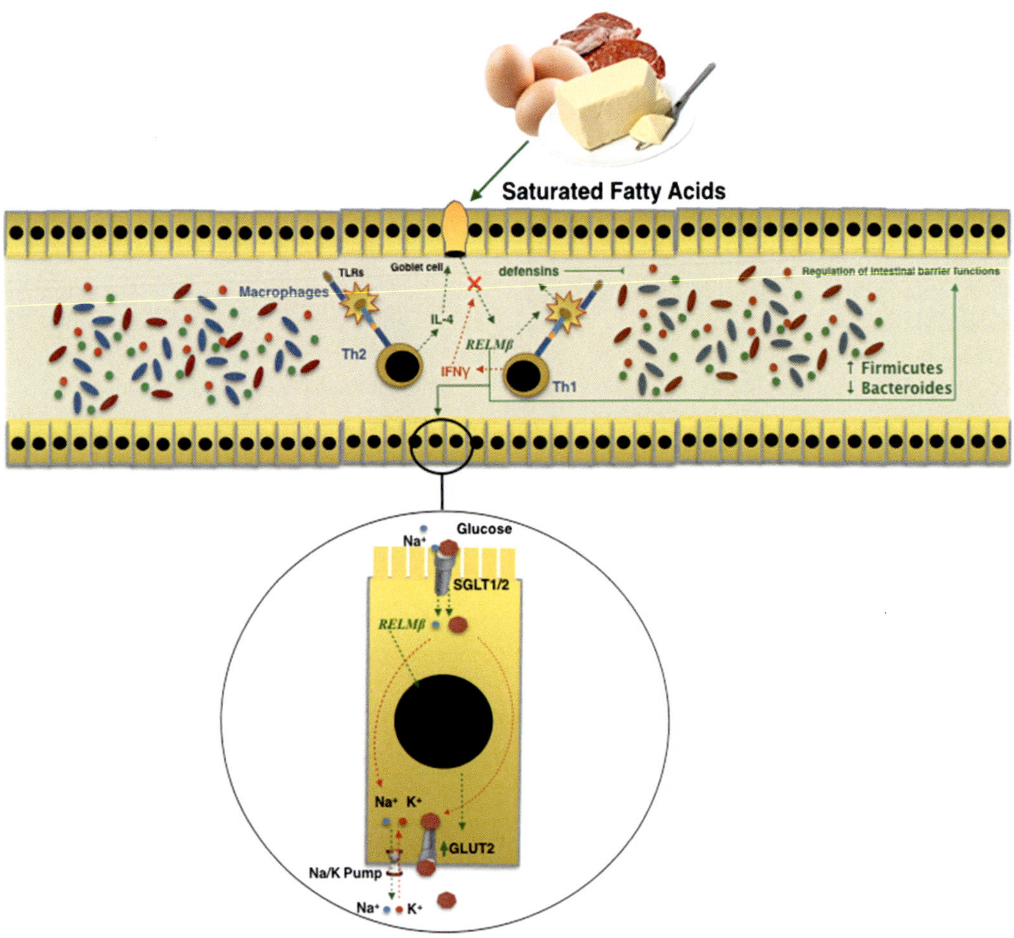

Fig. 7.2 RELMβ is produced by goblet cells in the gut in response to microbial intestinal colonization. Saturated fatty acids in a high-fat diet directly induced expression of RELMβ. The action carried out by RELMβ on both the intestinal microbiota and the glucose homeostasis may explain the link between diet and modification of the intestinal microbiota in obesity and metabolic syndrome

gives a specific response (humoral and cell-mediated immunity) with the activation of the immune response regulated by Th1, Th2, Th17, and Th1/Th17 cells. Innate immunity represents a defensive system with an important barrier function via several mechanisms: epithelial barrier, tight junctions, antimicrobial peptides such as cathelicidins and defensins. It includes various cells: neutrophils, basophils, eosinophils, mast cells, monocytes, macrophages, dendritic cells (DCs), NK and NK-T cells, B1 cells and $\gamma\delta$ T cells with the pathogen recognition receptors (PRRs). PRRs can be expressed on the cell surface or intracellularly. They recognize highly conserved antigens from bacteria, microbial-associated molecular patterns (MAMPs), and other pathogens, pathogen-associated molecular patterns (PAMPs). PRR activation by MAMPs, causing recruitment of down-stream signaling molecules, results in activation of NFkB transcription factor leading to increased production of pro-inflammatory cytokines [35].

Several families of innate receptors are involved in the recognition of PAMPs. They include toll-like receptors (TLRs), staying on the surface of the cellular membrane and intracellularly on a range of different cell types [36]; nucleotide oligomerization domains (NODs); inflammasomes, large intracellular cytoplasmic multi-protein complexes composed of one of several NOD-like receptors (NLRs) and pyrin and HIN domain-containing protein family (PYHIN: including NLRP1, NLRP3, NLRC4, and AIM2) playing a central role in innate immunity; C-type lectin receptors (CLRs) such as dectin-1, and RNA-sensing RIG-like helicases such as RLRs; RIG-I and MDA5; and cytosolic dsDNA sensors (CDSs). They are cytoplasmic receptors critical for host antiviral responses [37, 38] and for diverse MAMPs or death-associated molecular protein ligands released in response to cell necrosis or tissue injury: damage-associated molecular patterns (DAMPs) or alarmins.

The DAMPs contribute to "sterile inflammation" [39] via activation of TLR. Most DAMPs are substances that are normally sequestered within cells but released in response to injury. Degradation products of extracellular matrix or glycocalyx are heat shock proteins (HSP) (10), IgG chromatin complex (11), versican (12), high-mobility group box 1 (HMGB1), heparan sulfate (14), hyaluronan, uric acid, and others.

The two best characterized families of PRRs are TLRs and nucleotide oligomerization domains (NODs)-leucine-rich repeat (LRR) family (CATERPILLER family), which are intracellular receptors [37, 38]. The ligands identified for TLRs include PAMPs and DAMPs.

In the gut, TLRs and NODs are involved in maintaining mucosal and commensal homeostasis. The functional activity of the TLRs and NOD2 is very important for a healthy gut, as they are involved in host defense and tissue repair responses. Correction functioning of TLRs and NOD2 enhances barrier protection and antimicrobial activity, reduces bacterial invasion, confers tolerance, and promotes healing. When homeostasis between commensal and mucosal immunity is perturbed, TLRs and NOD2 signaling can result in an exaggerated proinflammatory responses through cytokine and chemokine production. Altered expression of TLRs induces intestinal barrier destruction, an increase in the passage of endotoxins, loss of tolerance, and antimicrobial activity with enhanced bacterial invasion [40].

Gram-negative bacteria present the LPS that binds TLR4, whereas Gram-positive bacteria have proteoglycans (PGN) and lipoteichoic acids that bind TLR2.

7.3.1.1 Gut Microbiota, Gut Barrier Integrity, and Chronic Low-Grade Inflammation

The gut barrier consists of an epithelial monolayer and its intercellular junctional system, mucus, and mucosal immune system.

Intestinal epithelial barrier integrity is an important factor in innate immunity function. It is essentially controlled by a complex system of junction proteins (tight junctions, zonula adherens, gap junctions, and desmosomes). The apical junction system is represented by tight junctions (TJs) and the zonula adherens. Together, the TJs and zonula adherens form the "apical junction complex" (AJC). In addition to providing a barrier to noxious molecules, TJs can also operate as pores for the permeation of ions, solutes, and water, as appropriate. The interplay among the tetra-span proteins (occludin, claudin, and tricellulin) [41] and specific claudin isoforms (claudin-2, 7, 12, and 15) determines selective barrier permeability. Single-span transmembrane proteins, on the other hand, are mostly junctional adhesion molecules. Belonging to the immunoglobulin superfamily, junctional adhesion molecules participate in the regulation and maintenance of the TJ barrier in an active way. These proteins are associated with peripheral membrane (plaque) proteins such as zonula occludens (ZO) proteins 1, 2, and 3 (Fig. 7.3) [42].

On the intracellular side of the plasma membrane, these proteins contribute to anchoring the junctional protein complex to the actin component of the cytoskeleton, making it sensitive to all factors acting both on the latter and on mitochondrial oxidative phosphorylation, such as FANS and propionic pump inhibitors [43].

The AJC complex is regularly remodeled by interactions with external stimuli: food, pathogenic bacteria, and microbiota components.

The mucosal integrity is guaranteed by the continuity of the epithelial cells and the junctional structure. Additionally, Paneth cells are a specialized type of secretory epithelial cells that inhabit the mucosal surface of the small intestine and produce high quantities of defensins, and other antimicrobial and antibiotic peptides that are very important for correct and ambient intestinal homeostasis [44]. With Paneth cell secretion, the goblet cells are also important for the production of the mucus consisting of a set of glycosylated molecules and enzymes. The mucus comprises two stratified layers: the external layer creates an ideal culture medium for microbial colonization, the inner layer, a denser layer, contains relatively few bacteria and exerts a protective function for the host [44].

The augmented paracellular permeability of the small intestine allowed the passage (leakage) of small quantities of microbes, and endotoxins in the circulation, such as LPS [45]) and peptidoglycan [46], with a secondary activation of the inflammatory response in target tissues such as liver, adipose tissue, coronary vessels, and articulations by triggering PRRs. It follows the

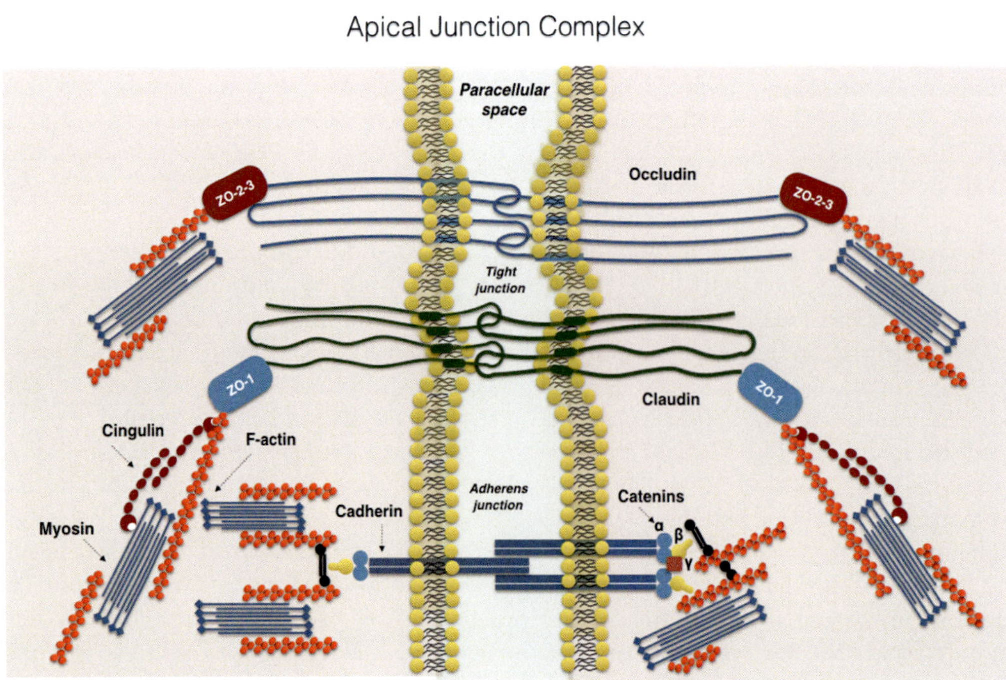

Fig. 7.3 The apical junction complex. A simplified diagram of the molecular composition of tight junctions and adherens junctions

onset of various diseases that together develop the framework of the MS.

The increased intestinal permeability promotes LPS absorption, which leads to a state of low-grade metabolic endotoxemia characterized by serum LPS concentration 10–50 times lower than the typical values for septicemia. This induces a state of chronic low-grade inflammation (CLGI) known as leaky gut syndrome (LGS).

Several studies suggest that the host–microbiota relationship might lead to the modulation of the gut barrier function [15, 47, 48].

The gut microbiota may modulate the intestinal barrier integrity via several mechanisms. The intestinal microbiome, by its metabolism of vegetable polysaccharides and short-chain fatty acids (SCFAs) production can regulate the GLP-2 production, improving mucosal barrier function. In effect, administration in mice of prebiotics increases the production of GLP2 in the jejunum and colon via both autocrine and paracrine regulatory loops, reducing metabolic endotoxemia, hepatic inflammation, and oxidative stress markers [47].

The role of microbiota in the modulation of gut permeability could also be mediated by the action of SCFAs on fatty acid synthase (FAS), an essential enzyme for de novo lipogenesis of the intestinal epithelial cells. FAS helps to maintain the mucus barrier by regulating mucin 2, the dominant mucin in the colon and an important component of the mucus. Indeed, specific modulation of gut microbiota composition with prebiotics, as inulin, improves gut barrier integrity, reduces metabolic endotoxemia, and lowers inflammation [49].

Diabetes, hyperlipidemia, obesity, insulin resistance, hypertension, cardiovascular disease, and arteriosclerosis are metabolic illnesses configuring the metabolic syndrome characterized by systemic CLGI [50]. Several findings correlate the altered intestinal permeability with the state of metabolic endotoxemia and consequent systemic low-grade inflammation [51] linked with a gradual deterioration of the organs involved in the inflammatory process.

The HF diet caused an increment of intestinal permeability by microbiota as demonstrated by the use of antibiotic treatment that abolished diet-induced gut permeability [13, 15]. Indeed, it is now well accepted that HF diet-induced metabolic diseases are associated with low-grade inflammation occurring, among other tissues, in adipose depots. This inflammatory process can cause an increase in inflammatory cytokine production and it is also characterized by increased macrophage infiltration [52].

Several research works demonstrate that an HF diet and consequent microbiota composition changes can contribute to the disruption of the TJ proteins (zonula occludens-1 and occludin) involved in the gut barrier function [51]. Moreover, some studies have demonstrated that intestinal luminal exposure to oleic acid can cause intestinal epithelial damage [53]. These effects induced by an HF diet could be mediated through the microbiota and TLR-2.

This condition plays an important regulatory role in tight junctions associated with intestinal epithelial barrier integrity. TLR-2 deficiency predisposes to alterations of TJ-modulated barrier function leading to the perpetuation of mucosal inflammation [40, 54]. Caricilli et al. [55] demonstrated that TLR2 knockout mice present an increase in LPS absorption secondary to decreased expression of TJ protein zonula occludens (ZO)-1 in the ileum with consequent disorder of gut barrier functions. This could be determined by a decrease in *Bifidobacterium* spp. The authors observed TLR2 knockout mice with a decrease in *Bifidobacterium* spp., supporting the lower expression of zonula occludens 1 (ZO-1). After gut microbiota transplantation from TLR2 knockout to *Bacillus*-monoassociated wild-type mice, Caricilli et al. [55] observed a reduction in the expression of ZO-1 in the ileum of the recipients, suggesting that the expression of this protein might be regulated by the particular microbiota present in the gastrointestinal tract of TLR2 knockout mice.

An HF diet promotes intestinal absorption of bacterial endotoxins by different mechanisms demonstrated in several findings. LPS can cross the intestinal barrier by transcellular transport through intestinal epithelial cells and/or intestinal-epithelial microfold cells (M-cells). These specialized epithelial cells are present in the intestinal epithelium; they are also permeable to bacteria and macromolecules, and able to express gut antigens via the underlying lymphoid tissue.

Amar et al. [56] demonstrated that an HF diet induces a "low-grade bacteremia" by an augmented bacterial translocation from the intestinal mucosal barrier. The authors showed that both the adipose tissue and the blood from diabetic mice fed with an HF diet contain living bacteria. They originated from the intestine and were linked to low-grade inflammation. Furthermore, intestinal mucosa from HF-fed mice exhibits properties that are different from the mucosa of normal chow-fed mice and which facilitate bacterial adherence. Using a labeled *E. coli* bacterial strain with a fluorophore and an ampicillin reporter gene, Amar et al. [56] believed that an HF diet led to an increase in the *E. coli* co-localization with dendritic cells (DCs) in the intestinal lamina propria. The bacteria, probably remaining inside the DCs, then rapidly disseminated into mesenteric adipose tissue (MAT) and corresponding mesenteric lymph nodes (MLN). However, the presence of various bacteria in MAT and corresponding MLN represents a physiological mechanism that is exacerbated during HF diet-induced metabolic diseases. It is noteworthy that an HF diet increases the accumulation of Gram-negative bacteria that produce LPS, which are highly inflammatogenic molecules, by triggering TLR4 in different tissue.

Toll-like receptors are expressed on the apical surface of enterocytes, where they recognize the MAMPs and active binding and internalizing of these endotoxins [57]. Indeed, the enterocytes can internalize Gram-negative bacteria through TLR4, which mediates phagocytosis and translocation of Gram-negative bacteria in vivo [58]. Furthermore, LPS may be internalized by enterocytes via a myeloid differentiation protein-2 (MD-2)-dependent mechanism [58]. In fact, MD-2 has been recognized as a key molecule for LPS signaling [59].

An HF diet seems to favor absorption of LPS because these have a great affinity for chylomicrons. There is a possibility that LPS could be associated with chylomicrons within the enterocyte and then secreted from cell-associated pools in a chylomicron-dependent manner. This condition could induce continuous postprandial low-grade endotoxemia finally resulting in low-grade inflammation [60] Indeed, TLR4 binding LPS could pass through the intestinal barrier assembled in chylomicrons [61]. Additionally, LPS is internalized in enterocytes through a TLR4 and is transported to the Golgi compartment and finally secreted from the basolateral surface into chylomicrons (Fig. 7.4) [62].

7.3.2 The Extraintestinal Causes of Increased Gut Permeability

7.3.2.1 Stress Impairs Gut Permeability

Numerous environmental factors are able to impair the gut permeability. Many of those act both through stress and activation of the hypothalamic–pituitary–adrenal (HPA) axis. Indeed, both cognitive and noncognitive stressors activate HPA axis inducing many important effects on gut. Noncognitive stressors, similar to pathogens, activate stress by IL-1β, IL-6, and TNFα secretion throughout inflammatory cells induction. These cytokines directly stimulate hypothalamus corticotropin-releasing factor (CRF) secretion, activating the HPA axis. In this way LGCI induces stress and increases LGS levels. Also, prolonged cognitive (psychological) stressors, such as chronic work stress, are linked to higher levels of cytokines IL-6 and TNFα [63]. Stressed mice demonstrate enhanced splenic macrophage microbicidal activity, a sign of increased innate immunity activity [64]. Exposure to cognitive stressors also increases cytokine production via LPS-stimulated splenic macrophages through the effects of stress on gut permeability to MAMPs [64].

The role of microbiota in this phenomena is demonstrated by the absence of this effect in germ-free mice. Furthermore, antibiotic treatment attenuating the stressor-induced splenic macrophage reactivity and preventing the increased circulating levels of bacterial peptidoglycan (PGN), suggest that translocation of microbiota-derived PGN might promotes innate immune system activation.

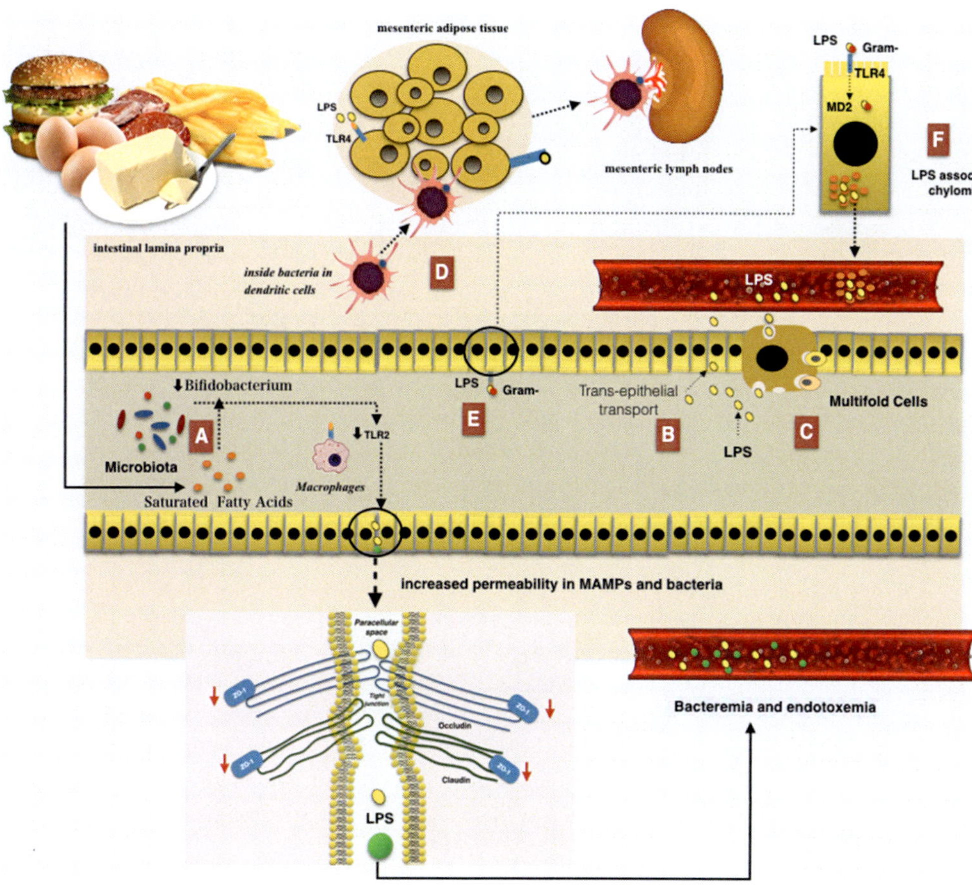

Fig. 7.4 The relationship between a high-fat (HF) diet and augmented gut permeability to bacteria and microbial-associated molecular patterns (MAMPs): (**a**) A reduced number of *Bifidobacterium* could induce TLR2 expression and then a reduction in the expression of zonula occludens 1 (ZO-1) would result in alterations of tight junction (TJ)-modulated barrier function, leading to the perpetuation of mucosal inflammation. (**b**) Lipopolysaccharides (LPS) can cross the intestinal barrier via transcellular transport through the intestinal epithelial cells. (**c**) LPS can also cross the intestinal barrier via transcellular transport through microfold cells. (**d**) An HF diet led to an increase in the *E. coli* co-localization with dendritic cells (DCs) in the intestinal lamina propria. The bacteria, probably remaining inside the DCs, are then rapidly disseminated into mesenteric adipose tissue and corresponding mesenteric lymph nodes. (**e**) The TLR is expressed on the apical surface of enterocytes and mainly recognize the MAMPs, where it is capable of binding and internalizing purified endotoxin and bacteria. Furthermore LPS may be internalized by enterocytes through a myeloid differentiation protein-2 (MD-2)-dependent mechanism. (**f**) LPS have a great affinity for chylomicrons and thus could be associated with them within the enterocytes and then secreted from cell-associated pools in a chylomicron-dependent manner

Several indications have demonstrated increased sympathetic nervous system (SNS) activity as being responsible for enhanced innate immune activity [65].

Exposure to stress results in alteration of the MGBA inducing important alteration in gut physiology: (1) alteration in gastrointestinal motility; (2) increase in visceral perception; (3) changes in gastrointestinal secretion; (4) increase in intestinal permeability; (5) negative effects on regenerative capacity of gastrointestinal mucosa and mucosal blood flow; (6) alteration of interactions between the immune system of the host and microbiota, inducing dysbiosis [66].

The brain interacts with the gut through multiple pathways, including the vagal and splanchnic pathways, HPA axis, and other connections.

All of these comprised the gut–brain axis (GBA) and for its important interplay with microbiota: the microbiota–gut–brain axis (MGBA). Indeed, as stress modifies the bacterial flora of the gut, inducing an immunological alteration of the GALT, at the same time, microbiota may have an important effect on the GBAm acting on modulation of the motility.

The involvement of the MGBA in the stress is particularly induced by corticotrophin releasing factor (CRF). The CRF family peptides are expressed both in the CNS and within the gut. Here, CRF plays an important role in many biological actions: inflammation modulation, visceral hypersensitivity (increasing pain perception), augmentation of gut permeability, and motility modulation.

An important pathogenetic role in induction of the gut alteration in stress is played by the mast cells. These cells, which have receptors for CRF on their surface, translate many signals of stress to the intestine [67]. Several studies demonstrate that CRF induces mast cell activation, causing the release of many pro-inflammatory mediators, including de novo synthesized mediators such as prostaglandins and leukotrienes, or preformed granule-housed mediators, including histamine, serine proteases, tryptase, chymase, and finally cytokines such as TNFα [68]. By the release of these mediators, mast cells induce increased intestinal permeability [68, 69]. In an animal model, Overman et al. [70] demonstrated that the gut barrier damage induced by mast cell activation via CRF is mediated by TNFα and proteases. Furthermore, CRF-mast cell signaling pathways and increased intestinal permeability require critical input from the enteric nervous system. In an animal model CRF could inhibit NLRP6 inflammasome signaling, which, with NLRP3, is important in the maintenance of healthy microbiota through the secretion of IL-18 [71]. The consequent alteration of microbiota composition stimulates CCL5 expression in intestinal epithelial cells, resulting in augmented permeability and adsorption of bacterial products and microorganism passage through the paracellular space. Administration of probiotics prevents stress-induced mucosal damage, demonstrating the pathogenetic role of dysbiosis caused by inhibition of NLRP6 via CRF (Fig. 7.5).

Stress induces a very important change in microbiota composition, in neurotransmitter and proinflammatory cytokine levels with direct and indirect effects on the same microbiota. Bailey et al. [65] demonstrated that stressor exposure has an impact on the stability of the microbiota and leads to bacterial translocation across the gut barrier. Mice subjected to chronic stress, which increases circulating cytokines and primes the innate immune system for enhanced reactivity, showed significant changes in the community structure of the microbiota with a decrease in *Bacteroides* and an increase in *Clostridium*. The stressed mice also showed increased circulating levels of IL-6 and MCP-1, which correlated significantly with stressor-induced changes to three bacterial genera (*Coprococcus*, *Pseudobutyrivibrio*, and *Dorea*). Mice treated with antibiotics did not show increased IL-6 and MCP-1 levels; dysbiosis is the primary cause of increased circulating cytokine levels.

The evidence suggests a paradigm in which stressor exposure alters homeostatic interactions among the intestinal microbiota, the mucosal immune system and balance in the MGBA. This leads to gut barrier damage and to translocation of MAMPs and pathogenic and/or commensal microbes from the lumen of the intestines to the interior of the host, where they trigger systemic inflammatory responses, inducing LGCI and anxiety-like behavior.

7.3.2.2 Iatrogenic Damage of Intestinal Permeability

Several therapeutic treatments may impair gut permeability. These include radiotherapy and many pharmacological therapies using antibiotic, chemotherapeutic, immunosuppressive drugs and nonsteroidal anti-inflammatory drugs (NSAIDs). These play a fundamental pathogenetic role in damage of the gut barrier. Indeed, these are over-the-counter drugs that are also widely used by heart patients. According to AIFA (Italian agency for drugs) statistics, the defined daily dose (DDD) of prescribed NSAIDs

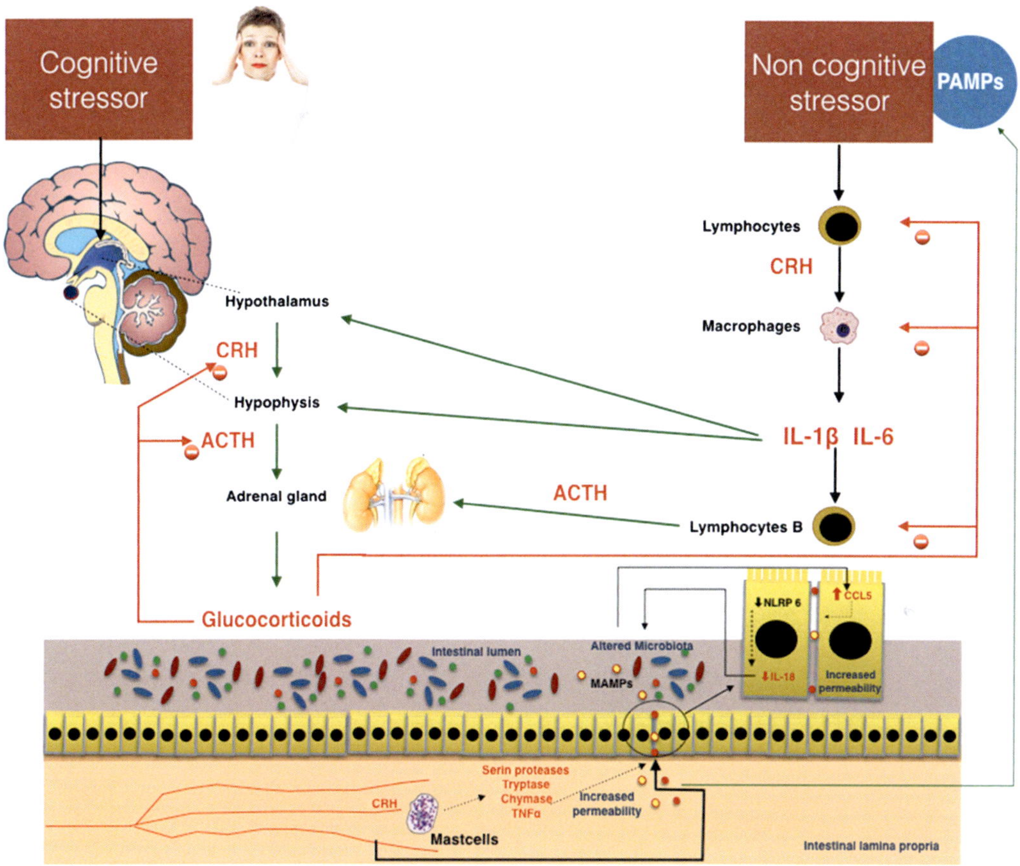

Fig. 7.5 Possible effects of cognitive and noncognitive stressors on gut permeability. Important effects altering intestinal permeability are mediated by corticotropin-releasing hormone (CRH), which is directly stimulated by cognitive stress and indirectly by noncognitive stressors through the mediation of proinflammatory cytokines IL-6 and IL1β. In the gut, CRH activates secretion of proteases and TNFα in mast cells. These substances damage the intestinal barrier, inducing increased permeability. The passage of pathogen-associated molecular patterns (PAMPs) and bacteria in the blood circulation increases the stress, favoring the development of systemic low-grade inflammation. *ACTH* adrenocorticotropic hormone

per 1,000 inhabitants per day in 2014 in Italy was 22.8.[1] This indicates that 2.28% of the Italian population (about 1,360,000 people) receive a daily prescription of NSAIDs from physicians. Recent studies demonstrate that damage of the mucosal barrier induced by NSAIDs is exacerbated by the use of proton pump inhibitors (PPIs).

It is generally accepted that the use of NSAIDs is frequently prone to side effects on the gastrointestinal system. Early pathogenetic events include a "topical" phase in addition to the inhibition of cyclooxygenase, followed by a multistage pathogenetic event in which intestinal permeability is impaired until awareness of gastric ulcers and intestinal erosions [72, 73]. NSAIDs can determine significant damage to the intestinal mucosa causing both increased intestinal permeability and erosive lesions through pathogenetic mechanisms acting at topical and systemic levels. Somasundaram et al. [73] demonstrated that within 1 h after administration of indomethacin rat intestine is damaged at the brush border of intestinal cells and their mitochondria are vacuolated. NSAIDs act at two

[1] Source: Agenzia Italia del Farmaco: L'uso dei farmaci in Italia—Rapporto nazionale anno 2014.

levels: (1) systemic, inhibiting cyclooxygenase and reducing the modulatory effects of PGs on intestinal homeostasis; (2) local, independent of the effect on cyclooxygenase and induced by the acidity of NSAIDs and its ability to uncouple oxidative phosphorylation and inhibit electron transportation into the mitochondria. NSAID administration results in a slowing down of mitochondrial respiration via uncoupling oxidative phosphorylation, as shown by the reversal of effect depending on the concentration. Indeed, NSAIDs stimulate mitochondrial respiration (uncoupled oxidative phosphorylation) at concentrations between 30 and 1,500 μM, depending on the particular NSAID studied, and inhibit respiration at higher concentrations [73].

Side effects of NSAIDs on the gut barrier are increased when they are associated with a low dose of aspirin, as in heart patients with chronic articular pain. In these cases, the intestinal damage score is higher than using NSAIDs alone. Surprisingly, the intestinal damage score rises when NSAIDs are associated with PPI and much higher if administered with PPIs and low-dose aspirin [74].

7.3.2.3 Gluten and Gut Permeability

During the past few years there has been a remarkable increase in the popularity of a gluten-free diet. Many people believe that it improves their health and leads to the disappearance of symptoms related to different diseases that share an inflammatory state. This attracted the interest of researchers to a disorder related to the ingestion of gluten or gluten-containing cereals, namely nonceliac gluten sensitivity (NCGS). This disorder was originally described in the 1980s [75] and is characterized by intestinal and extra-intestinal symptoms related to the ingestion of gluten-containing food in subjects who are not affected by either celiac disease (CD) or wheat allergy (WA). Thus, NCGS is a de facto gluten-related disorder. Indeed, to enable a consensus on new nomenclature and the classification of gluten-related disorders, a panel of experts first met in London in February 2011. The meeting resulted in a series of definitions and developed a diagnostic algorithm that has recently been published [76].

The most important pathogenetic mechanism induced by gluten is related to its capacity to increase gut barrier permeability. Although a recent study conducted by Sapone et al. [77] demonstrated in NCGS patients the absence of increased gut permeability, gluten is one of the more powerful factors able to trigger zonulin release and innate immune response.

Zonulin system (ZS) is an immunologically related, endogenous modulator of epithelial TJs [78]. Tripathi et al. [79] characterized zonulin as pre-haptoglobin2 (pre-HP2); to date, only regarded as an inactive precursor for HP2, one of two genetic variants of human haptoglobins (HP1 and HP2). The physiological role of this pathway is not completely clear. It appears to be involved in several functions, including TJ regulation responsible for the movement of fluid, macromolecules, and leukocytes between the bloodstream and the intestinal lumen, and vice versa [80]. Another potential physiological role is in innate immunity protecting against microorganism colonization of the proximal intestine [81]. The structure of zonulin is similar to several growth factors, which like zonulin, affect TJ integrity [82]. Indeed, zonulin activates epidermal growth factor receptor (EGFR), causing TJ disassembly, and then augments gut permeability [79]. *Zonulin as pre-HP2*, in its intact configuration, could activate EGFR through direct binding and/or through protease activated receptor 2 (PAR2), a transmembrane receptor that modulates inflammatory responses and acts as a sensor for proteolytic enzymes generated during infection. Intestinal tryptase IV induces structural changes in the molecule, altering its ability to bind to EGFR, but enabling its function as a hemoglobin scavenger. Meanwhile, it becomes an inflammatory marker [83]. Barone et al. [84] demonstrated that gliadin acts like EGF on actin cytoskeleton, with effects very similar to those induced by zonulin. Therefore, gliadin induces zonulin release by intestinal cells and whole intestinal tissues through CXCR3 binding (Fig. 7.6) [27, 28, 81].

Gluten is a complex macromolecule consisting of a globular protein, gliadin, and a fibrous protein, glutenin.

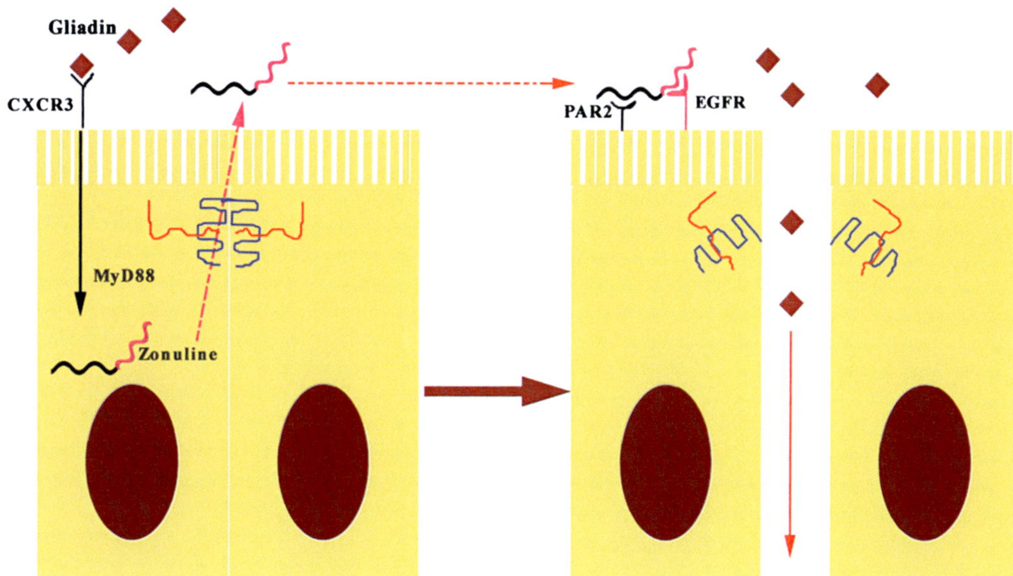

Fig. 7.6 The pathogenetic effects of gliadin on gut permeability are mediated by zonulin. The fragments 11–130 and 151–170 of gluten binding to CXCR3 activates zonulin secretion via MyD88, enabling paracellular translocation of gliadin through the effects of zonulin on the TJ, increasing paracellular permeability. *EGFR* epidermal growth factor receptor

There are at least 50 toxic epitopes in gluten peptides with cytotoxic (*peptide fragment 31–43*), immunomodulatory (*33-mer gliadin fragment* – 57–89 peptide and *IL8-releasing peptide* – fragment 261–277), and gut-permeating activities (CXCR3-binding *zonulin-releasing peptide* fragments 11–130 and 151–170) [85].

The permeabilizing effects of gliadin peptides in vivo was confirmed in patients with active *celiac disease* (CD) and non-CD control patients, when analyzing their intestinal tissue after gliadin challenge [86]. The Fasano group studies suggests that gluten induces changes in gut permeability and activation of innate immunity response comes before that of adaptive immunity [87].

According Fasano, gliadin ingestion throughout *IL8-releasing peptide* induces [88] IL-8 release and recruitment of neutrophils in the intestinal lamina propria in CD patients. Together, *CXCR3-binding zonulin-releasing fragments* activates *zonulin* secretion through MyD88 pathway enabling paracellular translocation of gliadin. Consequently, *33-mer* gliadin and other immunomodulatory peptides of gliadin interact with macrophages of gut submucosa [89]. This interaction via MyD88 induces Th1-type cytokine secretion, resulting in mononuclear cell infiltration of intestinal submucosa. The presence of *IFNγ* and *TNFα* augments epithelial and endothelial gut permeability [90].

In genetically predisposed subjects (*DQ2+* and *DQ8+*) gliadin antigen presentation by dendritic cells to Th cells in intestinal lamina propria induces the loss of oral tolerance and switch to *Th1/Th17* response. The migration of gliadin-loaded DCs in mesenteric lymph nodes leads to migration of $CD4^{-}$ $CD8^{-}$ $\gamma\delta$, and $CD4^{-}$ $CD8^{+}$ $\alpha\beta$ T cells to the gut, where they cause inflammation in patients with *CD*.

7.3.3 CLGI in Cardiovascular Disease

The role of *CLGI* in the pathogenesis of arteriosclerosis and other *CVDs* is now clear and accepted. Currently, the main challenge in atherosclerosis research is the identification of disease-specific *PAMPs* or *DAMPs* able to give innate immune responses in the arterial wall, and finally to promote plaque development [91]. In 1999, Wiedermann demonstrated how subclinical endotoxemia constitutes a strong risk factor for the development of carotid atherosclerosis, particularly among smokers [92]. The same study revealed that plasma from individuals with prevalent atherosclerosis of the carotid arteries could activate endothelium, promoting leukocyte transmigration; this suggested the role of systemic pro-inflammatory mediators. Furthermore, plasma collected from patients without atherosclerosis at the time of enrollment in the study was tested for its capacity to induce endothelial cell activation and transmigration of leukocytes. Increased plasma-induced endothelial cell activation was associated with an increased risk for the development of atherosclerotic lesions such as revealed by subsequent follow-up data on new lesion formation after 5 years. These data indicated that plasma-mediated endothelium activation by interaction with leukocytes promotes the development of atherosclerotic lesions. Plasma collected from patients without atherosclerosis at the time of enrollment in the study resulted in being able to induce endothelial cell activation and transmigration of leukocytes in those subjects who had subsequently developed atherosclerotic lesions [93].

It has long been recognized that in sepsis caused by Gram-negative bacteria, plasma endotoxins are elevated and able to evoke inflammatory cells, such as monocytes and macrophages, and in endothelial and smooth muscle cells numerous proinflammatory responses, including up-regulation of adhesion molecule expression, increased production of *cytokines, reactive oxygen species (ROS), and reactive nitrogen species, prostaglandins, and tissue factor, loss* of monolayer integrity and barrier function, and apoptosis. However, endotoxin levels observed during sepsis are far greater than the low-level endotoxemia that has been associated with atherosclerosis. The Bruneck study demonstrated that subjects with levels of 50 pg/mL or greater were recognized as being at an increased risk for the development of atherosclerosis. This level of endotoxin can induce inflammatory responses in human *monocytes* and *macrophages* and intact human blood vessels exhibit profound responsiveness to endotoxins (cytokine release, superoxide production, and monocyte adhesion). Low oxidative stress modulates endothelial gene expression, which induces atherogenic factors, forming early atherosclerotic plaque [94].

Serum lipoproteins, especially high-density lipoprotein (HDL), play a major role in the clearance of circulating endo- toxin [95]. *HDL* binds *LPS* and transports them to the liver hepatocytes and hepatic macrophages provide LPS clearance and its final biliary excretion [95]. Low-density lipoprotein (LDL) is generally believed to be much less effective than *HDL* at removing endotoxin from the blood. Moreover, in a study conducted in human volunteers, infusion of *HDL* was associated with reduced *LPS-mediated* release of TNF-α, IL-6, and IL-8 [96].

Innate immunity throughout its receptor system plays an important role. Endotoxins are able, via TLR activation, to promote different types of proinflammatory responses strictly connected to the pathogenesis of atherosclerosis. In phagocytic cells, endotoxins potently induce *ROS* production by stimulating *NADPH oxidase* activity. This enzyme is present in other vascular cells, too, such as *endothelial cells, smooth cells,* fibroblasts, and may participate in the induction of cytokine expression, *smooth muscle cell* growth and apoptosis. It can play an important role in the pathogenesis of hypertension and atherosclerosis [97]. The oxidant process induced by *ROS* induces a vicious circle via lipid peroxidation with formation of *lipoperoxides* that behave like *ROS*, amplifying oxidative damage. The oxLDL acts as a *TLR4* agonist on macrophages. Indeed, the formation of the plaque is initiated through the uptake of *LDL* from blood by endothelial cells, and the oxidation of LDL by reactive oxygen species within the vessel wall. Subsequently, the oxLDL is phagocytized by macrophages through scavenger receptors (such as *CD36* and *macrophage scavenger receptor class A* (*SR-A*) leading to macrophage transformation into lipid-laden activated foam cells. *Foam cells* produce proinflammatory cytokines and *matrix metalloproteinases* and express costimulatory molecules for T-cell activation (such as CD40). The recruitment of lymphocytes at the inflammatory site of the vessel induces the production of IgM-specific antibodies for *oxLDL* during atherogenesis. The formation of immune complexes could have protective effects on foam cell formation. Indeed, these antibodies may be able to cross the endothelial monolayer to reach the atherosclerotic plaques. There, they bind to antigens on the surface of *oxLDL*, form immune complexes, and block the uptake of oxLDL by macrophages.

The stimulation of *TLR4* on vascular smooth cells induces an increased *LDL* and extracellular matrix deposition in the plaque. *IFN-α* enhances *TLR4* signaling and thereby the consequent production of *TNF-α*, *IL-12*, and matrix *metalloproteinase* 9 (MMP9) with amplification of the inflammatory process [98].

Induction of proinflammatory cytokines and chemokines by PRR stimulation is associated with plaque pathogenesis. *LPS binding protein*, *CD14*, *toll-like receptor-4* (*TLR-4*), and *MD-2* at the cell membrane initiate the inflammatory cascade that throughout NF-kB recruits proinflammatory cytokines and chemokines at the inflammatory site [99–101]. Of the earliest cytokine discoveries among those implicated in the pathogenesis of arteriosclerosis, there is macrophage migration inhibitory factor (MIF), which has since been shown to be expressed by *monocytes/macrophages*, *T* cells, *B* cells, and by endocrine and epithelial cells [102]. *MIF* exerts both autocrine and paracrine effects on TLR-4 expression. In addition to the induction of *MIF*, endotoxins can contribute either directly or indirectly to increased release of other cytokines including *IFNγ*, *IL-1*, *IL-6*, *IL-8*, *TNFα*, and *granulocyte-macrophage colony- stimulating factor* (*GMCSF*), along with *platelet-activating factor* (*PGF*) [103]. It is very important that endotoxin also contributes to the increased expression of the *TNF receptor* [104].

Of the chemokines induced by triggering *PRRs* via endotoxins, *MCP-1* and *IL-8* appear to play critical roles in atherosclerosis. The first is highly expressed in human atherosclerotic plaques and plays a crucial role in *monocyte* recruitment into subendothelial lesions of vessels [105]. *MCP-1* induction is sensitive to very low levels of endotoxin (1 ng/mL) [106, 107]. *IL-8* is known to be chemotactic for *neutrophils*. *IL8* activates *NADPH* oxidase in these cells and increases production of *ROS*, initiating the oxidative process [108]. This cytokine also plays a role as a chemotactic factor, recruiting at the site of the lesion *monocytes* and *T-lymphocytes* that are prevalent in the fibrous cap of atherosclerotic lesions, where they may be involved in the pathogenesis of acute coronary syndromes. Low levels of endotoxin induce *IL8* release and confirm the role of low-grade endotoxemia in the pathogenesis of CLGI in CVD.

The release of chemokines attracts inflammatory cells to inflammatory sites of the vessel wall where *monocytes*, *neutrophils*, and *T lymphocytes* arrive. The "rolling" of leukocytes on the endothelial surface is mediated by *selectins* (*P* and *E selectins*) [109] (that are not normally expressed on endothelial cells, but their expression can be transcriptionally induced by cytokines, bacterial endotoxins, and other mediators [110]). Next, "firm adhesion" of leukocytes is permitted by the binding of *β_2-integrins* expressed on leukocytes to *cellular adhesion molecules* (*CAMs*), such as *intercellular adhesion molecule-1* (*ICAM-1*), *vascular cell adhesion molecule* (*VCAM-1*), which are expressed on the apical surface of the endothelium [109]. After adhesion, leukocytes cross the endothelium via interactions between *PECAM-1* molecules, which are expressed by both cell types [111]. The process of transmigration of the inflammatory cells is modulated by endotoxins at multiple steps. They activate *β_2-integrins*, upregulate *E-selectin* and *CAMs*, in addition to increasing phosphorylation of *platelet endothelial cell adhesion molecule-1* (*PECAM-1*), the release *platelet adhesion factor* (*PAF*), and the expression of its receptor on endothelial cells [109, 112].

A central role in plaque formation is played by *macrophages* in which there is excessive accumulation of lipids, resulting in foam cell formation. *TLR4* stimulation by *LPS* and/or *FFA* has been shown to contribute to early-stage intimal foam cell accumulation. *Intimal smooth muscle cells* surround and penetrate early lesions, where

TLR4 signaling, enhanced by hypercholesterolemia, promotes lesion progression by stimulation of *acyl-coenzyme A, cholesterol acyltransferase-1 mRNA* expression, cytoplasmic *cholesterol ester* accumulation, and *MCP-1* mRNA and protein expression in a *TLR4*-dependent manner [113]. The modulation of endotoxin-induced cellular activation could be one mechanism for the antiatherogenic effects of high HDL levels. Indeed, a recent study in humans has shown that *HDL* reduces plasma levels of *TNF-α* and expression of *CD11b* on monocytes [114].

T lymphocytes seep through the intima vessels by binding to *VCAM-1* and secondary to *interferon gamma-induced protein–10* (*IP-10*), *monokine induced by gamma interferon* (*MIG*), and *interferon-inducible T cell alpha chemoattractant* (*I-TAC*) induced by *CLGI* [115–118]. Activated lymphocytes in intima produce inflammatory cytokines, including the *CD40 ligand* (*CD154*), member of the *TNF superfamily* of molecules. Ligation of *CD40* by *CD154* on endothelial cells induces *ROS* production and expression of adhesion molecules such as *E-selectin*, *ICAM-1*, and *VCAM-1*, amplifying chemotactic processes. This also induces production of extracellular matrix-degrading *MMPs*, and the potent procoagulant *tissue factor* (*TF*) (also known as *platelet tissue factor*, *factor III*, *thromboplastin*, or *CD142*), which initiates the coagulation cascade, enhancing the thrombogenicity of the lipid core present in the plaque (Fig. 7.7) [119, 120].

7.4 Integrated Treatment of LGS and CLGI in Cardiometabolic Syndrome

The fundamental roles of the microbiome and gut in the pathogenesis of LGCI and cardiovascular diseases correlated with cardiometabolic syndrome (CMS) justify the necessity of an integrated treatment targeting the complexity of the problem. The evidence for the interactions between microbiota epigenetic regulation and its immunoregulatory effects on the host, induced to hypothesize the use of probiotics and prebiotics or symbiotics for the treatment of metabolic and immunological alterations, altered gut permeability, both responsible for CMS pathogenesis. Gut microbiota can be considered an important target in the management of diseases induced by LGCI, such as CMS.

The microbiota can be manipulated by prebiotics, probiotics, and antibiotics. Probiotics affect the microbiota directly by modulating its bacterial content, and indirectly through bacteriocins produced by the probiotic bacteria. Both prebiotics and probiotics induce health-promoting effects through their ability to antagonize pathogenic bacteria and to modulate immune and metabolic responses of the host [121].

7.4.1 Prebiotics

Dietary interventions influencing microbial composition may therefore be considered an option in the engagement against metabolic syndrome [122]. Indeed, several studies showed that in humans, the addition of nondigestible carbohydrates (fructo-oligo-saccharides: FOS) to the diet also protects against body weight gain, adipose mass increase, and plasmatic triacylglycerol accumulation induced by a high-fat diet [123]. Furthermore, FOS has been shown to promote satiety in healthy humans [123] and a recent study reported that FOS increased gut permeability [124]. FOS should be administered in nutraceutical treatment in association with substances that improve the intestinal barrier as colostrum and glutamine, which have important prebiotic effects.

Prebiotics are nondigestible/fermentable carbohydrates and fibers, such as galacto-oligosaccharides and inulin-type fructans or arabinoxylans, and fructo-oligosaccharides (FOS). They act as selective stimulators of metabolic activities and the growth of limited number of bacteria, such as probiotics. In several experimental models of obesity, dietary supplementation with prebiotics showed beneficial effects: reducing adiposity and improving the gut

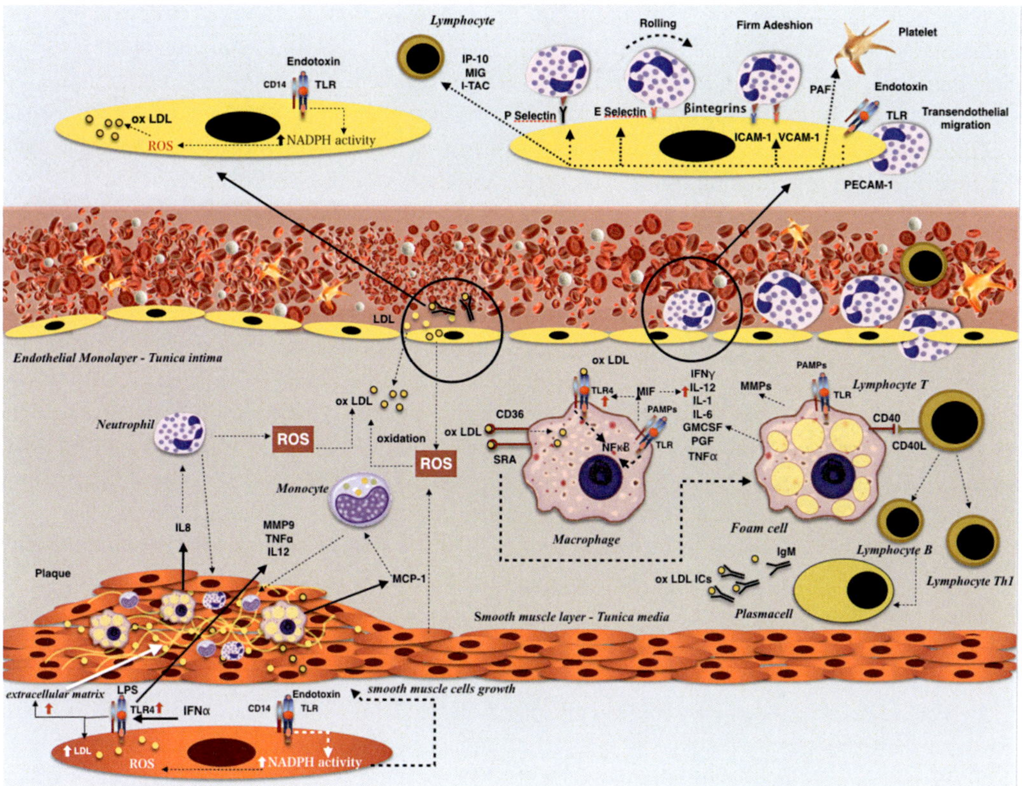

Fig. 7.7 The pathogenetic mechanism of plaque formation. Today the role of *CGLI* in plaque formation is commonly accepted by the scientific community. The activation of innate immunity by *PAMPs*, in low-grade endotoxemia, fires the inflammation response through *PRR* stimulation. This triggers the oxidative metabolism in endothelial and smooth cells, leading to *ROS* formation. These oxidize *LDL*, causing the formation of *oxLDLs* that are phagocytized by macrophages transforming them into foam cells. These cells produce metalloproteinases, chemokines, cytokines, and chemotactic factors, expanding the inflammatory process and favoring plaque formation. *TLR4* stimulation by *LPS* and/or *FFA* has been shown to contribute to early-stage intimal foam cell accumulation, confirming the role played by low-grade endotoxemia favored by increased intestinal permeability in the pathogenesis of atherosclerosis. *LDL* low density lipoprotein, *oxLDL* oxidized LDL, *NADPH* nitrate reductases, *TLR* toll like receptor, *IP-10* interferon γ-induced protein-10, *MIG* monokine induced by γ-interferon, *I-TAC* interferon-inducible T cell α-chemoattractant, *SRA* macrophage scavenger receptor class A, *IFN-γ* interferon γ, *IL-12* interleukin 12, *IL-1* interleukin 1, *IL-6* interleukin 12, *GCSF* granulocyte–macrophage colony stimulating factor, *PGF* platelet-activating factor, *TNF-α* tumor necrosis factor α, *MMPs* matrix metalloproteinases, *PAMPs* pathogen associated molecular patterns, *ICs* immune complexes, *MIF* macrophage migration inhibitory factor, *MCP-1* monocyte chemotactic protein-1, *MMP-9* matrix metalloproteinase, *IFN-α* interferon α

permeability, low-grade inflammation, and glycemic levels in the host [47, 125].

The different patterns of intestinal fermentation determine the type and amount of SCFA production. These patterns are determined by carbohydrate intake and by microbiota composition that, in turn, is influenced the by type of diet. Indeed, long-term ingestion of fermentable dietary fibers increases luminal concentrations of SCFAs [124]. These modify the neuroendocrine profile of the gut, influencing gene expression. In the rat proximal colon dietary supplementation with FOS for 4 weeks increases the density of L cells expressing FFA2 and GLP-1, but did not affect the fecal content or the density of enterochromaffin (EC) cells producing 5-HT. Furthermore, several studies demonstrate that supplementation with FOS upregulates the expression of *neurogenin 3* and *NeuroD*, factors able to promote the differentiation of enteroendocrine cells. Otherwise, dietary supplementation with cellulose, an insoluble dietary fiber, increases fecal content and augments the density of EC cells in the rat colon compared with those in rats fed a fiber-free diet.

Everard et al. [49] demonstrated that gut microbiota controls leptin action and prebiotics treatment can improve leptin sensitivity in diet-induced obese and type 2 diabetic mice and is probably responsible for an increase in plasma GLP-1 levels. The effects of prebiotics on humans have been partially confirmed. Prebiotic supplementation (5–20 g per day) changes the composition of the gut microbiota and increases plasma GLP-1 levels [126]. This effect has been associated with other clinical modifications: lower postprandial glycemia [13, 127]; an increased sense of satiety and a decreased feeling of hunger and energy intake [13, 123, 126, 127]; and a reduction in visceral fat mass [13, 123, 126, 127].

A recent clinical trial demonstrated beneficial effects of the prebiotics on the host metabolism. In the Parnell and Reimer study, during dietetic supplementation for 3 months (21 g/day), with a short chain inulin-type fructan, they found a reduction of food intake, gain in body weight, and development of fat mass in obese subjects. This supports the evidence that prebiotics promote weight maintenance. The authors found higher plasma *PYY* levels after meal, and a decrease in ghrelin over a 6-h meal tolerance test [127]. In healthy individuals, fructan-type prebiotics in dietetic supplementation (16 g/day for 2 weeks) also demonstrated the ability to stimulate the release of anorexigenic peptides, *GLP-1*, *PYY*, and *GIP*, with a secondary reduction of glycemic response and energy intake [13].

The same effects on *GLP-1* and *PYY* were associated with a decrease in orexigenic neuropeptide ghrelin, occurring in obese animals treated with inulin-type fructans [128]. The activation of intestinal GLP-1 producing cells drives the improvement of glycemic and insulin response in rats and mice receiving diet supplementation. These results suggest an increase in L cells in the jejunum and in the colon mucosa and demonstrate that the metabolic effects of diet supplementation with inulin fructans-type are mediated through the modulation of the neuroendocrine function of the *MGBA*. Furthermore, the over-secretion of *GLP-2* by *L cells*, induced in obese animals fed with inulin-type fructans, correlates with improvement of *LGI*, as demonstrated by decreased circulating levels of *LPS* and proinflammatory cytokines in obese mice. The positive effects observed in prebiotics-treated animals can also depend on the activation of the endocannabinoid system in the gut and adipose tissue. These effects seems to interfere with intestinal permeability, increasing the absorption of LPS, the expression and the activity of *ZO-1* and *occludin*, two fundamental proteins in the constitution of TJs.

An *HF* diet causes dysbiosis in animal models secondary to a decrease in the number of bifidobacteria in the intestinal microbiota [27, 28]. Modification of the composition of intestinal microbiota with changes in the metabolic and immunological state of the host can induce a *CLGI* state and the development of MS. Several studies demonstrate positive effects of treatment with prebiotics on host health in animal models and in clinic trials, but the relevance of specific intestinal microbial species/phyla ameliorating *MS* in prebiotic treatment with *inulin fructans-type* remains unrecognized. Thus, we can hypothesize that the improving effects of prebiotic treatment on *MS* might be mediated by positive effects on bifidobacteria species.

The effects enacted by prebiotics on the metabolism of the host could also be induced through an adaptive process of the host to energy sparing, owing to the production of *SCFAs* via the increased fermentative activity of the intestinal microbiota, which has been supplanted by other biochemical events occurring in the gut subsequent to changes in the microbiota. Indeed, fermentation end products, especially *SCFAs*, are believed to engage the epigenetic regulation of inflammatory reactions via free fatty acid receptor (*FFARs*) and other short chain fatty acid receptors. Furthermore, in a recent work, Remely et al. [122] claimed that a different composition of gut microbiota in obesity and type 2 diabetes patients can affect the epigenetic regulation of genes. The interactions between the microbiota and epigenetic regulation of the host may involve not only short chain fatty acids binding to *FFARs*. Remely et al. [122] observed in some patients a lower methylation in the promoter region of *FFAR3*, associated with a lower abundance of *Faecalibacterium prausnitzii*.

7.4.2 Probiotics

The modification of the gut microbiota can also achieved by the administration of probiotics. These are: "live microbial feed supplements which beneficially affect the host animal by improving its intestinal microbial balance" [129]. The most common probiotics are: *Bifidobacterium, Lactobacillus, Saccharomyces, Streptococcus, and Enterococcus.* The mechanisms whereby probiotic bacteria may have an impact on the microbiota include: competition for dietary ingredients as growth substrates; bioconversion of carbohydrates into fermentation products with inhibitory properties; production of growth substrates, such as *EPS* or vitamins, for other bacteria; direct antagonism by bacteriocins; competitive exclusion of pathogenic microorganisms for binding sites; improved barrier function; reduction of inflammation, thus altering intestinal properties for colonization and persistence within; stimulation of innate immune response [130].

Probiotics such as *Lactobacillus casei*, *paracasei*, and *acidophilus* with *Bifidobacterium animalis* can survive and grow in the gastrointestinal tract at a 20–40 % rate of survival after oral administration, as they are able to increase their development in the gut [131].

Probiotics demonstrated anti-inflammatory effects: *Lactobacillus casei* is negatively associated with *NF-κB p50/p65* activation, which is induced by *LPS* through *TLR4* activation and positively associated with *PPARγ* activation [132].

These effects are also indirectly induced by probiotics improving the gut permeability and consequently reducing bacterial translocation and *LPS* passage across the intestinal barrier. Indeed, certain members of the gut microbiota, including strains of *Lactobacillus plantarum* [133], *Escherichia coli* [134], and *Bifidobacterium lactis* [135], are capable of directly improving the expression of the TJ proteins occludin and ZO-1, increasing intestinal barrier functions. Furthermore, some studies demonstrate that metabolic bacteremia is modified by a treatment using the probiotic strain *Bifidobacterium animalis ssp. lactis 420*, which reduced the mucosal adherence and bacterial translocation of Gram-negative bacteria from the *Enterobacteriaceae* group [56]. Several lactobacilli have been reported to enhance barrier function and/or protect against barrier disruption by pathogens in vitro [136]. Different strains of *Lactobacillus plantarum* (*DSM 2648*, *MB452*, *299v*) have been reported to prevent the reduction in gut barrier function caused by the pathogenetic role of *E. coli* when cocultured with the pathogen [133]. This could be due to inhibition of the pathogen or enhancement of the barrier function by modulating TJ composition, such as demonstrated by Well et al. perfusing *L. plantarum* into the duodenum in human volunteers. After perfusion, the authors showed increased localization of occludin and *ZO-1* in the epithelial *TJs* of tissue biopsies.

Probiotics can antagonize LPS and bacterial endotoxin products by *extracellular polysaccharides* (*EPS*) of pathogenic bacteria. These consist of sugar residues bound to the cell surface of Gram-positive/-negative bacteria, or secreted as soluble/insoluble polymers. Probiotic-derived *EPS* are counterparts of LPS, ets. They are heat-resistant; thus the degradation temperature is 260 °C [137].

Wu et al. [25] demonstrated that the supplementation of *EPS* isolated from *Bifidobacterium longum* results in immunomodulatory effects (5 g/mL of *EPS*) in macrophages by inducing *IL-10* and suppressing *LPS*-induced macrophage growth inhibition and release of *TNF-α* secretion, furthering the antimicrobial effects on pathogenic bacteria (80 g/mL of *EPS*). Vinderola et al. [138] showed that oral administration of *EPS* (100 mg/kg body weight/day of *Lactobacillus kefiranofaciens* for 2–7 days) induced modulation of systemic immunity by stimulating the release of *IgA* and cytokines such as *IL-6, IL-10*, and *IL-12* into gut lamina propria and into the circulating blood of *BALB/c mice*. *EPS* from *Lactobacillus paracasei* exercises immunomodulatory, anti-inflammatory, and dose-dependent antioxidant effects. *Lactobacillus* species-derived *EPS* (kefiran), able to prevent in hypercholesterolemic rabbits fed a diet with 1 % w/w *kefiran*, demonstrated the same effects.

Probiotics such as *Bifidobacterium bifidum*, *Lactobacillus acidophilus*, and *Streptococcus faecalis* also have the capacity to reduce the severity of stress-induced gut pathological conditions and reverse fecal microbiota alterations. The same effect was not observed if probiotics were dispensed at the start of the stress condition [139].

Many studies have demonstrated the role of probiotics in metabolic alterations in typical diseases of *CMS*. Some of these effects are mediated by the production of *conjugated linoleic acid* (*CLA*), a group of *octadecadienoic acids* that are naturally present in foods derived from ruminant animals such as meat and dairy products. The group includes some unsaturated fatty acids isomers of *linoleic acid* (*ω-6, C18:2*). A few of these, with a trans double bond, have biological effects [140]. Some *Lactobacillus* (*lactic acid bacteria—LAB*) species such as *Lactococcus lactis*, *Lactobacillus acidophilus*, *L. plantarum*, and *Bifidobacterium animalis* produced *CLA* in vitro and in vivo in mice [141]. *CLA* producing *Lactobacillus* species such as *L. casei* and *L. plantarum* demonstrated anti-inflammatory effects along with increased PPARγ expression [141]. Indeed, *CLA* is a possible *PPARγ* agonist and has been demonstrated to have antioxidant, anti-inflammatory, anti-atherogenic, and anti-obesity effects [142]. This showed a dose-dependent effect associated with redox-sensitive transcription factors *PPARγ* and NFk-B in human endothelial cells [142, 143]. These transcription factors seem to modulate oxidative stress and inflammation in a coordinated fashion, depending on microenvironmental factors [144]. Bassaganya-Riera et al. demonstrated that *CLA* produced by probiotics in vivo should remain within the intestinal lumen acting as a *PPARγ* agonist locally, whereas orally supplemented *CLA* seems to be absorbed and has a systemic effect [145].

The metabolic anti-obesity effects of *CLA* seem to be induced by: a reduction of energy intake through appetite suppression; induction of energy expenditure in white adipose tissue, muscles, and liver tissue; reduction of lipogenesis or adipogenesis; induction of lipolysis; induction of adipocyte apoptosis [146]. The effects of *CLA* in humans affected by obesity are supported by two meta-analyses by Whigham et al. [147].

In a recent study, *Lactobacillus paracasei*, was shown to be able to increase the gene expression for *angiopoietin-like 4* (*ANGPTL 4*), the circulating lipoprotein lipase inhibitor influencing lipid metabolism.

Probiotics promote gut barrier functions. *Lactobacillus paracasei* and *Lactobacillus plantarum* normalize intestinal paracellular permeability via thier bacterial products [133]. *L. plantarum* increases the expression levels of intestinal epithelial cell genes involved in the whole TJ signaling pathway. Then, probiotics counteract the effects of stress on intestinal permeability.

7.4.3 Treatment of Gut Permeability

Augmented gut permeability is one of the most important pathogenetic mechanisms of LGCI. The treatment of altered intestinal mucosal permeability should be made a priority in the patient affected by CVD and MS.

7.4.3.1 Colostrum in the Treatment of Altered Intestinal Mucosal Permeability

Colostrum is first secretion produced by the mammary glands of mammals (including humans) in late pregnancy or just before giving birth. Colostrum can be considered to be the most important natural prebiotic. It prepares the intestinal environment for bacterial colonization of the gut by nursing.

The composition of colostrum is different from that of normal maternal milk. It is high in antibodies specific to many human pathogens, including *E. coli*, *Cryptosporidium parvum*, *Shigella flexneri*, *Salmonella species*, and *Staphylococcus* species. It also consists of immunomodulatory components and defensive factors such as *lysozyme*, *defensins*, *cathelicidins*, *lactoperoxidase*, *lactoferrin*, and *hemopexin* [148], which also have important antioxidant effects binding free *heme* in the circulation [149]. The antioxidant capacity is guaranteed by the presence of *retinol*, *tocopherol*, and *β-carotene* vitamins.

The concentrations of cytokines (*IL-1β*, *IL-6*, *TNF-α* and *IFN-γ*) in colostrum are significantly higher than those in mature milk and have significant immunomodulatory activity [150] and effects also in patients with immunodeficiency. Case reports and clinical trials suggest that antibodies extracted by bovine colostrum might be of use for the treatment of chronic diarrhea in people with immune deficiency syndromes [151].

Furthermore, bovine colostrum is an available source of growth factors such as the *epidermal growth factor receptor ligand family* (*EGFRLF*), *TGFα, the TGFβ family IGF1 and their binding* proteins, *growth hormone* (*GH*) and its releasing factor (*GHRF*), and *platelet-derived growth factor* (*PDGF*) [152], helping to reduce gastrointestinal injury such as that demonstrated in studies conducted in rats and mice [153, 154] and confirmed in human research [154].

The *EGFRLF* includes a group of polypeptides, with the common property of binding to the *EGF receptor* (also known as the *c-erb1 receptor*): *EGF* itself, *TGF-α*, *mammary-derived growth factor II* (*MDGF-II*). EGF stimulates cell proliferation and migration and also influences crypt fission, an identified mechanism by which new crypts are produced. The *EGF* in colostrum may therefore play a role in preventing bacterial translocation and stimulating gut growth in suckling neonates.

Tumor growth factor (*TGF*)-*α* plays a complementary role to *TGF-β*, controlling the balance between proliferation and differentiation in the intestinal epithelium. Although *TGF-α* acts as a mucosal-integrity peptide, maintaining normal epithelial function in the nondamaged mucosa [155], *TGF-β* in colostrum demonstrated the ability to prevent indomethacin-induced gastric injury in rats [156], suggesting that it might play a key role in maintaining gastrointestinal integrity.

IGF-1 promotes cell proliferation and differentiation, and its concentration in bovine colostrum is very high. It is relatively stable to both heat and acidic conditions, surviving in ambient gastric acidity and maintaining its biological activity. *IGF-I* promotes protein enhancement, acting as an anabolic agent mediating the growth-promoting activity of *growth hormone* (*GH*). Bovine colostrum also consists of IGF-II at a lower concentration than *IGF-I*. Also, I*GF-II* has the same anabolic activity. *IGF-I* and *-II* in colostrum are present in both free and bound forms.

Platelet-derived growth factor (*PDGF*) is an acid-stable molecule synthesized by platelets and macrophages. Administration of exogenous *PDGF* has been shown to facilitate ulcer healing when administered orally to animals although, to date, it is believed that most of the *PDGF-like* mitogenic activity in colostrum milk is derived from *bovine colostral growth factor*, which has structural homology of amino-acid sequences with *PGDF* [157].

Growth hormone (*GH*) and *GHRF* are present in bovine colostrum. *GH* receptors have been reported to be present throughout the human gastrointestinal tract.

Recent findings demonstrate that peptides in colostrum act on the *Fas*/*Fas* ligand (*FasL*) signaling system. *Fas* is a member of the *tumor necrosis factor* and *nerve growth factor receptor family* expressed in various cells, including the gastrointestinal mucosa. Colostrum peptides may influence the rate of programmed cell death (*apoptosis*) within the gut, acting via *FasL*. Indeed, the presence of soluble *Fas* in milk acts as an alternative receptor site for any *FasL* produced within the mucosa by activated immune cells, thereby reducing the rate of mucosal apoptosis [158].

A recent work demonstrated the effects of the administration of bovine colostrum, associated with *Morinda citrifolia* (*Noni*) extract, on epithelial cell turn-over, inflammatory events, and intestinal junctional systems management in an in vitro model of intestinal epithelium, based on the *Caco-2 cell* line. The association between colostrum and noni stimulated cell turn-over and activate the gene expression of *IL-8*, which are two important mechanisms for repairing the gut barrier [159].

7.4.3.2 Glutamine in the Treatment of Altered Mucosal Intestinal Permeability

Glutamine (*GLN*) is the preferential substrate for enterocytes, and it works in concert with other amino acids, such as leucine and arginine, to maintain gut barrier integrity and function [160]. It is an important target of *MGBA* imbalance. Indeed, gut permeability augmentation induces bacterial translocation, increased passage of *PAMPs*, and cytokine release. Subsequent HPA activation, induced by cytokines such as *IL1β* and *IL-6*, leads to the increased secretion of cortisol, which stimulates release of glutamine from skeletal muscle and lungs into the circulating glutamine pool. Then, *GLN* is taken up from the circulation to repair damage to the intestinal barrier. Indeed, cortisol increases glutaminase activity in enterocytes, leading to increased breakdown and utilization of *GLN* in the small intestine [161].

Glutamine plays an important role in the maintenance of intestinal barrier function in various animal models and critically in human bodies. Studies conducted in vitro by intestinal cell monolayers indicated that *GLN* can maintain transepithelial resistance and decrease gut permeability. *GLN* may act to attenuate gut injury and potential subsequent gut-derived systemic inflammatory response. A very likely activity could be induced by an *EGF* receptor-dependent mechanism with important effects on proteins involved in the intracellular junctional complex [162]. The role of *GLN* in the maintenance of gut barrier function is demonstrated by the effects of nutritional depletion on increased intestinal permeability [163]. Particularly, *GLN* has the ability to protect stomach and gut mucosa from damage induced by *NSAIDs* [164].

Glutamine influences a variety of different molecular pathways, although the major proportion of glutamine energy is generated through the tricarboxylic cycle and thus depends on oxidative phosphorylation. The first two steps in the metabolism of *GLN*, i.e., the conversion of *GLN* to *glutamate* and further deamination to *α-ketoglutarate*, yields one molecule, *NADPH*. In contrast to *NADH*, which generates *ATP* through oxidative phosphorylation, blocked by *NSAID*, *NADPH* is not converted to *ATP* in oxidative phosphorylation, but is used directly in many endergonic reactions, producing alternative fuel. In addition to its role as a fuel, the beneficial effect of glutamine in *NSAID*-induced damage may result from the fact that it provides amide nitrogen for nucleotide biosynthesis [165].

Acknowledgements A special thanks to Valentina Cagnetta (MD) for assisting me in the manuscript editing.

Competing interests Enrico Biffi declares a conflict of interest as he serves as a medical consultant for GUNA S.p.a. and Profenix Srl.

References

1. Bäckhed F, Manchester JK, Semenkovich CF, Gordon JI (2007) Mechanisms underlying the resistance to diet-induced obesity in germ-free mice. Proc Natl Acad Sci USA 104:979–984
2. Lyte M (2014) Microbial endocrinology and the microbiota-gut-brain axis. Adv Exp Med Bill 817:3–24
3. Qin R, Li J, Raes M, Arumugam KS, Burgdorf C, Manichanh T, Nielsen N, Pons F, Levenez F, Yamada T, MetaHIT Consortium et al (2010) A human gut microbial gene catalogue established by metagenomic sequencing. Nature 464:59–65
4. Peterson J, Garges S, Giovanni M, McInnes P, Wang L, Schloss JA, Bonazzi V, McEwen JE, Wetterstrand KA, Deal C et al (2009) The NIH human microbiome project. Genome Res 19:2317–2323
5. Costello EK, Lauber CL, Hamady M, Fierer N, Gordon JI, Knight R (2009) Bacterial community variation in human body habitats across space and time. Science 326:1694–1697
6. Dethlefsen L, Huse S, Sogin ML, Relman DA (2008) The pervasive effects of an antibiotic on the human gut microbiota, as revealed by deep 16S rRNA sequencing. PLoS Biol 6, e280
7. Willing BP, Russell SL, Brett Finlay B (2011) Shifting the balance: antibiotic effects on host–microbiota mutualism. Nat Rev Microbiol 9:233–243

8. Pace NR, Stahl DA, Lane DJ, Olsen GJ (1985) Analyzing natural microbial populations by rRNA sequences. ASM News 51:4–12
9. Arumugam M et al (2011) Enterotypes of the human gut microbiome. Nature 473:174–180
10. Claesson MJ, Jeffery IB, Conde S, Power SE, O'Connor EM, Cusack S, Harris HM, Coakley M, Lakshminarayanan B, O'Sullivan O et al (2012) Gut microbiota composition correlates with diet and health in the elderly. Nature 488:178–184
11. Koren O, Spor A, Felin J, Fak F, Stombaugh J, Tremaroli V, Behre CJ, Knight R, Fagerberg B, Ley RE, Bäckhed F (2011) Human oral, gut, and plaque microbiota in patients with atherosclerosis PNAS 108 [Suppl 1]:4592–4598
12. Stoll LL, Denning GM, Weintraub NL (2006) Endotoxin, TLR4 signaling and vascular inflammation: potential therapeutic targets in cardiovascular disease. Curr Pharm Des 32(12):4229–4245
13. Cani PD, Lecourt E, Dewulf EM, Sohet FM, Pachikian BD, Naslain D, De Backer F, Neyrinck AM, Delzenne NM (2009) Gut microbiota fermentation of prebiotics increases satietogenic and incretin gut pep- tide production with consequences for appetite sensation and glucose response after a meal. Am J Clin Nutr 90:1236–1243
14. Ley RE, Turnbaugh PJ, Klein S, Gordon JI (2006) Microbial ecology: human gut microbes associated with obesity. Nature 444:1022–1023
15. Cani PD, Bibiloni R, Knauf C, Waget A, Neyrinck AM, Delzenne NM, Burcelin R (2008) Changes in gut microbiota control metabolic endotoxemia-induced inflammation in high-fat diet-induced obesity and diabetes in mice. Diabetes 57(6):1470–1481
16. Creely SG, McTernan PG, Kusminski CM, Fischer M, Da Silva NF, Khanolkar M, Evans M, Harte AL, Kumar S (2006) Lipopolysaccharide activates an innate immune system response in human adipose tissue in obesity and type 2 diabetes. Am J Endocrinol Metab 292:E740–E747
17. Frazier TH, DiBaise JK, McClain CJ (2011) Gut microbiota, intestinal permeability, obesity-induced inflammation, and liver injury. JPEN J Parenter Enteral Nutr 35 [5 Suppl]:14S–20S
18. Schwiertz A, Taras D, Schafer K, Beijer S, Bos NA, Donus C, Hardt PD (2010) Microbiota and SCFA in lean and overweight healthy subjects. Obesity (Silver Spring) 18:190–195
19. Ravussin Y, Koren O, Spor A, Leduc C, Gutman R, Stombaugh J, Knight R, Ley RE, Leibel RL (2012) Responses of gut microbiota to diet composition and weight loss in lean and obese mice. Obesity 20:738–747
20. Armougom F, Henry M, Vialettes B, Raccah D, Raoult D (2009) Monitoring bacterial community of human gut microbiota reveals an increase in lactobacillus in obese patients and methanogens in anorexic patients. PLoS One (9) 4:e7125
21. Million M, Angelakis E, Maraninchi M, Henry M, Giorgi R, Valero R, Vialettes B, Raoult D (2013) Correlation between body mass index and gut concentrations of Lactobacillus reuteri, Bifidobacterium animalis, Methanobrevibacter smithii and Escherichia coli. Int J Obes 37 (11):1460–1466
22. Leibold MA, Holyoak M, Mouquet N, Amarasekare P, Chase JM, Hoopes F, Holt RD, Shurin B, Law R, Tilman D, Loreau M, Gonzalez A (2004) The metacommunity concept: a framework for multi-scale community ecology. Ecol Lett 7:601
23. Hildebrandt MA, Hoffmann C, Sherrill-Mix SA, Keilbaugh SA, Hamady M, Chen YY, Knight R, Ahima RS, Bushman F, Wu GD (2009) High fat diet determines the composition of the murine gut microbiome independently of obesity. Gastroenterology 137(5):1716–1724
24. De Filippo C, Cavalieri D, Di Paola M, Ramazzotti M, Poullet JB, Massart S, Collini S, Pieraccini G, Lionetti P (2010) Impact of diet in shaping gut microbiota revealed by a comparative study in children from Europe and rural Africa. Proc Natl Acad Sci USA 107(33):14691–14696
25. Wu GD, Chen J, Hoffmann C, Bittinger K, Chen YY, Keilbaugh SA, Bewtra M, Knights D, Walters WA, Knight R, Sinha R, Gilroy E, Gupta K, Baldassano R, Nessel L, Li H, Bushman FD, Lewis JD (2011) Linking long-term dietary patterns with gut microbial enterotypes. Science 334:105–108
26. Cani PD, Neyrinck AM, Fava F, Knauf C, Burcelin RG, Tuohy KM, Gibson GR, Delzenne NM (2007) Selective increases of bifidobacteria in gut microflora improve high-fat-diet-induced diabetes in mice through a mechanism associated with endotoxaemia. Diabetologia 50:2374–2383
27. Wang F, Schwarz BT, Graham WV, Wang Y, Su L, Clayburgh DR, Abraham C, Turner JR (2006) IFN-gamma-induced TNFR2 expression is required for TNF-dependent intestinal epithelial barrier dysfunction. Gastroenterology 131:1153–1163
28. Wang Z, Xiao G, Yao Y, Guo S, Lu K, Sheng Z (2006) The role of bifidobacteria in gut barrier function after thermal injury in rats. J Trauma 61:650–657
29. Hosoi T, Okuma Y, Matsuda T, Nomura Y (2005) Novel pathway for LPS-induced afferent vagus nerve activation: possible role of nodose ganglion. Auton Neurosci 120:104–107
30. He W, Wang ML, Jiang HQ, Steppan CM, Shin ME, Thurnheer MC, Cebra JJ, Lazar MA, Wu GD (2003) Bacterial colonization leads to the colonic secretion of RELM/FIZZ2, a novel goblet cell-specific protein. Gastroenterology 125:1388–1397
31. Nair MG, Guild KJ, Artis D (2006) Novel effector molecules in type 2 inflammation: lessons drawn from helminth infection and allergy. J Immunol 177:1393–1399

32. Artis D, Wang ML, Keilbaugh SA, He W, Brenes M, Swain GP, Knight PA, Donaldson DD, Lazar MA, Miller HR, Schad GA, Scott P, Wu GD (2004) RELM/FIZZ2 is a goblet cell-specific immune effector molecule in the gastrointestinal tract. Proc Natl Acad Sci USA 101:13596–13600
33. Hogan SP, Seidu L, Blanchard C, Groschwitz K, Mishra A, Karow ML, Ahrens R, Artis D, Murphy AJ, Valenzuela DM, Yancopoulos GD, Rothenberg ME (2006) Resistin-like molecule β regulates innate colonic function: barrier integrity and inflammation susceptibility. J Allerg Clin Immunol 118:257–268
34. Fujio J, Kushiyama A, Sakoda H, Fujishiro M, Ogihara T, Fukushima Y, Anai M, Horike N, Kamata H, Uchijima Y, Kurihara H, Asano T (2008) Regulation of gut-derived resistin-like molecule β expression by nutrients. Diabetes Res Clin Pract 79:2–10
35. Tlaskalová-Hogenová H, Stepánková R, Hudcovic T, Tucková L, Cukrowska B, Lodinová-Zádníková R, Kozáková H, Rossmann P, Bártová J, Sokol D, Funda DP, Borovská D, Reháková Z, Sinkora J, Hofman J, Drastich P, Kokesová A (2004) Commensal bacteria (normal microflora), mucosal immunity and chronic inflammatory and autoimmune diseases. Immunol Lett 93:97–108
36. Kamdar K, Nguyen V, DePaolo RW (2013) Toll-like receptor signaling and regulation of intestinal immunity. Virulence 4:207–212
37. Inohara N, Nuñez G (2003) NODs: intracellular proteins involved in inflammation and apoptosis. Nat Rev Immunol 3(5):371–382
38. Sanderson IL, Walker WA (2007) TLRs in the Gut I. The role of TLRs/Nods in intestinal development and homeostasis (2007) TLRs in the Gut I. The role of TLRs/Nods in intestinal development and homeostasis. Am J Physiol Gastrointest Liver Physiol 292 (1):G6–10
39. Chen GY, Nuñez G (2010) Sterile inflammation: sensing and reacting to damage. Nat Rev Immunol 12(10):826–837
40. Cario E (2005) Bacterial interactions with cells of the intestinal mucosa: toll like receptors and nod2. Gut 54:1182–1193
41. Tsukita S, Furuse M (1999) Occludin and claudins in tight-junction strands: leading or supporting players? Trends Cell Biol 9:268–273
42. Stevenson BR, Siliciano JD, Mooseker MS, Goodenough DA (1986) Identification of ZO-1: a high molecular weight polypeptide associated with the tight junction (zonula occludens) in a variety of epithelia. J Cell Biol 103:755–766
43. Biffi E (2014) Dalla disbiosi alla low grade chronic inflammation.– Effetti del Colostro Noni sul turnover delle cellule epiteliali, sugli stati infiammatori e sull'integrità dei sistemi giunzionali della mucosa intestinale. La Med Biol 4:77–83
44. Liévin-Le MV, Servin AL (2006) The front line of enteric host defense against unwelcome intrusion of harmful micro-organisms: mucins, antimicrobial peptides, and microbiota. Clin Microbiol Rev 19:315–337
45. Guttman JA, Samji FN, Li Y, Vogl AW, Finlay BB (2006) Evidence that tight junctions are disrupted due to intimate bacterial contact and not inflammation during attaching and effacing pathogen infection in vivo. Infect Immun 74:6075–6084
46. Tabata T, Tani T, Endo Y, Hanasawa K (2002) Bacterial translocation and peptidoglycan translocation by acute ethanol administration. J Gastroenterol 37:726–731
47. Cani PD, Delzenne NM (2009) The role of gut microbiota in energy metabolism and metabolism disease. Curr Pharm Des 15:1546.1558
48. De La Serre CB, Ellis CL, Lee J, Hartman AL, Rutledge JC, Raybould HE (2010) Propensity to high-fat diet-induced obesity in rats is associated with changes in the gut microbiota and gut inflammation. Am J Physiol Gastrointest Liver Physiol 299:440–448
49. Everard A, Lazarevic V, Derrien M, Girard M, Muccioli GM, Neyrinck AM, Possemiers S, Van Holle A, François P, De Vos WM, Delzenne NM, Schrenzel J, Cani PD (2011) Responses of gut microbiota and glucose and lipid metabolism to prebiotics in genetic obese and diet-induced leptin-resistant mice. Diabetes 60:2775–2786
50. Ross R (1999) Atherosclerosis is an inflammatory disease. Am Heart J 138:S419–420
51. Cani PD, Osto M, Geurts L, Everard A (2012) Involvement of gut microbiota in the development of low-grade inflammation and type 2 diabetes associated with obesity. Gut Microbes 3:279–288
52. Weisberg SP, Hunter D, Huber R, Lemieux J, Slaymaker S, Vaddi K, Charo I, Leibel RL, Ferrante AW (2006) Jr CCR2 modulates inflammatory and metabolic effects of high-fat feeding. J Clin Invest 116:115–124
53. Velasquez OR, Henninger K, Fowler M, Tso P, Crissinger KD (1993) Oleic acid-induced mucosal injury in developing piglet intestine. Am J Physiol 264:G576–G582
54. Cario E, Gerken G, Podolsky DK (2007) Toll-like receptor 2 controls mucosal inflammation by regulating epithelial barrier function. Gastroenterology 132:1359–1374
55. Caricilli AM, Picardi PK, de Abreu LL, Ueno M, Prada PO, Ropelle ER, Hirabara SM, Castoldi Â, Vieira P, Camara NO, Curi R, Carvalheira JB, Saad MJ (2011) Gut microbiota is a key modulator of insulin resistance in TLR 2 knockout mice. PLoS Biol 9, e1001212
56. Amar J, Chabo C, Waget A, Klopp P, Vachoux C, Bermudez-Humaran LG, Smirnova N, Berge M, Sulpice T, Lahtinen S, Ouwehand A, Langella P, Rautonen N, Sansonetti PJ, Burcelin R (2011) Intestinal mucosal adherence and translocation of commensal bacteria at the early onset of type 2 diabetes:

Molecular mechanisms and probiotic treatment. EMBO Mol Med 2011(3):559–572
57. Otte JM, Cario E, Podolsky DK (2004) Mechanisms of cross hyporesponsiveness to Toll-like receptor bacterial ligands in intestinal epithelial cells. Gastroenterology 126:1054–1070
58. Neal MD, Leaphart C, Levy R, Prince J, Billiar TR, Watkins S, Li J, Cetin S, Ford H, Schreiber A, Hackam DJ (2006) Enterocyte TLR4 mediates phagocytosis and translocation of bacteria across the intestinal barrier. J Immunol 176:3070–3079
59. Lotz M, Gutle D, Walther S, Menard S, Bogdan C, Hornef MW (2006) Postnatal acquisition of endotoxin tolerance in intestinal epithelial cells. J Exp Med 203:973–984
60. Erridge C, Attina T, Spickett CM, Webb DJ (2007) A high-fat meal induces low-grade endotoxemia: evidence of a novel mechanism of postprandial inflammation. Am J Clin Nutr 86:1286–1292
61. Ghoshal S, Witta J, Zhong J, de Villiers W, Eckhardt E (2009) Chylomicrons promote intestinal absorption of lipopolysaccharides. J Lipid Res 50:90–97
62. Hornef MW, Frisan T, Vandewalle A, Normark S, Richter-Dahlfors A (2002) Toll-like receptor 4 resides in the Golgi apparatus and colocalizes with internalized lipopolysaccharide in intestinal epithelial cells. J Exp Med 195:559–570
63. Kiecolt-Glaser JK, Preacher KJ, MacCallum RC, Atkinson C, Malarkey WB, Glaser R (2003) Chronic stress and age-related increases in the proinflammatory cytokine IL-6. Proc Natl Acad Sci USA 100:9090–9095
64. Allen RG, Lafuse WP, Galley JD, Ali MM, Ahmer BMM, Bailey MT (2012) The intestinal microbiota are necessary for stressor-induced enhancement of splenic macrophage microbicidal activity. Brain Behav Immun 26:371–382
65. Bailey MT (2014) Influence of stressor-induced nervous system activation on the intestinal microbiota and the importance for immunomodulation. Adv Exp Med Biol 817:255–276
66. Konturek PC, Brzozowski T, Konturek SJ (2011) Stress and the gut: pathophysiology, clinical consequences, diagnostic approach and treatment options. J Physiol Pharmacol 62(6):591–599
67. Farhadi A, Fields JZ, Keshavarzian A (2007) Mucosal mast cells are pivotal elements in inflammatory bowel disease that connect the dots: stress, intestinal hyperpermeability and inflammation. World J Gastroenterol 13:3027–3030
68. Santos J, Yates D, Guilarte M, Vicario M, Alonso C, Perdue MH (2008) Stress neuropeptides evoke epithelial responses via mast cell activation in the rat colon. Psychoneuroendocrinology 33:1248–1256
69. Saunders PR, Santos J, Hanssen NP, Yates D, Groot J, Perdue MH (2002) Physical and psychological stress in rats enhances colonic epithelial permeability via peripheral CRH. Dig Dis Sci 47:208–215
70. Overman EL, Rivier JE, Moeser AJ (2012) CRF induces intestinal epithelial barrier injury via the release of mast cell proteases and TNF-α. PLoS One 7, e39935
71. Sun Y, Zhang M, Chen CC, Gillilland M, Sun X, El-Zaatari M, Huffnagle GB, Young VB, Zhang J, Hong SC, Chang YM, Gumucio DL, Owyang C, Kao JY (2013) Stress-induced corticotropin-releasing hormone-mediated NLRP6 inflammasome inhibition and transmissible enteritis in mice. Gastroenterology 144:1478–1487
72. Bjarnason I, Takeuchi K (2009) Intestinal permeability in the pathogenesis of NSAID-induced enteropathy. J Gastroenterol 44:23–29
73. Somasundaram S, Hayllar J, Rafi S, Wrigglesworth J, Macpherson A, Bjarnason I (1995) The biochemical basis of NSAID-induced damage to the gastrointestinal tract: a review and a hypothesis. Scand J Gastroenterol 30:289–299
74. Wallas JL (2013) Mechanisms, prevention and clinical implications of nonsteroidal anti-inflammatory drug-enteropathy. World J Gastroenterol 19 (12):1861–1876
75. Cooper BT, Holmes GK, Ferguson R, Thompson RA, Allan RN, Cooke WT (1981) Gluten-sensitive diarrhea without evidence of celiac disease. Gastroenterology 81:192–194
76. Sapone A, Bai JC, Ciacci C, Dolinsek J, Green PHR, Hadjivassiliou M, Kaukinen K, Rostami K, Sanders DS, Schumann M, Ullrich R, Villalta D, Volta U, Catassi C, Fasano A (2012) Spectrum of gluten-related disorders: consensus on new nomenclature and classification. BMC Med 10:13
77. Sapone A, Lammers KM, Mazzarella G, Mikhailenko I, Carteni M, Casolaro V, Fasano A (2010) Differential mucosal IL-17 expression in two gliadin-induced disorders: gluten sensitivity and the autoimmune enteropathy celiac disease. Int Arch Allergy Immunol 152:75–80
78. Wang W, Uzzau S, Goldblum SE, Fasano A (2000) Human zonulin, a potential modulator of intestinal tight junctions. J Cell Sci 113:4435–4440
79. Tripathi A, Lammers KM, Goldblum S, Shea-Donohue T, Netzel-Arnett S, Buzza MS, Antalis TM, Vogel SN, Zhao A, Yang S, Arrietta MC, Meddings JB, Fasano A (2009) Identification of human zonulin, a physiological modulator of tight junctions, as prehaptoglobin-2. Proc Natl Acad Sci USA 106:16799–804
80. Fasano A (2001) Pathological and therapeutical implications of macromolecule passage through the tight junction. In: Tight Junctions. CRC, Boca Raton, FL, pp 697–722
81. El Asmar R, Panigrahi P, Bamford P, Berti I, Not T, Coppa GV, Catassi C, Fasano A (2002) Host-dependent activation of the zonulin system is involved in the impairment of the gut barrier function following bacterial colonization. Gastroenterology 123:1607–1615

82. Jin M, Barron E, He S, Ryan SJ, Hinton DR (2002) Regulation of RPE intercellular junction integrity and function by hepatocyte growth factor. Invest Ophthalmol Vis Sci 43:2782–2790
83. Fasano A (2011) Zonulin and its regulation of intestinal barrier function: the biological door to inflammation, autoimmunity, and cancer. Physiol Rev 91:151–175
84. Barone MV, Gimigliano A, Castoria G, Paolella G, Maurano F, Paparo F, Maglio M, Mineo A, Miele E, Nanayakkara M, Troncone R, Auricchio S (2007) Growth factor-like activity of gliadin, an alimentary protein: implications for coeliac disease. Gut 56:480–488
85. Nikulina M (2004) Wheat gluten causes dendritic cell maturation and chemokine secretion. J Immunol 173:1925–1933
86. Drago S, El AR, Di PM, Grazia CM, Tripathi A, Sapone A, Thakar M, Iacono G, Carroccio A, D'Agate C, Not T, Zampini L, Catassi C, Fasano A (2006) Gliadin, zonulin and gut permeability: effects on celiac and non-celiac intestinal mucosa and intestinal cell lines. Scand J Gastroenterol 41:408–419
87. Fasano A (2009) Surprises from celiac disease. Sci Am 301:54–61
88. Lammers KM, Khandelwal S, Chaudhry F, Kryszak D, Puppa EL, Casolaro V, Fasano A (2011) Identification of a novel immunomodulatory gliadin peptide that causes interleukin-8 release in a chemokine receptor CXCR3-dependent manner only in patients with coeliac disease. Immunology 132:432–440
89. Thomas KE, Fasano A, Vogel SN (2006) Gliadin stimulation of murine macrophage inflammatory gene expression and intestinal permeability are MyD88-dependent: role of the innate immune response in celiac disease. J Immunol 176:2512–2521
90. Zufferey C, Erhart D, Saurer L, Mueller C (2009) Production of interferon-γ by activated T-cell receptor-αβ CD8αβ intestinal intraepithelial lymphocytes is required and sufficient for disruption of the intestinal barrier integrity. Immunology 128:351–359
91. Witztum JL, Lichtman AH (2014) The influence of innate and adaptive immune responses on atherosclerosis. Annu Rev Pathol 9:73–102
92. Wiedermann CJ, Kiechl S, Dunzendorfer S, Schratzberger P, Egger G, Oberhollenzer F, Willeit J (1999) Association of endotoxemia with carotid atherosclerosis and cardiovascular disease. Prospective results from the Bruneck study. J Am Coll Cardiol 34:1975–1981
93. Schratzberger P, Kiechl S, Dunzendorfer S, Kahler CM, Patsch JR, Willeit J, Wiedermann CJ (2000) Plasma-induced endothelial activation associated with incident atherosclerosis: prospective results from the Bruneck Study. J Cardiovasc Risk 7:285–291
94. Alekperov ÉZ, Nadzhafov RN (2010) Contemporary concepts of the role of inflammation in atherosclerosis. Kardiologiia 50(6):88–91
95. Read TE, Harris HW, Grunfeld C, Feingold KR, Kane JP, Rapp JH (1993) The protective effect of serum lipoproteins against bacterial lipopolysaccharide. Eur Heart J 14 [Suppl K]:125–129
96. Pajkrt D, Doran JE, Koster F, Lerch PG, Arnet B, van der Poll T, ten Cate JW, van Deventer SJH (1996) Antiinflammatory effects of reconstituted high-density lipoprotein during human endotoxemia. J Exp Med 184:1601–1608
97. Li WG, Miller FJ Jr, Zhang HJ, Spitz DR, Oberley LW, Weintraub NL (2001) H(2)O(2)-induced O (2) production by a non-phagocytic NAD(P)H oxidase causes oxidant injury. J Biol Chem 276:29251–29256
98. Spirig R, Tsui J, Shaw S (2012) The emerging role of TLR and innate immunity in cardiovascular disease. Cardiol Res Pract 2012:181394. doi:10.1155/2012/181394
99. Libby P, Okamoto Y, Rocha VZ, Folco E (2010) Inflammation in atherosclerosis. Nature 420:868–874
100. Mantovani A, Dejana E (1989) Cytokines as communication signals between leukocytes and endothelial cells. Immunol Today 10:370–375
101. Pant S, Deshmukh A, Gurumurthy GS, Pothineni NV, Watts TE, Romeo F, Mehta JL (2014) Inflammation and atherosclerosis—revisited. J Cardiovasc Pharmacol Ther 19:170–178
102. Calandra T (2003) Macrophage migration inhibitory factor and host innate immune responses to microbes. Scand J Infect Dis 35:573–576
103. Diks SH, van Deventer SJH, Peppelenbosch MP (2001) Lipopolysaccharide recognition, internalisation, signalling and other cellular effects. J Endotoxin Res 7:335–348
104. Strieter RM, Remick DG, Ham JM, Colletti LM, Lynch JP 3rd, Kunkel SL (1990) Tumor necrosis factor-α gene expression in human whole blood. J Leukoc Biol 47:366–370
105. Harrington JR (2000) The role of MCP-1 in atherosclerosis. Stem Cells 18:65–66
106. Rice JB, Stoll LL, Li W-G, Denning GM, Weydert J, Charipar E, Richenbacher WE, Miller FJ Jr, Weintraub NL (2003) Low level endotoxin induces potent inflammatory activation of human blood vessels: inhibition by statins. Arterioscler Thromb Vasc Biol 23:1576–1582
107. Stoll LL, Denning GM, Li WG, Rice JB, Harrelson AL, Romig SA, Gunnlaugsson ST, Miller FJ Jr, Weintraub NL (2004) Regulation of endotoxin-induced proinflammatory activation in human coronary artery cells: expression of functional membrane-bound CD14 by human coronary artery smooth muscle cells. J Immunol 173:1336–1343
108. Daniels RH, Finnen MJ, Hill ME, Lackie JM (1992) Recombinant human monocyte IL-8 primes

NADPH-oxidase and phospholipase A_2 activation in human neutrophils. Immunology 75:157–163
109. Shen Y, Sultana C, Arditi M, Kim KS, Kalra VK (1998) Endotoxin-induced migration of monocytes and PECAM-1 phosphorylation are abrogated by PAF receptor antagonists. Am J Physiol 75:E479–E486
110. Eppihimer MJ, Wolitzky B, Anderson DC, Labow MA, Granger DN (1996) Heterogeneity of expression of E- and P-selectins in vivo. Circ Res 79:560–569
111. Newman PJ (1994) The role of PECAM-1 in vascular cell biology. Ann N Y Acad Sci 714:165–174
112. Vestweber D (2007) Adhesion and signaling molecules controlling the transmigration of leukocytes through endothelium. Immunol Rev 218:178–196
113. Higashimori M, Tatro JB, Moore KJ, Mendelsohn ME, Galper JB, Beasley D (2011) Role of toll-like receptor 4 in intimal foam cell accumulation in apolipoprotein E-deficient mice. Arterioscler Thromb Vasc Biol 31:50–57
114. Shaw JA, Bobik A, Murphy A, Kanellakis P, Blombery P, Mukhamedova N, Woollard K, Lyon S, Sviridov D, Dart AM (2008) Infusion of reconstituted high-density lipoprotein leads to acute changes in human atherosclerotic plaque. Circ Res 103:1084–1091
115. Heller EA, Liu E, Tager AM, Yuan Q, Lin AY, Ahluwalia N, Jones K, Koehn SL, Lok VM, Aikawa E, Moore KJ, Luster AD, Gerszten RE (2006) Chemokine CXCL10 promotes atherogenesis by modulating the local balance of effector and regulatory T cells. Circulation 113:2301–2312
116. Match F, Sauty A, Iarossi AS, Sukhova GK, Neote K, Libby P, Luster AD (1999) Differential expression of three T lymphocyte-activating CXC chemokines by human atheroma-associated cells. J Clin Investig 104:1041–1050
117. Van Wanrooij EJA, De Jager SCA, Van Es T, De Vos P, Birch HL, Owen DA, Watson RJ, Biessen EAL, Chapman GA, Van Berkel TJC, Kuiper J (2008) CXCR3 antagonist NBI-74330 attenuates atherosclerotic plaque formation in LDL receptor-deficient mice. Arterioscler Thromb Vasc Biol 28:251–257
118. Veillard NR, Steffens S, Pelli G, Lu B, Kwak BR, Gerard C, Charo IF, Mach F (2005) Differential influence of chemokine receptors CCR2 and CXCR3 in development of atherosclerosis in vivo. Circulation 112:870–878
119. Mach F, Schönbeck U, Sukhova GK, Bourcier T, Bonnefoy JY, Pober JS, Libby P (1997) Functional CD 40 Ligand is expressed on human 50. Vascular endothelial cells, smooth muscle cells, and macrophages: implications for CD40-CD40 ligand signaling in atherosclerosis. Proc Natl Acad Sci USA 94:1931–1936
120. Schönbeck U, Mach F, Sukhova GK, Herman M, Graber P, Kehry MR, Libby P (2000) CD40 ligation induces tissue factor expression in human vascular smooth muscle cells. Am J Pathol 156:7–14
121. Yan F, Polk DB (2011) Probiotics and immune health. Curr Opin Gastroenterol 27:496–501
122. Remely M, Aumuellera E, Merolda C, Dworzaka S, Hippea B, Zannera J, Pointnera A, Brathb H, Haslberger AG (2014) Effects of short chain fatty acid producing bacteria on epigenetic regulation of FFAR3 in type 2 diabetes and obesity. Gene 1 (537):85–92
123. Cani PD, Joly E, Horsmans Y, Delzenne NM (2006) Oligofructose promotes satiety in healthy human: a pilot study. Eur J Clin Nutr 60:567–572
124. Ten Bruggencate SJ, Bovee Oudenhoven IM, Lettink Wissink ML, Van der Meer R (2005) Dietary fructooligosaccharides increase permeability in rats. J Nutr 135:837–842
125. Neyrinck AM, Delzenne NM (2010) Potential interest of gut microbial changes induced by non-digestible carbohydrates of wheat in the management of obesity and related disorders. Curr Opin Clin Nutr Metab Care 2010(13):722–728
126. Verhoef SP, Meyer D, Westerterp KR (2011) Effects of oligofructose on appetite profile, glucagon-like peptide 1 and peptide YY3-36 concentrations and energy intake. Br J Nutr 106:1757–1762
127. Parnell JA, Reimer RA (2009) Weight loss during oligofructose supplementation is associated with decreased ghrelin and increased peptide YY in overweight and obese adults. Am J Clin Nutr 89:1751–1759
128. Takemura N, Okubo T, Sonoyama K (2010) Lactobacillus plantarum strain No. 14 reduces adipocyte size in mice fed high-fat diet. Exp Biol Med (Maywood) 235:849–856
129. Fuller R (1989) Probiotics in man and animals. J Appl Bacteriol 66:365–378
130. O'Toole PW, Cooney JC (2008) Probiotic bacteria influence the composition and function of the intestinal microbiota. Interdiscipl Perspect Infect Dis 2008:175285
131. Roessler A, Forssten SD, Glei M, Ouwehand AC, Jahreis G (2011) The effect of probiotics on faecal microbiota and genotoxic activity of faecal water in patients with atopic dermatitis: a randomized, placebo-controlled study. Clin Nutr 2011 (31):22–29
132. Eun CS, Han DS, Lee SH, Jeon YC, Sohn JH, Kim YS, Lee J (2007) Probiotics may reduce inflammation by enhancing peroxisome proliferator activated receptor gamma activation in HT-29 cells. Korean J Gastroenterol 49:139–146
133. Anderson RC, Cookson AL, McNabb WC, Kelly WJ, Roy NC (2010) Lactobacillus plantarum DSM 2648 is a potential probiotic that enhances intestinal barrier function. FEMS Microbiol Lett 309:184–192

134. Ukena SN, Singh A, Dringenberg U, Engelhardt R, Seidler U, Hansen W, Bleich A, Bruder D, Franzke A, Rogler G, Suerbaum S, Buer J, Gunzer F, Westendorf AM (2007) Probiotic Escherichia coli Nissle 1917 inhibits leaky gut by enhancing mucosal integrity. PLoS One 2, e1308
135. Putaala H, Salusjarvi T, Nordstrom M, Saarinen M, Ouwehand AC, Hansen EB, Rautonen N (2008) Effect of four probiotic strains and Escherichia coli O157:H7 on tight junction integrity and cyclo-oxygenase expression. Res Microbiol 159:692–698
136. Wells JM, Konstaninov S, Konings I, Karczewski J (2011) Effects of probiotic and commensals on epithelial barrier function. Int J Probiot Prebiot 2008 3 (3):127–132
137. Ismail B, Nampoothiri KM (2010) Production, purification and structural characterization of an exopolysaccharide produced by a probiotic Lactobacillus plantarum MTCC9510. Arch Microbiol 192:1049–1057
138. Vinderola G, Perdigon G, Duarte J, Farnworth E, Matar C (2006) Effects of the oral administration of the exopolysaccharide produced by Lactobacillus kefiranofaciens on the gut mucosal immunity. Cytokine 36:254–260
139. Bailey MT, Dowd SE, Galley JD, Hufnagle AR, Allen RG, Lyte M (2011) Exposure to a social stressor alters the structure of the intestinal microbiota: implications for stressor-induced immunomodulation. Brain Behav Immun 25:397–407
140. Lawson RE, Moss AR, Givens DI (2001) The role of dairy products in supplying conjugated linoleic acid to man’s diet: a review. Nutr Res Rev 1(4):153–172
141. Ewaschuk JB, Walker JW, Diaz H, Madsen KL (2006) Bioproduction of conjugated linoleic acid by probiotic bacteria occurs in vitro and in vivo in mice. J Nutr 136:1483–1487
142. Nakamura YK, Omaye ST (2009) Conjugated linoleic acid isomers’ roles in the regulation of PPARγ and NF-κBDNA binding and subsequent expression of antioxidant enzymes in human umbilical vein endothelial cells. Nutrition 25:800–811
143. Nakamura YK, Dubick MA, Omaye ST (2012) Modulation of oxidative stress by gamma-glutamylcysteine (GGC) and conjugated linoleic acid (CLA) in human umbilical vein endothelial cells. Food Chem Toxicol 50:1854–1859
144. Nakamura YK, Omaye ST (2010) Lipophilic compound-mediated gene expression and implication for intervention in reactive oxygen species (ROS)-related diseases: mini-review. Nutrients 2:725–736
145. Bassaganya-Riera J, Viladomiu M, Pedradosa M, De Simone C, Carbo A, Shaykhutdinov R, Jobin C, Arthur JC, Corl BA, Vogel H, Storr M, Hontecillas R (2012) Probiotic bacteria produce conjugated linoleic acid locally in the gut that targets macrophage PPARγ to suppress colitis. PLoS One 7, e31238
146. Kennedy A, Martinez K, Schmidt S, Mandrup S, Lapoint K, McIntosh MK (2010) Antiobesity mechanisms of action of conjugated linoleic acid. J Nutr Biochem 21:171–179
147. Whigham LD, Watras AC, Schoeller DA (2007) Efficacy of conjugated linoleic acid for reducing fat mass: a meta-analysis in humans. Am J Clin Nutr 85:1203–1211
148. Pakkanen R, Aalto J (1997) Growth factors and antimicrobial factors of bovine colostrum. Int Dairy J 7:285–297
149. Zaczyńska E, Kocięba M, Śliwińska E, Zimecki M (2014) Bovine lactoferrin enhances proliferation of human peripheral blood lymphocytes and induces cytokine production in whole blood cultures. Adv Clin Exp Med 6(23):871–876
150. Hagiwara K, Kataoka S, Yamanaka H, Kirisawa R, Iwai H (2000) Detection of cytokines in bovine colostrum. Vet Immunol Immunopathol 76:183–190
151. Rump JA, Arndt R, Arnold A, Bendick C, Dichtelmuller H, Franke M, Helm EB, Jager H, Kampmann B, Kolb P, Kreuz W, Lissner R, Meigel W, Ostendorf P, Peter HH, Plettenberg A, Schedel I, Stellbrink HW, Stephan W (1992) Treatment of diarrhoea in human immunodeficiency virus-infected patients with immunoglobulins from bovine colostrum. Clin Investigator 70:588–594
152. Elfstrand L, Lindmark-Mansson H, Paulsson M, Nyberg L, Àkesson B (2002) Immunoglobulins, growth factors and growth hormone in bovine colostrum and the effects of processing. Int Dairy J 12:879–887
153. Kim J, Jeon W, Chun H, Kim Y, Yun J (2004) Effects of bovine colostrum in diclofenac induced gut injured rat model. Korean J Med 67:49–57
154. Playford RJ, MacDonald CE, Calnan DP, Floyd DN, Podas T, Johnson W, Wicks AC, Bashir O, Marchbank T (2001) Co-administration of the health food supplement, bovine colostrum, reduces the acute non-steroidal anti-inflammatory drug-induced increase in intestinal permeability. Clin Sci 100:627–633
155. Playford RJ (1995) Leading article: peptides and gastrointestinal mucosal integrity. Gut 37:595–597
156. Marchbank T, Playford RJ (1998) Bovine colostrum or TGF (a major bioactive constituent of colostrum) are prophylactic against indomethacin induced injury. Gut 42 [Suppl]:A68
157. Shing YW, Klagsbrun M (1987) Purification and characterization of a bovine colostrum-derived growth factor. Mol Endocrinol 1:335–338
158. Srivastava MD, Sahai Srivastava BI (1999) Soluble Fas and soluble Fas ligand proteins in human milk: possible significance in the development of immunological tolerance. Scand J Immunol 49:51–54

159. Cardani D (2014) Effetti del colostro noni sul turnover delle cellule epiteliali, sugli stati infiammatori e sull'integrità dei sistemi giunzionali della mucosa intestinale. Minerva Gastroenterol Dietol 60(1):71–78
160. Marc RJ, Wu G (2009) Glutamine, arginine, and leucine signaling in the intestine. Amino Acids 37:111–122
161. Wilmore DW, Smith RJ, O'Dwyer ST, Jacobs DO, Ziegler TR, Wang XD (1988) The gut: a central organ after surgical stress. Surgery 104:917–923
162. Li N, Lewis P, Samuelson D, Liboni K, Neu J (2004) Glutamine regulates Caco-2 cell tight junction proteins. Am J Physiol Gastrointest Liver Physiol 287:G726–G733
163. Hulsewe KW, van der Hulst RW, van Acker BA, von Meyenfeldt MF, Soeters PB (2004) Inflammation rather than nutritional depletion determines glutamine concentrations and intestinal permeability. Clin Nutr 23:1209–1216
164. Hond ED, Peeters M, Hiele M, Bulteel V, Ghoos Y, Rutgeerts P (1999) Effect of glutamine on the intestinal permeability changes induced by indomethacin in humans. Aliment Pharmacol Ther 13:679–685
165. Souba WW (1991) Glutamine: a key substrate for the splanchnic bed. Ann Rev Nutr 11(285):308

Endocrine System and Cardiovascular Disease

8

Carlo Maria Rotella, Ilaria Dicembrini, and Laura Pala

Endocrine dysfunction may have a significant impact on the cardiovascular system. Restoration of normal endocrine function often results in a reversal of adverse cardiovascular changes.

8.1 Pineal Gland and the Cardiovascular System

The hormones of the pituitary gland send signals to other endocrine glands to stimulate or inhibit their own hormone production. Under the control of the hypothalamus, the pituitary gland ensures that all the body's functions express at the best their interactions. Considering hormones secreted by the anterior pituitary, disorders of prolactin, growth hormone (GH), and adrenocorticotropic hormone (ACTH) may be associated with cardiac diseases. Although hyperprolactinemia itself does not have a clear effect on the cardiovascular system, there is a possible association between long-term treatment with dopamine agonists and cardiac valve abnormalities [1]. An excess of GH causes a specific derangement of cardiomyocytes, leading to abnormalities in cardiac muscle structure and function that induce a specific cardiomyopathy. In the early phase of acromegaly, the excess of GH and IGF-I induces a hyperkinetic syndrome characterized by increased heart rate and increased systolic output. Concentric hypertrophy is the most common feature of cardiac involvement in acromegaly. This abnormality is currently associated with diastolic dysfunction and impaired systolic function, ending in chronic heart failure. In addition, abnormalities of cardiac rhythm and valves have also been described in acromegaly. Successful control of acromegaly induces a decrease in the left ventricular mass and an improvement in diastolic function, whereas the effects of GH/IGF-I suppression on systolic function are more variable. An early diagnosis and prompt effective treatment are important for reversing acromegalic cardiomyopathy [2]. On the other hand, GH deficiency is associated with increased body fat and central adiposity, dyslipidemia, endothelial dysfunction, and insulin resistance. GH replacement therapy can result in increased lean body mass and decreased visceral adipose tissue and total and low-density lipoprotein cholesterol (LDL-C) levels [3]. The excess of ACTH secretion induces in hypercortisolism or Cushing's syndrome a clinical condition leading to hypertension, central obesity, diabetes, and insulin resistance; these conditions produce an increased cardiovascular risk [4].

C.M. Rotella (✉) • I. Dicembrini • L. Pala
Department of Biomedical, Experimental and Clinical Sciences, University of Florence Medical School, Florence, Italy
e-mail: carlomaria.rotella@unifi.it

M. Fioranelli (ed.), *Integrative Cardiology*, DOI 10.1007/978-3-319-40010-5_8

8.2 Thyroid and the Cardiovascular System

All organs and tissues are influenced by thyroid hormones. Actions of thyroid hormone result in cardiovascular hemodynamic changes in overt hyperthyroidism that include decreased systemic vascular resistance, increased heart rate, increased cardiac preload, and increased cardiac output [5]. In hyperthyroidism, systemic vascular resistance is reduced because of the thyroid hormone–mediated relaxation of vascular smooth muscle cells and increased endothelial nitric oxide (NO) production. Moreover, this reduction stimulates the renin–angiotensin–aldosterone system, leading to increased plasma volume and increased cardiac preload. Thyroid hormone also promotes an increase in blood volume via upregulation of erythropoietin secretion, enhancing cardiac preload. Enhancement in contractility and in resting heart rate further contributes to the increase in cardiac output. Treatment of hyperthyroidism reverses these hemodynamic changes [6].

Extensive evidence indicates that the cardiovascular system responds to minimal, but persistent changes in circulating thyroid hormone levels, which are typical of individuals with subclinical thyroid dysfunction. Subclinical hyperthyroidism is associated with increased heart rate, atrial arrhythmias, increased left ventricular mass, impaired ventricular relaxation, reduced exercise performance, and increased risk of cardiovascular mortality. Sinus tachycardia occurs in approximately 40% of cases of overt hyperthyroidism and resolves after restoration of euthyroidism. Subclinical hyperthyroidism is also associated with an increased heart rate.

Atrial fibrillation is the second most common arrhythmia in overt hyperthyroidism, its prevalence increasing with age [7]. Hypothyroidism is associated with accelerated atherosclerosis and coronary artery disease that may be ascribed to diastolic hypertension, impaired endothelial function, and hypercholesterolemia. This increase in diastolic pressure is the result of increased systemic vascular resistance and increased arterial stiffness. It resolves with T4 replacement therapy [8].

Subclinical hypothyroidism is associated with impaired left ventricular diastolic function and systolic dysfunction. Preliminary clinical investigations suggest that administration of thyroid hormone greatly ameliorates these patients' clinical condition, highlighting the potential role of thyroid hormone treatment in patients with acute and chronic cardiovascular disease [9]. Moreover, electrocardiography (ECG) changes in hypothyroidism include sinus bradycardia and low-voltage complexes that justify the ventricular conduction abnormalities reported in hypothyroidism [6]. An interesting review discusses the appropriate thyroid function tests to establish a suspected diagnosis, and the treatment modalities necessary to restore patients to a euthyroid state, and also reviews the alterations in thyroid hormone metabolism that accompany chronic congestive heart failure and the approach to the management of patients with amiodarone-induced alterations in thyroid function tests [10]. There is increasing evidence that the endocrine system may be dysfunctional in patients with heart failure. T3 and T4 concentrations in the patients were significantly lower with respect to normal values in patients with idiopathic dilated cardiomyopathy [11]. No significant variance was observed among patients with cardiac catheterization, ST-elevation myocardial infarction (STEMI), non-STEMI, unstable angina, and atrial fibrillation with respect to FT4, FT3, and thyroid-stimulating hormone (TSH) levels during coronary care unit hospitalization based on their profile data (Fig. 8.1) [12].

Amiodarone, a benzofuranic iodine-rich antiarrhythmic drug, causes thyroid dysfunction in 15–20% of treated patients, including both hypothyroidism and thyrotoxicosis. Amiodarone-induced hypothyroidism results from persistent iodine-induced inhibition of thyroid gland function and is more prevalent in patients with preexisting thyroid autoimmunity. Amiodarone could also induce thyrotoxicosis of two forms: iodine-induced hyperthyroidism or destructive

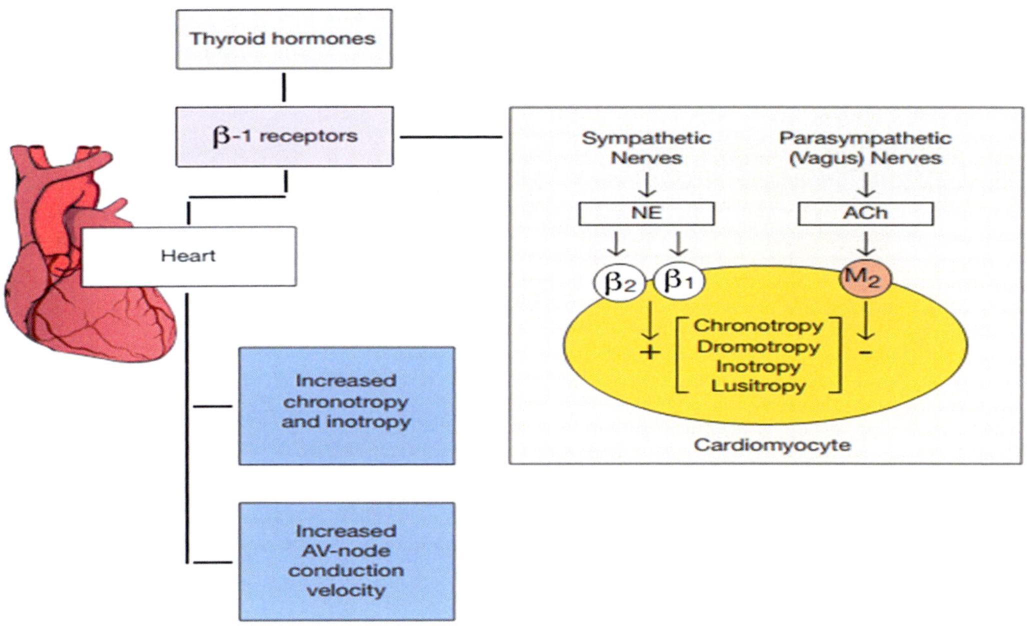

Fig. 8.1 The effect of thyroid hormones on the heart

thyroiditis. Type 1 results in the synthesis and release of excess thyroid hormone, whereas type 2 results in the release of preformed thyroid hormone from the inflamed thyroid gland [13].

8.3 Parathyroid and the Cardiovascular System

Parathyroid hormone regulates the body's calcium levels. Hypercalcemia induces cardiac effects including syncope from arrhythmias, whereas hypoglycemia may result in refractory hypotension or arrhythmias. Calcium plays a key role in heart muscle contraction and relaxation. Hypocalcemic heart failure is a rare and potentially reversible disturbance, which reflects its intrinsic relationship. In this clinical condition, the ECG shows severe global left ventricular dysfunction, normal coronary arteries at cardiac catheterization, severe hypocalcemia, and new-onset hypoparathyroidism. This condition completely normalizes after metabolic stabilization considering hypocalcemia as a cause of reversible myocardial dysfunction. Hypercalcemia,

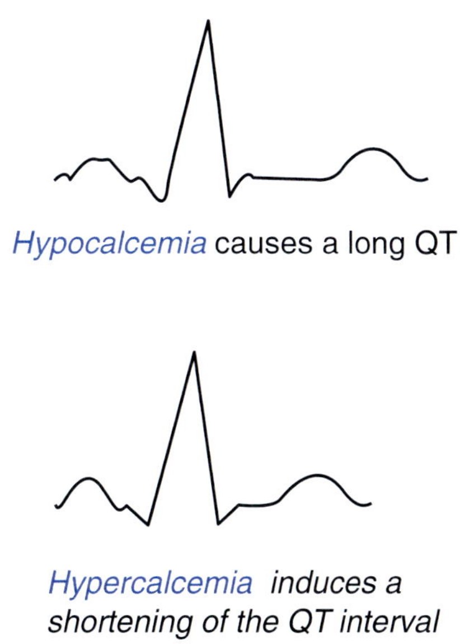

Fig. 8.2 Electrocardiographic alterations induced by hypocalcemia and hypercalcemia

acute and chronic, is known to have effects on the heart and the vascular system that are potentially life-threatening. Some of these effects include accelerated atherosclerosis, uncontrolled hypertension, structural effects, and progressive cardiac dysfunction. Figure 8.2 shows the ECG modifications induced by hypocalcemia and hypercalcemia. Hypocalcemia causes a long QT, whereas hypercalcemia induces a shortening of the QT interval.

8.4 Adrenal Gland and the Cardiovascular System

Of all the hormones secreted by the adrenal glands, those involved in cardiovascular regulation are glucocorticoids, mineralocorticoids, and adrenomedullary hormones. Glucocorticoids released by the adrenal cortex include hydrocortisone, commonly known as cortisol, which regulates mechanisms inducing the conversion of fats, proteins, and carbohydrates to energy. It also helps in the regulation of blood pressure and cardiovascular function. The principal mineral corticoid is aldosterone, which maintains the balance of salt and water and helps to control blood pressure. The hormones of the adrenal medulla are released after the sympathetic nervous system is stimulated, which occurs during stress, and stimulate the heart rate. Epinephrine, well-known as adrenaline rapidly responds to stress by increasing the heart rate and rushing blood to the muscles and brain. Norepinephrine works with epinephrine in response to stress, causing vasoconstriction, increasing blood pressure. Hypercortisolism is associated with hypertension, central obesity, insulin resistance, dyslipidemia, and alterations in the clotting and platelet functions. Patients with hypercortisolism may have impaired fasting glucose, impaired glucose tolerance, hyperinsulinemia, insulin resistance, and/or diabetes mellitus. Cushing's syndrome has been associated with increased lipoprotein(a), decreased HDLc, and increased triglycerides. The duration of cortisol excess correlates with the degree of dyslipidemia seen. Cortisol also increases the synthesis of several coagulation factors, stimulating endothelial production of von Willebrand factor and concomitantly increasing factor VIII. Hypercortisolism may also enhance platelet aggregation and reduce plasma fibrinolytic capacity [4]. Moreover, hyperaldosteronism causes maladaptive cardiac remodeling and has been associated with heart failure, cardiac fibrosis, and diastolic dysfunction [14]. Aldosterone has also been shown to promote collagen deposition, activate inflammatory cells, and stimulate fibroblast proliferation [15]. Surgical and medical treatments may be effective in reducing left ventricular mass, with decreases in blood pressure and plasma aldosterone levels predictive of response to therapy. At the very least, excess catecholamine action in pheochromocytoma can lead to cardiomyopathy, ischemic heart disease, myocardial stunning, and cardiogenic shock. Echocardiogram may reveal left ventricular dilatation with a diffuse decrease in contractility, left atrial dilatation with increased end-diastolic pressure, reduced ejection fraction, and septal hypertrophy. In the setting of intravascular volume depletion and impaired diastolic filling, patients may present with an outflow obstruction that mimics hypertrophic obstructive cardiomyopathy [16].

8.5 Diabetes Mellitus and the Cardiovascular System

In patients affected by diabetes, atherosclerotic cardiovascular disease is the leading cause of morbidity and mortality and represents the major determinant of direct and indirect costs related to the disease. Diabetes is associated with a two- to four-fold increased mortality risk for heart disease together, with significantly higher mortality after myocardial infarction and a worse overall prognosis in coronary heart disease [17]. The common conditions coexisting with diabetes (e.g., hypertension and dyslipidemia) are clear major risk factors for atherosclerotic cardiovascular disease, and the chronic hyperglycemia itself confers a further independent risk [18]. However, the contribution of glucose-lowering to the reduction of macrovascular complications appears to be controversial.

In type 1 diabetes, follow-up results from a large randomized clinical trial suggest that the improvement of metabolic control, obtained through intensive insulin treatment, might prevent cardiovascular events in the long term [19]. On the other hand, despite some encouraging results, the large clinical trials designed to test the efficacy of tight glycemic control in patients affected by type 2 diabetes, with near-normal glycemic control for a median of 3.5–5 years failed to show a significant reduction of cardiovascular events within that period [20]. The increase in iatrogenic hypoglycemia incidence strictly related to antidiabetic therapies at high hypoglycemic risk (e.g., sulfonylureas and insulin) may represent a plausible explanation by determining adrenergic activation, oxidative stress, and cardiac repolarization, leading to cardiac ischemia or fatal arrhythmia [21].

Moreover, concerns have been raised regarding the fact that different glucose-lowering drugs, irrespective of their action on glycemic control, may exert different effects on the cardiovascular risk profile. Although available clinical data ruled out any overall harmful cardiovascular effect of metformin unless when it is added to sulfonylureas, sulfonylureas themselves, insulin, and thiazolidinediones have been suspected of negative cardiovascular effects, although some results were not confirmed by subsequent investigations [22]. To date, the Food and Drug Administration requires preapproval and post-approval studies for all new antidiabetic drugs to rule out excess cardiovascular risk. Despite growing in vivo and in vitro evidence for the cardiovascular benefits, only neutral effects on cardiovascular risk have been demonstrated for incretin-based therapy (e.g., GLP-1 receptor agonist and dipeptidyl peptidase, DPP-44 inhibitors) through large clinical trials with cardiovascular endpoints [23, 24]. The diverging results regarding the relationship between DPP-4 inhibitors and heart failure require further investigation.

More recent data coming from the EMPA-REG Outcome study [25] showed that therapy with sodium-glucose cotransporter 2 inhibitors, the newest antidiabetic drug class, significantly reduced cardiovascular risk in type 2 diabetic patients at high cardiovascular risk. Empagliflozin, then, is the first antidiabetic drug associated with cardiovascular positive effects, with a 38% reduction in cardiovascular death. Further studies to investigate whether this treatment will have similar effects in lower-risk diabetic patients are required.

Recommendations for cardiovascular disease and risk management from the American Diabetes Association pointed out that large benefits are seen only when multiple risk factors are addressed simultaneously. As a consequence, diabetes care implies a multifactorial management of cardiovascular risk, which includes multiple therapeutic goals beyond glycemic control.

8.6 Obesity and the Cardiovascular System

Obesity has been shown to have several negative effects through thrombogenic, atherogenic, oncogenic, hemodynamic, and neurohumoral pathways and has been linked to several chronic diseases, such as diabetes, hypertension, dyslipidemia, and cardiovascular disease, together with malignancies. Overweight and obesity constitute the fifth leading risk for global death according to the World Health Organization. At least, 2.8 million subjects die each year for complications related to overweight/obesity. Moreover, the 44% of diabetes and 23% of ischemic heart disease burden can be attributed to an excess of adipose tissue [26].

Obesity, according to the World Health Organization, is defined by a body fat representation >25% in men and >35% in women at bioelectrical impedance analysis. In clinical practice, overweight and obesity are traditionally diagnosed if body mass index (BMI) is $\geq$26 and $\geq$30 kg/m^2 respectively. However, several studies have shown a paradoxical relationship between BMI and all-cause and/or cardiovascular mortality, identifying a higher survival rate in overweight in comparison with normal weight or obesity [27–31].

Thus, obesity cannot be adequately ruled out by the BMI calculation, which showed a low sensitivity, missing more than 50% of people with excessive fat mass [32]. Further studies demonstrated a significant association between visceral adiposity, better than BMI, mortality, and cardiovascular disease. Waist circumference as a surrogate measure of abdominal adipose tissue has been placed as one of the main contributors to the metabolic syndrome by the National Cholesterol Education Program Adult Treatment Panel III in 2001 [33] and then as the core feature of the diagnostic criteria proposed by the International Diabetes Federation in 2005.

A possible mechanism linking obesity with cardiovascular disease is subclinical low-grade inflammation. The adipose tissue is recognized as an endocrine organ, capable of synthesizing a large number of biologically active cytokines that regulate metabolic homeostasis. Obesity, and in particular, excess visceral adiposity, results in many qualitative changes in the cellular composition of the tissue itself, including alterations in the number and phenotype of the adipocytes, infiltration by immune, vascular, and structural cells, thus determining a relevant dysregulation of the secretion of those cytokines referred to as adipokines. The overexpression of the pro-inflammatory adipokines (leptin, TNF, IL-6, resistin, retinol-binding protein 4 [RbP4], lipocalin 2, IL-18, angiopoietin-like protein 2 [ANGPTL2], CC-chemokine ligand 2 [CCL2], CXC-chemokine ligand 5 [CXCL5], and nicotinamide phosphoribosyltransferase [NAmPT]), together with impairment of the anti-inflammatory ones (adiponectin and secreted frizzled-related protein 5 [SFRP5]), leads to the development of a chronic inflammatory state [34]. This condition contributes to metabolic dysfunction, which has a deleterious effect on the cardiovascular system, leading to the development of endothelial dysfunction, myocardial ischemia, and cardiomyopathy.

Moreover, recent data have pointed to the important role of a multi-organ cross talk also involving cytokines and other peptides secreted from skeletal muscles in response to exercise with local effects within the muscle or by targeting distant organs. Such proteins are recognized as myokines (e.g., IL-6 and irisin) and represent important contributors of the beneficial metabolic effects of exercise [35]. Skeletal muscle plays a critical role in the glucose metabolism and peripheral insulin sensitivity, and its impairment is commonly related to the increase in adipose tissue, leading to a condition defined as sarcopenic obesity. Adipose tissue excess could underlie the development of sarcopenia. A possible role of vitamin D in sarcopenia has been postulated in two studies, demonstrating that serum 25-hydroxy vitamin D was negatively correlated with appendicular (legs and arms) fat mass and positively associated with appendicular muscle mass, both evaluated through DEXA analysis [36].

Thus, the use of traditional anthropometric measures and lifestyle modifications to characterize and adequately manage patients affected by obesity could be misleading.

8.7 Gonads and the Cardiovascular System

8.7.1 Male

In the cardiovascular system, androgens display predominantly genomic effects, but there is also evidence for nongenomic effects. Genomic effects involve the transcription of specific segments of DNA through the binding of testosterone or dihydrotestosterone to the androgen receptor, which is widely expressed in the cardiovascular system, particularly in vascular smooth muscle, endothelial cells, myocardial fibers, and macrophages. The nongenomic effects of androgens are rapid compared with the genomic effects and include the activation of kinase signaling cascades and the modulation of intracellular calcium levels. Moreover, testosterone also exerts indirect effects through the activation of estrogen receptors, after aromatization into estradiol by the aromatase (P450a) enzyme [37].

A decreased testosterone level in men during aging is a condition defined as hypogonadism.

Observational studies have suggested an association between low endogenous testosterone levels and a high cardiometabolic risk (increased blood pressure, dyslipidemia, insulin resistance, atherosclerosis, thrombosis), in addition to a modest increase in total and cardiovascular mortality. All the evidence currently available shows no unequivocal relationship between low testosterone and atherosclerosis [37]. Potential confounding factors cannot be excluded; moreover, low testosterone could be related to a poor state of health.

Testosterone replacement therapy is associated with many improvements regarding sexual function, bone mineral density, body fat mass, and muscle mass and strength, together with possible positive effects on lipid and glucose metabolism. Two studies have recently been published analyzing the effect of hormonal replacement therapy in men affected by hypogonadism. The first found that hormonal replacement therapy significantly reduced mortality during a mean follow-up period of 40.5 months (10.3 vs 20.7% in controls; $p < 0.0001$) [38]. Even after multivariate adjustment, testosterone treatment was associated with a decreased risk of death. The second study examined retrospectively the effect on all-cause mortality in men with type 2 diabetes and found significant survival benefits [39].

Systematic meta-analyses confirmed no adverse effects of testosterone replacement on cardiovascular mortality and morbidity [40].

8.7.2 Female

Sexual female hormones are important for maintaining the health and normal functions of several organs, such as the brain, bone, and cardiovascular system.

Cardiovascular diseases are the leading cause of mortality and morbidity in both men and women. It should be pointed out that women of reproductive age show a three- to five-fold lower rate of mortality for myocardial infarction than men, but this difference disappears with aging [41]. Cardiovascular diseases are generally infrequent in young women, and this has been explained, at least in part, by the protective vascular effects of endogenous estrogen. Estrogens exert protective effects on the cardiovascular system through beneficial effects on the lipid metabolism, and more direct actions on arterial vessels via inhibition of atherosclerotic plaque formation. Moreover, positive effects on endothelium, vascular smooth muscle, autonomic nervous function, nitric oxide, and the renin–angiotensin system have been described. At menopause, the protective effects of estrogen are lost and cardiovascular risk significantly increases. In symptomatic perimenopausal women aged 60 years and younger, hormonal replacement therapy has been shown to provide significant benefits (a reduction in menopausal symptoms and urogenital symptoms) and it has also been shown to reduce the cardiovascular risk [42].

Hormone replacement therapy can be administered orally or most commonly by use of a transdermal patch. At equivalent dosages, the oral route of administration via first-induced hepatic metabolism seems to have more beneficial effects on cholesterol metabolism than transdermal administration in terms of lowering LDL-C and increasing high-density lipoprotein cholesterol (HDL-C). However, transdermal administration is related to a significant reduction of triglycerides, in comparison with oral estrogen [43]. However, in women treated with oral estrogen compared with transdermal formulations, no significant differences in cardiovascular mortality and morbidity outcomes have been determined [42]. Overall, with regard to the cardiovascular risk profile, the route of administration of estrogen probably has less impact than the dose administered.

References

1. Schade R, Andersohn F, Suissa S, Haverkamp W, Garbe E (2007) Dopamine agonists and the risk of cardiac-valve regurgitation. N Engl J Med 356:29–38
2. Vitale G, Pivonello R, Lombardi G, Colao A (2004) Cardiac abnormalities in acromegaly. Pathophysiology and implications for management. Treat Endocrinol 3(5):309–318

3. Attanasio AF, Do M, Erfurth EM, Tan M, Ho KY, Kleinberg D et al (2010) Prevalence of metabolic syndrome in adult hypopituitary growth hormone (GH)-deficient patients before and after GH replacement. J Clin Endocrinol Metab 95:74–81
4. Faggiano A, Pivonello R, Spiezia S, De Martino MC, Fillippella M, Di Somma C et al (2003) Cardiovascular risk factors and common carotid artery caliber and stiffness in patients with Cushing's disease during active disease and 1 year after disease remission. J Clin Endocrinol Metab 88:2527–2533
5. Kahaly GJ, Dillman WH (2005) Thyroid hormone action in the heart. Endocr Rev 26:704–728
6. Klein I, Danzi S (2007) Thyroid disease and the heart. Circulation 116:1725–1735
7. Northcote RJ, MacFarlane P, Kesson CM, Ballantyne D (1986) Continuous 24-hour electrocardiography in thyrotoxicosis before and after treatment. Am Heart J 112:339–344
8. Biondi B, Klein I (2004) Hypothyroidism as a risk factor for cardiovascular disease. Endocrine 24:1–13
9. Fazio S, Palmieri EA, Lombardi G, Biondi B (2004) Effects of thyroid hormone on the cardiovascular system. Recent Prog Horm Res 59:31–50
10. Irwin Klein MD, Danzi S (2007) Thyroid disease and the heart. Circulation 116:1725–1735
11. Naderi N, Heidarali M, Barzegari F, Ghadrdoost B, Amin A, Taghavi S (2015) Hormonal profile in patients with dilated cardiomyopathy. Res Cardiovasc Med 4(3):e27631
12. Qari A (2015) Thyroid hormone profile in patients with acute coronary syndrome. Iran Red Crescent Med J 17(7):e26919
13. Barbesino G (2010) Drugs affecting thyroid function. Thyroid 20:763–770
14. Galetta F, Bernini G, Franzoni F, Bacca A, Fivizzani I, Tocchini L (2009) Cardiac remodeling in patients with primary aldosteronism. J Endocrinol Invest 32:739–745
15. Rizzoni D, Paiardi S, Rodella L, Porteri E, De Ciuceis C, Rezzani R et al (2006) Changes in extracellular matrix in subcutaneous small resistance arteries of patients with primary aldosteronism. J Clin Endocrinol Metab 91:2638–2642
16. Galetta F, Franzoni F, Bernini G, Poupak F, Carpi A, Cini G et al (2010) Cardiovascular complications in patients with pheochromocytoma: a mini-review. Biomed Pharmacother 64:505–509
17. Donahoe SM, Stewart GC, McCabe CH et al (2007) Diabetes and mortality following acute coronary syndromes. JAMA 298:765–775
18. Aronson D, Edelman ER (2016) Coronary artery disease and diabetes mellitus. Heart Fail Clin 12 (1):117–133
19. Nathan DM, Cleary PA, Backlund JY, Genuth SM, Lachin JM, Orchard TJ, Raskin P, Zinman B, Diabetes Control and Complications Trial/Epidemiology of Diabetes Interventions and Complications (DCCT/EDIC) Study Research Group (2005) Intensive diabetes treatment and cardiovascular disease in patients with type 1 diabetes. N Engl J Med 353 (25):2643–2653
20. Aronson D, Edelman ER (2014) Coronary artery disease and diabetes mellitus. Cardiol Clin 32(3):439–455
21. Yakubovich N, Gerstein HC (2011) Serious cardiovascular outcomes in diabetes: the role of hypoglycemia. Circulation 123:342–348
22. Mannucci E, Dicembrini I, Lauria A, Pozzilli P (2013) Is glucose control important for prevention of cardiovascular disease in diabetes? Diabetes Care 36 [Suppl 2]:S259–S263
23. Pfeffer MA, Claggett B, Diaz R, Dickstein K, Gerstein HC, Køber LV, Lawson FC, Ping L, Wei X, Lewis EF, Maggioni AP, McMurray JJ, Probstfield JL, Riddle MC, Solomon SD, Tardif JC, ELIXA Investigators (2015) Lixisenatide in patients with type 2 diabetes and acute coronary syndrome. N Engl J Med 373(23):2247–2257
24. Son JW, Kim S (2015) Dipeptidyl peptidase 4 inhibitors and the risk of cardiovascular disease in patients with type 2 diabetes: a tale of three studies. Diabetes Metab J 39(5):373–383
25. Zinman B, Wanner C, Lachin JM, EMPAREGOUTCOME Investigators et al (2015) Empagliflozin, cardiovascular outcomes, and mortality in type 2 diabetes. N Engl J Med; 374(11):1094
26. World Health Organization. Fact Sheet No. 311. Available from: http://www.who.int/mediacentre/factsheets/fs311/en/index.html
27. Romero-Corral A, Montori VM, Somers VK, Korinek J, Thomas RJ, Allison TG, Mookadam F, Lopez-Jimenez F (2006) Association of bodyweight with total mortality and with cardiovascular events in coronary artery disease: a systematic review of cohort studies. Lancet 368:666–678
28. McGee DL (2005) Body mass index and mortality: a meta-analysis based on person-level data from twenty-six observational studies. Ann Epidemiol 15:87–97
29. Flegal KM, Graubard BI, Williamson DF, Gail MH (2007) Cause-specific excess deaths associated with underweight, overweight, and obesity. JAMA 298:2028–2037
30. Yusuf S, Hawken S, Ounpuu S, Bautista L, Franzosi MG, Commerford P, Lang CC, Rumboldt Z, Onen CL, Lisheng L et al (2005) Obesity and the risk of myocardial infarction in 27,000 participants from 52 countries: a case–control study. Lancet 366:1640–1649
31. Price GM, Uauy R, Breeze E, Bulpitt CJ, Fletcher AE (2006) Weight, shape, and mortality risk in older persons: elevated waist-hip ratio, not high body mass index, is associated with a greater risk of death. Am J Clin Nutr 84:449–460
32. Romero-Corral A, Somers VK, Sierra-Johnson J, Thomas RJ, Collazo-Clavell ML, Korinek J, Allison TG, Batsis JA, Sert-Kuniyoshi FH, Lopez-Jimenez F (2008) Accuracy of body mass index in diagnosing obesity in the adult general population. Int J Obes (Lond) 32:959–966
33. National Cholesterol Education Program (NCEP) Expert Panel on Detection, Evaluation, and Treatment

of High Blood Cholesterol in Adults (Adult Treatment Panel III) (2002) Third Report of the National Cholesterol Education Program (NCEP) Expert Panel on Detection, Evaluation, and Treatment of High Blood Cholesterol in Adults (Adult Treatment Panel III) final report. Circulation 106(25):3143–3421

34. Ouchi N, Parker JL, Lugus JJ, Walsh K (2011) Adipokines in inflammation and metabolic disease. Nat Rev Immunol 11(2):85–97
35. Pedersen L, Hojman P (2012) Muscle-to-organ cross talk mediated by myokines. Adipocyte 1(3):164–167
36. Rotella CM, Dicembrini I (2015) Measurement of body composition as a surrogate evaluation of energy balance in obese patients. World J Methodol 5(1):1–9
37. Ruige JB, Ouwens DM, Kaufman JM (2013) Beneficial and adverse effects of testosterone on the cardiovascular system in men. J Clin Endocrinol Metab 98 (11):4300–4310
38. Shores MM, Smith NL, Forsberg CW, Anawalt BD, Matsumoto AM (2012) Testosterone treatment and mortality in men with low testosterone levels. J Clin Endocrinol Metab 97:2050–2058
39. Muraleedharan V, Marsh H, Kapoor D, Channer KS, Jones TH (2013) Testosterone deficiency is associated with increased risk of mortality and testosterone replacement improves survival in men with type 2 diabetes. Eur J Endocrinol 169:725–733
40. Corona G, Maseroli E, Rastrelli G, Isidori AM, Sforza A et al (2014) Cardiovascular risk associated with testosterone-boosting medications: a systematic review and meta-analysis. Expert Opin Drug Saf 13:1327–1351
41. The ESHRE Capri Workshop Group (2006) Hormones and cardiovascular health in women. Hum Reprod Update 12:483–497
42. Stevenson JC (2011) A woman's journey through the reproductive, transitional and postmenopausal periods of life: impact on cardiovascular and musculo-skeletal risk and the role of estrogen replacement. Maturitas 70(2):197–205
43. Baksu B, Davas I, Agar E et al (2007) Do different delivery systems of estrogen therapy influence serum lipids differently in surgically menopausal women? J Obstet Gynaecol Res 33:346–352

9 Cardiovascular Aging

Leda Galiuto and Gabriella Locorotondo

9.1 Introduction

Cardiovascular disease (CVD) is the leading cause of death worldwide and its prevalence increases with age. Increasing life expectancy and improved health care have progressively led to an expanding proportion of elderly patients requiring cardiovascular treatment. It has been estimated that the number of cardiac surgical patients >80 years old has increased up to 24-fold over the past two decades [1, 2]; thus, CVD currently represents a major financial burden to the healthcare system.

The notion that age itself is a major risk factor for developing CVD is by now well established and widely acknowledged. This is not only because the prevalence of atherosclerosis, valvular dysfunction, and their consequences increases dramatically with age, but also because cardiovascular risk factors tend to develop and worsen over time in both sexes. Most advancements in the knowledge of pathophysiological mechanisms determining CVD in the past decades have contributed to shifting the concept of atherosclerosis from a "degenerative" to an "inflammatory" disease. Inflammation and aging are nowadays considered two sides of the same coin: according to the "inflammaging" paradigm, survival of human beings would be an effective balance between oxidative stress and reparative structural and molecular processes. In light of this view, it is conceivable that the relationship between the cardiovascular system and aging is deeper than is commonly known: indeed, as recently demonstrated at histological and molecular levels, the cardiovascular system itself modifies over time and gets older. Arterial rigidity, the hallmark of cardiovascular aging, is an independent cardiovascular risk factor caused by diverse pathological clinical variables: hyperlipidemia, diabetes mellitus, arterial systemic hypertension, and smoking, and by some physiological factors (aging, female sex, and black race). Underlying mechanisms that contribute to the decline in cell and tissue functions with age are nowadays almost entirely known; they include increased levels of reactive oxygen species, DNA damage, accumulation of dysfunctional organelles, and oxidized proteins and lipids. These all contribute to a progressive decline in the normal physiological function of the cell and to the onset of age-related conditions. Cardiac homeostasis and the ability to adapt to stress are subordinated to the continuous control of cell quality. Autophagy is an important quality control pathway, and its reduction is a major contributor to the aging process, although its enhanced activity delays aging by counteracting age-associated accumulation of protein aggregates and damaged organelles in cells.

L. Galiuto (✉) • G. Locorotondo
Catholic University of the Sacred Heart, Rome Policlinico Agostino Gemelli Foundation, Rome, Italy
e-mail: leonarda.galiuto@unicatt.it

M. Fioranelli (ed.), *Integrative Cardiology*, DOI 10.1007/978-3-319-40010-5_9

Over the past 30 years, research on aging has emphasized the distinction between the amount of time spent alive, the amount of time being healthy, and the amount of time able to perform activities of daily living without difficulty. These characterize different dimensions of the aging process, as individuals may vary in their health or ability status even if living the same number of years. Inequalities in the able state and healthy life expectancy among sexes, races, and geographical areas have been described: white women spend the longest time alive, the longest time healthy, and the longest time able to perform activities of daily living, followed by white men, nonwhite women, and nonwhite men. However, regardless of starting age, individuals of the same race and sex groups spent similar amounts of time in an unhealthy or unable state [3]. The cellular processes that contribute to aging are attractive targets for therapeutic interventions that can delay or prevent the development of age-related diseases. The possibility of delaying aging of the cardiovascular system, thus potentially reducing the incidence of CVD, is a fascinating goal of current scientific research. If such a goal were achieved, it would have a great impact on people economically and with regard to survival. Novel prevention and treatment strategies are under investigation, and progress in the knowledge of pathophysiological mechanisms on the basis of age-related changes in the cardiovascular system has been made.

9.2 Changes of Cardiovascular System Related to Age

With increasing age, cardiovascular system develops structural and functional changes at the level of both the heart and vessels, which finally lead to reduced physiological reserves. In such a condition, patients typically do not show signs of impaired hemodynamic performance at rest, but manifest reduced resistance in response to physical stresses. Age-related changes of cardiovascular system may manifest at different levels (Table 9.1):

1. *Structural level.* Aging may involve systemic arterial vessels, coronary arteries, and myocardium with different pathophysiological mechanisms and related consequences:
   a) *Systemic arterial vessels.* Morphology and function of arterial vessels change with aging. Some changes have a genetic basis, others occur as a result of intrinsic cellular or systemic stimuli. Genetic predisposition determines racial differences, with accelerated arterial aging among African–Caribbean individuals. Moreover, age-related artery change is more pronounced in women, reflecting intrinsic differences in arterial properties between sexes: although men have more prominent, accelerated aging over time compared with women, there are complex effects of hormone deficiency and replacement therapy on CVD. Postmenopausal women exhibit higher aortic rigidity and lower vascular compliance in relation to men, which has a significant impact on their mortality and is probably caused by estrogen deprivation. Even though the smaller diameter of the aortic root has been considered responsible for women's increased pulse pressure, there is strong evidence that the vascular wall composition is the most important factor responsible for it. Overall, with increasing age, large arteries are known to dilate and thicken their walls, particularly because of wall matrix changes and an increase in elastolytic and collagenolytic activity and in smooth muscle tone. In particular, vessel aging leads to intimal and medial thickening (vascular remodeling), and to the gradual loss of arterial elasticity: reduced medial smooth muscle cell number, increased collagen deposition, and fracture of the elastin lamellae are common characteristics of aging vessels. Overall, these changes may lead to vessel dilation and increased lumen size. Increased collagen and decreased elastin content are promoted, at least in part by

Table 9.1 Summary of the most important changes in the cardiovascular system related to age and their functional consequences

Level	Changes	Consequences
Structural		
Systemic arterial vessels	Intimal and medial thickening of large artery walls Changes in wall matrix (increase in elastolytic and collagenolytic activity, increased collagen deposition, fracture of the elastin lamellae, with gradual loss of arterial elasticity) Reduced medial smooth muscle cell number and changes in their tone Increased secretion of proinflammatory cytokines and increased uptake of plasma lipoproteins by endothelial and smooth muscle cells	Elevated systolic arterial pressure and pulse-wave velocity, augmentation of aortic impedance and cardiac mechanical afterload. Atherosclerosis
Myocardium	Alterations of intracellular molecular and biochemical pathways Stiffening of myocardial cells, mural connective tissue and valves, decreased number of myocytes, increased myocyte size, increased rate of myocyte apoptosis, and blunted adrenoceptor-mediated contractile and inotropic response Fibrotic remodeling (reactive fibrosis and replacement/reparative fibrosis, perivascular fibrosis)	Decreased mechanical and contractile efficiency. Increased left ventricular stiffness Decreased coronary blood flow Impaired relaxation and diastolic dysfunction
Coronary arteries	Endothelium-dependent dilation of large epicardial and resistance coronary vessels becomes blunted Basal and stimulated release of nitric oxide by the coronary endothelium decreases. Coronary vasoconstrictor effect of endothelin-1 increases	Coronary flow reserve gradually impairs as result of both abnormal vasodilatory capacity and elevated cardiac work at baseline
Cellular	Stiffening of vascular smooth muscle cells Differential expression of proteins involved in the mechanical regulation of vascular function Changes in cell proliferative potential, increased propensity to undergo cell death, elevated DNA damage, and extensive telomere shortening and dysfunction, oxidative stress-related damage	Arterial rigidity Cell senescence
Ultrastructural	Accumulation of dysfunctional organelles, DNA mutations, oxidized proteins and lipids into endothelial and smooth muscle cells, cardiomyocytes and fibroblasts owing to impaired autophagy	Cell senescence

the age-associated increase in glycated proteins, matrix metalloproteinase enzyme activity, and trophic stimuli such as angiotensin II signaling. As a final result, vascular stiffness increases with advancing age [4–6], and is in turn the main cause of subsequent elevated systolic arterial pressure and pulse-wave velocity: pulse pressure waves reflect early and peak systolic pressure appears late. Hypertension can further stimulate collagen production with increased vessel stiffness and endothelial cell dysfunction. The final step is the augmentation of aortic impedance and cardiac mechanical afterload. Thus, arterial stiffening triggers a variety of cardiac adjustments, which are additional and similar to the age-related intrinsic changes in cardiac morphology and may, therefore, be expected to worsen cardiac performance. Moreover, aging endothelial and smooth muscle cells also show increased secretion of proinflammatory cytokines and increased uptake of plasma lipoproteins, which ultimately constitute the substratum of atherosclerosis (see below).

b) *Myocardium*. At the heart level, aging is known to determine numerous ionic, molecular, and biochemical changes [7] that affect protein function, mitochondrial oxidative phosphorylation, excitation–contraction coupling, calcium kinetics, myofilament activation, matrix composition and regeneration, cell growth and size, and the apoptosis process. Alterations of the intracellular molecular and biochemical pathways produce modifications in cardiac morphology, which ultimately have an impact on cardiac function. Decreased mechanical and contractile efficiency, stiffening of myocardial cells, mural connective tissue and valves, a decreased number of myocytes, increased myocyte size, an increased rate of myocyte apoptosis, and blunted-adrenoceptor-mediated contractile and inotropic response are all distinctive signs of cardiac aging [8]. Pathological fibrosis in the aging mouse heart is associated with dysregulated resident mesenchymal stem cells arising from reduced stemness and aberrant differentiation into dysfunctional inflammatory fibroblasts. Fibroblasts derived from aging mesenchymal stem cells secrete higher levels of collagen type 1, which directly contributes to fibrosis, monocyte chemoattractant protein-1, which attracts leukocytes from the blood, and interleukin-6, which facilitates the transition of monocytes into myeloid fibroblasts. The intrinsic change in the mesenchymal stem cell phenotype acquired by advanced age is specific to the heart, as mesenchymal stem cells originating from the bone wall or fibroblasts derived from them are free of these alterations [9]. Two types of fibrotic remodeling can potentially occur in the myocardium: reactive fibrosis (also known as diffuse fibrosis), which describes the expansion of existing collagen fibers without a significant loss of myocytes, and replacement/reparative fibrosis, or scar formation (focal fibrosis), which occurs when collagen is newly deposited in the place of necrotic/apoptotic myocytes. Diffuse, reactive fibrosis is a typical feature of the aging heart. However, some amount of replacement fibrosis may also occur; myocyte apoptosis and necrosis increase with age. Conversely, neither reactive nor reparative fibrosis correlates with age in patients with idiopathic dilated cardiomyopathy. The significance of these fibrotic patterns is likely diverse, as the nature or quality of the collagen network may have a differential impact on myocardial stiffness or signal propagation. It is known that reactive fibrosis increases left ventricular stiffness. Accumulation of collagen surrounding blood vessels in the heart is named perivascular fibrosis and may precede or act as an extension of reactive fibrosis. Perivascular fibrosis increases in the aging heart. In patients with non-ischemic heart failure, perivascular fibrosis is associated with decreased coronary flow of the left anterior descending artery, and such impaired coronary blood flow has been demonstrated to correlate with elevated left ventricular wall stress in patients with heart failure. Perivascular fibrosis occurring during aging may have local or paracrine effects on the surrounding myocardium, which in turn could contribute to cardiac dysfunction in elderly subjects. In particular, myocardial fibrosis may be a contributing factor for impaired relaxation and diastolic dysfunction. From this point of view, excess collagen, rather than myocyte hypertrophy, causes myocardial stiffness. Indeed, in experimental models of hypertension-induced diastolic heart failure, collagen deposition, hypertrophic remodeling, and myocardial stiffness are abrogated by an angiotensin II receptor antagonist. In a clinical human setting, contradictory findings have been shown: in some studies of hypertensive patients, those presenting with diastolic heart failure were older and had higher levels of serum markers of collagen turnover; in others, no correlation has been found between diastolic dysfunction and collagen content in the aging heart [10].

c) *Coronary arteries.* Pathophysiological modifications related to aging have also been shown to involve also structure and function of coronary vasculature, which could affect myocardial perfusion. Coronary flow reserve is gradually impaired and such a reduction may be the result of abnormal vasodilator capacity, elevated cardiac work, and myocardial blood flow at baseline [11]. In particular, the endothelium-dependent dilation of large epicardial and resistance coronary vessels becomes blunted [12], basal and stimulated release of nitric oxide by the coronary endothelium decreases [13], and the coronary vasoconstrictor effect of endothelin-1 [14], whose plasma concentrations are raised in the elderly [15], increases, thus finally determining a reduction of the coronary vasodilatory reserve.

2. *Cellular level.* Contrary to the traditional paradigm, which associated vascular compliance only with extracellular matrix composition, vascular smooth muscle cells have been recently demonstrated to contribute, by visco-elasticity, to the vessels' overall mechanics. Under physiological conditions, the mechanical behavior of vascular smooth muscle cells varies according to the position in the arterial tree and intensity of regional mechanical forces, whereas, in the pathological scenario, their cytoplasm stiffening is associated with aging and arterial hypertension, causing arterial rigidity in the absence of extracellular matrix modifications. Thus, almost one-third of the differences found between stiff and distensible vessels are due to the differential expression of proteins involved in the mechanical regulation of vascular function, especially the components of the vascular smooth muscle cell cytoskeleton and extracellular matrix. Aging determines marked changes in vascular smooth muscle cells and inflammatory cells. First, the ability of cells to divide is lost with aging. Such an irreversible change depicts so-called cell senescence. Two types of cell senescence have been described: "replicative" senescence refers to exhaustion of the proliferative lifespan over time, a characteristic of aging, associated with critically shortened telomeres at the chromosomal ends, which then induce a DNA damage response. "Stress-induced premature" senescence is triggered by external stimuli, including oxidizing agents and radiation, which activate the intracellular senescence cascade prematurely. Prematurely and naturally aging cells share several characteristics: changes in cell proliferative potential, increased propensity to undergo cell death, elevated DNA damage, and extensive telomere shortening and dysfunction. In aging vessels, vascular smooth muscle cells undergo reduced proliferation and prolonged population doubling times. Although most of these cells are presumed to be derived from the vessel wall itself, a proportion of cells expressing smooth muscle or endothelial cell markers may be procured from bone marrow-derived progenitor cells and endothelial progenitor cells that migrate and integrate into the vessel wall. They may also be affected by aging, which determines impaired migration and adhesion, owing to the reduced expression of cell surface markers and cytokines for chemotaxis and increased oxidative stress and inflammation. Oxidative stress plays a major role in age-related damage of the cardiovascular system at the cellular level.

3. *Ultrastructural level.* Aging is depicted by the accumulation of dysfunctional organelles, DNA mutations, and oxidized proteins and lipids into endothelial and smooth muscle cells, cardiomyocytes, and fibroblasts: this phenomenon contributes to alteration of the normal physiological function of the cells. Under homeostatic conditions, abnormal constituents and organelles are eliminated through sequestration into double membrane vesicles, which subsequently deliver the content to a lysosome for degradation. This tightly regulated control of cell quality is ensured by the so-called autophagy, an intracellular pathway responsible for removing senescent and dysfunctional cellular

components. Its activation involves the coordination of multiple protein complexes at several different stages: activation, formation, and elongation of the phagophore, engulfment of the cargo, and delivery to the lysosome for degradation. Such a complex activity is regulated by both extra- and intracellular signals, which are centrally inhibited by the mammalian target of rapamycin (mTOR) and activated by 5′ AMP-activated protein kinase (AMPK). When activated, mTOR inhibits autophagy, throughout the PI3K/Akt signaling pathway [16]. Studies have shown that under nutrient-rich conditions, autophagy is depressed. In contrast, during nutrient-limiting conditions, autophagy is activated by the energy sensor AMPK. Once started, autophagy proceeds with the formation and elongation of a small vesicular sac (named phagophore), through lipid acquisition. Lipid sources for phagosomes may derive from the membrane of mitochondria, endoplasmic reticulum, and Golgi, or may be composed of membranes from multiple sources to avoid affecting the homeostasis of a specific subcellular compartment [17]. Probably, different types of autophagy induction lead to the formation of different types of phagosomes. The biogenesis and elongation of the phagosome is regulated by a number of conserved autophagy-related proteins and involves two ubiquitin-like conjugation systems. The growing phagophore elongates until it closes on itself, engulfing the cargo to be degraded. Then, the newly formed structure fuses with a lysosome to form the autolysosome, in which cargo and inner membrane of the autophagosome are subsequently degraded by the lysosomal hydrolases. Although few studies have directly assessed autophagic activity in aging tissues, it is widely accepted that autophagy declines with age and that this impairment is a major contributor to aging. Mice with impaired autophagic capability have an accelerated aging phenotype, including the development of left ventricular hypertrophy, decreased fractional shortening, and premature death [18]. This finding confirms that clearance of damaged proteins is an important cellular quality control mechanism that prevents premature aging, and autophagy may conceivably have an anti-aging effect on the cardiovascular system. There are many potential causes underlying the alterations in cardiovascular function with age, but the accumulation of cytotoxic proteins and dysfunctional organelles contributes to the development of age-related pathological conditions, such as skeletal muscle atrophy, neurodegeneration, and cardiac dysfunction. The underlying mechanisms for the reduction in autophagy in aging tissues are not well understood and probably involve numerous proteins. The most reliable hypothesis is that changes in metabolism and hormonal responses with age might be associated with transcriptional downregulation of autophagy, which could contribute to the age-dependent development of CVD observed. For instance, in rats, long-term excessive fat intake inhibits autophagic flux in the heart and is associated with myocyte apoptosis and cardiac dysfunction [19]. Under such conditions, reactive oxygen species (ROS), which are usually generated in the cell at low levels as a by-product of mitochondrial respiration and have signaling functions, are increased. Excessive ROS negatively affects cellular processes by modifying proteins and lipids and inducing DNA damage. When mitochondria become dysfunctional in aging cells, excessive ROS production contributes to impaired autophagy. If autophagic activity is reduced with age, dysfunctional mitochondria tend to be less frequently removed and to accumulate in aging myocytes.

More recent evidence has shown that microRNAs (miRNAs), which are small noncoding RNAs, post-transcriptionally controlling gene expression by inhibiting translation or inducing degradation of targeted mRNAs, can contribute in the regulation of longevity and senescence. In humans, comparisons of miRNA expression between peripheral blood mononuclear cells of young versus old individuals reveal the downregulation of various miRNAs. Several studies have addressed the regulation of miRNAs during culture-induced senescence of vascular cells. In human cell culture studies, miRNAs were detected in senescent endothelial cells: some miRNAs are up-regulated, others are down-regulated, whereas in the entire vessel wall miRNAs are generally up-regulated. These differences between the profiles of cultured endothelial cells and entire vessels likely reflect the different cellular compositions as, in whole vessels, smooth muscle cells and invaded inflammatory cells, but not endothelial cells, are the predominant cell types. Some specific miRNAs are well known to repress matrix proteins in the heart, and the increased expression of such miRNAs in the aorta of aged mice is associated with a decline in matrix protein expression, such as collagens and elastin, which is considered to contribute to aneurysm formation, a vascular disease typically associated with age. Potential development of therapeutic miRNA targeting strategies is currently further limited by the need to understand whether the deregulated miRNAs during aging are causes or effectors of the age-associated disease or if they may even act as compensatory feedback loops. The knowledge that miRNAs are involved in more complex regulatory pathways in competition with other competitive endogenous RNAs makes the scenario challenging. Given that such interactions likely depend on the number of molecules of each interacting species, new models that take into account quantitative biology are required to understand network modulation and finally develop therapeutic interventions [20].

9.3 Atherosclerosis and Cardiovascular Aging Enhance Each Other

A very strict link has been demonstrated between atherosclerosis and aging: cellular senescence is usually observed in patients with atherosclerosis and, in turn, cardiovascular risk factors may promote premature or accelerated vascular aging. Increasing evidence indicates a potential causative role of inflammation and oxidative stress at the basis of the association; thus, in the last few decades, atherosclerosis has been no longer considered merely a degenerative disease, but also an inflammatory disease. This assumption is derived from histological findings of augmented inflammatory milieu and senescent cells within atherosclerotic arterial walls. Atherosclerotic plaques are usually formed by accumulation of inflammatory cells (macrophages, T lymphocytes, dendritic cells, and mast cells), and both intracellular and extracellular lipids and debris, together with vascular smooth muscle cells, collagen, and elastin. Oxidized lipids are often concentrated in a necrotic core surrounded by a fibrous cap, composed predominantly of smooth muscle cells. Aged and atherosclerotic smooth muscle cells contain high levels of oxidative stress-induced damage, probably because of the combination of higher reactive oxygen species (ROS) generation and impaired antioxidant defense. Increased oxidized LDL (oxLDL) during atherogenesis also provokes a gradual loss of mitochondrial function. Mitochondrial DNA damage and dysfunction can increase ROS generation, creating a positive feedback loop. Moreover, ROS production can be regulated through mechanical stress, as endothelial cells under laminar shear stress up-regulate anti-oxidant enzymes. Turbulent flow at sites of plaque formation would thus reduce anti-oxidant capacity. In addition to directly promoting DNA damage, ROS can modulate atherosclerosis progression via other mechanisms: they can downregulate telomerase activity, thus directly promoting apoptosis; they can reduce the expression of survival signals, and can increase the expression of cell surface receptors required for the uptake of oxLDL. Direct experimental evidence shows that aging promotes proinflammatory changes in monocyte/macrophages that are relevant to atherosclerosis: both migration and activation of macrophages within plaques increase with age. Indeed, expression of leukocyte adhesion molecules on endothelial cells of atherosclerotic vessels is increased: such a feature promotes migration of monocytes from the blood stream to the arterial wall and is followed by the increased uptake of atherogenic lipoproteins with subsequent inflammation. Autopsies performed in patients who died owing to an acute coronary syndrome have shown that ruptured plaques are characterized by a thin cap, necrotic smooth muscle cells, and disrupted collagen and extra-cellular matrix. Thus, it has become conceivable that stability of the atherosclerotic plaque might depends on the thickness of the fibrous cap and the degree of cap inflammation. Rupture of atherosclerotic plaques is frequently subclinical, as smooth muscle cells repair the rupture and reorganize associated thrombus, by proliferating and synthesizing matrix. The final result is a progressive narrowing of the vessel lumen. Reparative processes may be altered by cellular senescence: shortened telomeres are evident in atherosclerosis, observed in plaque smooth muscle cells and endothelial cells, relative to the normal vessel wall, and in circulating endothelial progenitor cells. Additionally, leukocytes in patients with atherosclerosis show shorter telomeres compared with control subjects: this feature correlates inversely with cardiovascular disease risk in patients with subclinical diseases. Vascular smooth muscle cells, endothelial cells, macrophages, and circulating cells from the elderly and patients with atherosclerosis also share an increased amount of damaged DNA in both nuclei and mitochondria, compared with younger subjects and those without vascular disease. The accumulation of DNA damage may reflect both ongoing damage-inducing stimuli and defects in the repair process. When DNA damage is too diffuse to be repaired or when the repairing cascades are impaired, cell senescence and apoptosis occur. An increased rate of apoptosis can be found in vascular smooth muscle cells and other cells within atherosclerotic plaques. Notably, most cell death in atheromas takes place within the macrophage-rich necrotic core of the plaque.

On the other hand, acquired cardiovascular risk factors themselves contribute to premature vascular aging and cellular senescence. Smoking increases arterial stiffness and pulse pressure. Chronic high alcohol intake also increases arterial stiffness, whereas low to moderate and/or acute alcohol intake produces the opposite effect. Moreover, age- and diet-associated elevation of serum glucose is associated with both premature vascular stiffness and vascular cell senescence. Glucose participates in a spontaneous, non-enzymatic reaction known as glycation, which adds sugars to proteins and lipids to form reactive advanced glycation end products. This phenomenon is enhanced by aging, particularly in patients with atherosclerosis and metabolic disorders. Hyperglycemia and glycation products promote vascular stiffness through collagen stabilization and attenuated nitric oxide production in endothelial cells and by increasing vascular permeability and cell adhesion, enhancing smooth muscle cell migration, augmenting circulating lipoproteins for oxidation and their subsequent uptake by macrophages, and increasing inflammation and oxidative stress.

9.4 Can Cardiovascular Aging Be Delayed?

Interventions that target the underlying aging process can potentially delay or interrupt the development of age-related CVD [21]. Some anti-aging interventions are currently under investigation, which may involve different factors of the aging process.

1. *Inhibition of autophagy*. Evidence from experimental studies suggest the hypothesis that enhancing autophagy should counteract age-associated accumulations of protein aggregates and damaged organelles in cells [22]. Pharmacological activation of autophagy using the mTOR inhibitor rapamycin or spermidine has been demonstrated to significantly extend the life span of mice [23, 24]. Mice with reduced mTOR expression and enhanced autophagic flux in all tissues, including heart, lungs, skeletal muscle, and brain, have extended survival and exhibit anti-aging phenotypes, such as increased insulin sensitivity, leanness, and

improved motor function [25]. Experimental stimulation of autophagy may have an impact on cardiovascular function and health. Unfortunately, there are no current pharmacological interventions known to selectively increase autophagy.

2. *Cell-based therapy*. Implantation of autologous bone marrow-derived stem and progenitor cells is a potential treatment for age-related impairment of neovascularization in response to ischemia [26]. Cell-based therapies have been safely conducted and demonstrated beneficial effects in augmenting neovascularization in preclinical animal studies. The isolated stem cells are highly regenerative and may contain low amounts of cumulative ROS-related damage. On the contrary, human clinical trials involving administration of autologous bone marrow cells or progenitor cells from bone marrow or peripheral blood have provided conflicting results. It may be at least in part because patients who would undergo cell-based therapy are elderly, with increased ROS levels and reduced numbers of stem and progenitor cells with impaired regenerative potential. Studies have investigated different approaches to enhancing the therapeutic potential of stem and progenitor cells by modulating their redox regulation. The first strategy involved suppressing excessive oxidative stress by promoting the anti-oxidative potential: mesenchymal stem cell engraftment in the infarcted heart is enhanced by the co-injection of anti-oxidants, which mitigates ROS-induced inhibition of cell–matrix adhesion. Preconditioning stem cells, with either a brief period of ischemia/anoxia or repeated cycles of intermittent hypoxia/reoxygenation, increase post-engraftment cell survival or neovascular potential through the oxidative stress resistance mechanism. Another approach involved stimulating stem cells with a low dose of pro-oxidants: in vitro treatment of adipose-derived stroma cells with pharmacological inhibitors to generate mitochondrial ROS increases the secretion of proangiogenic factors and protects such cells against ROS-induced apoptosis. Although most of these enhancements are demonstrated in cells from young donors and recipients, some have been shown to be effective in aged cells and old recipients: hypoxic preconditioning of human adipose-derived stroma cells from donors over 50 years of age increases redox metabolism and promotes paracrine secretion. On the other hand, despite promising results, it has to be considered that, in the clinical scenario, elderly patients often suffer from comorbidities that affect neovascularization, such as diabetes, hypercholesterolemia, and advanced atherosclerosis. Therefore, it may be beneficial to develop cell-based therapies targeting combined pathophysiological conditions such as aging, metabolic disorders, and inflammatory diseases.

3. *Anti-oxidants*. Expression of natural antioxidants, such as ferritin and glutathione, is reduced by age and atherosclerosis. However, although antioxidants have been demonstrated to have significant anti-atherosclerosis effects in vitro and in animal models, their efficacy in humans is questionable. Vitamin E can reduce the uptake of oxLDL by macrophages and inhibit the subsequent inflammatory responses that stimulate atherosclerosis development, but there is now extensive evidence indicating that supplementing dietary?? with antioxidants has no significant effect on reducing cardiovascular risk. Statins primarily reduce the cholesterol level, but have been demonstrated to exert multiple effects, including improved endothelial function and reduced inflammation responses. In particular, statins target mechanisms involved into premature aging, thus leading to enhanced telomere protection, decreased DNA damage, and suppressed oxidative stress. Moreover, statins can delay replicative senescence of vascular smooth muscle cells in vivo in atherosclerosis. Angiotensin II increases ROS and promotes oxidative DNA damage. ACE inhibitors/ARBs, then, can

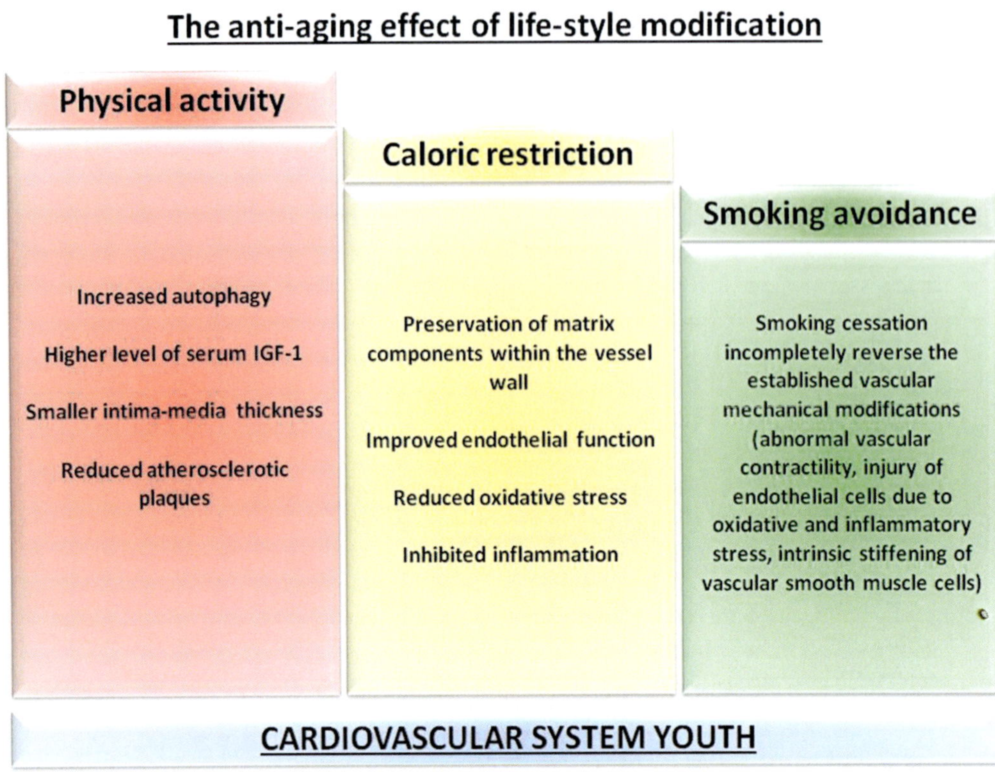

Fig. 9.1 Schema illustrating the most important lifestyle modifications, which have been demonstrated to significantly reduce entity and progression of cardiovascular aging. Pathophysiological bases are explained in lower boxes. For details, see text

reduce oxidative stress and subsequent DNA damage. Bradykinin, a hormone that mediates some of the vasoprotective effects of ACE inhibitors, protects endothelial cells from superoxide-induced senescence. However, at present, it is not known whether these drugs reduce premature aging in vivo.

4. *Lifestyle modifications*. Despite limited data in a human setting, many lifestyle modifications have been demonstrated that delay the aging process (Fig. 9.1). Exercise is known to have beneficial effects against cardiovascular diseases and aging [27, 28]. It can be partly or entirely attributed to increased autophagy in the heart [29]. In a recent large population study, higher exercise capacity remained a powerful predictor of survival, despite lower average exercise capacity at older ages, reinforcing its importance in patients of all ages. Fitness-associated biological age was a stronger predictor of survival than chronological age [30]. Soluble insulin-like growth factor-1 (IGF-1) has been found to be associated with coronary and carotid atherosclerotic burden and physical fitness in the oldest old: individuals with a higher level of serum IGF-1 had smaller right and left intima-media thickness, reduced atherosclerotic plaques, and greater walking speed compared with those with lower levels of circulating IGF-1 [31]. Nutritional status and diet are associated with age-related vascular changes and with atherosclerosis. Caloric restriction is a potent inducer of autophagy in the heart [32] and, when used as long-term treatment in aged mice, leads to preserved contractile function [33] and improved left ventricular diastolic function. In vivo beneficial effects of caloric restriction include preservation of matrix components within the vessel wall, improved

endothelial function by augmenting nitric oxide generation, reduced sensitivity to oxLDL, reduced oxidative stress by upregulating anti-oxidants and protecting mitochondrial function, and inhibited inflammation. Drugs and dietary supplements that mimic caloric restriction effects without affecting nutritional balance may be appropriate in most patients to delay the aging process. Nowadays, the plant polyphenol resveratrol, an activator of autophagy, is being explored as a potential therapeutic strategy. Studies have reported that resveratrol is cardioprotective and slows the progression of heart failure after myocardial infarction [34], pressure overload, [35] and chemotherapy-induced cardiotoxicity [36]. However, the beneficial effects of resveratrol on cardiac cells are dose-dependent. At lower doses, resveratrol enhances autophagy and has anti-apoptotic properties, whereas high doses attenuate autophagy and promote apoptosis [37].

Finally, it is known that smoking and female sex are independent predictors of vascular smooth muscle cell stiffness [38]. The exposure to tobacco is an independent risk factor for arterial rigidity. Unfortunately, exposure removal is ineffective at completely reversing the established vascular mechanical modifications. The abnormal vascular contractility observed in smokers is associated not only with the injury of endothelial cells due to oxidative and inflammatory stress, but also with intrinsic stiffening of vascular smooth muscle cells, which, taken together, are responsible for arterial rigidity. Indeed, vascular smooth muscle cells of smokers are stiffer than those of nonsmokers, regardless of the presence of the endothelium, suggesting that smoking might have a direct action on smooth muscle cells. There is evidence of increased activity of the matrix metalloproteinases in association with nicotine exposure and of increased production of PDGF, leading to chronic modifications in vascular smooth muscle cell cytoskeleton, following tobacco exposure.

References

1. Friedrich I, Simm A, Kötting J, Thölen F, Fischer B, Silber R-E (2009) Cardiac surgery in the elderly patient. Dtsch Arztebl Int 106:416–422
2. Seco M, Edelman JJB, Forrest P, Ng M, Wilson MK, Fraser J, Bannon PG, Vallely MP (2014) Geriatric cardiac surgery: chronology vs. biology. Heart Lung Circ 23:794–801
3. Thielke SM, Diehr PH, Yee LM, Arnold AM, Quiñones AR, Whitson HE, Jacob ME, Newman AB (2015) Sex, race, and age differences in observed years of life, healthy life, and able life among older adults in the cardiovascular health study. J Pers Med 5:440–451. doi:10.3390/jpm5040440
4. Lakatta EG (1999) Cardiovascular aging research: the next horizons. J Am Geriatr Soc 47(5):613–625
5. Lakatta E (1994) Aging effects on the vasculature in health: risk factors for cardiovascular disease. Am J Geriatric Cardiol 3(6):11–50
6. Priebe HJ (2000) The aged cardiovascular risk patient. Br J Anaesth 85(5):763–778
7. Folkow B, Svanborg A (1993) Physiology of cardiovascular aging. Physiol Rev 73(4):725–764
8. Olivetti G, Melissari M, Capasso JM, Anversa P (1991) Cardiomyopathy of the aging human heart. Myocyte loss and reactive cellular hypertrophy. Circ Res 68(6):1560–1568
9. Trial J, Entman ML, Cieslik KA (2015) Mesenchymal stem cell-derived inflammatory fibroblasts mediate interstitial fibrosis in the aging heart. J Mol Cell Cardiol 91:28–34. doi:10.1016/j.yjmcc.2015.12.017
10. Horn MA, Trafford AW (2015) Aging and the cardiac collagen matrix: novel mediators of fibrotic remodeling. J Mol Cell Cardiol 93:175–185
11. Czernin J, Muller P, Chan S et al (1993) Influence of age and hemodynamics on myocardial blood flow and flow reserve. Circulation 88(1):62–69
12. Egashira K, Inou T, Hirooka Y et al (1993) Effects of age on endothelium-dependent vasodilation of resistance coronary artery by acetylcholine in humans. Circulation 88(1):77–81
13. Amrani M, Goodwin AT, Gray CC, Yacoub MH (1996) Ageing is associated with reduced basal and stimulated release of nitric oxide by the coronary endothelium. Acta Physiol Scand 157(1):79–84
14. Goodwin AT, Amrani M, Marchbank AJ, Gray CC, Jayakumar J, Yacoub MH (1999) Coronary vasoconstriction to endothelin-1 increases with age before and after ischaemia and reperfusion. Cardiovasc Res 41(3):554–562
15. Miyauchi T, Yanagisawa M, Iida K et al (1992) Age- and sex-related variation of plasma endothelin-1 concentration in normal and hypertensive subjects. Am Heart J 123(4):1092–1093
16. Inoki T, Li Y, Zhu T, Wu J, Guan KL (2002) TSC2 is phosphorylated and inhibited by Akt and suppresses mTOR signalling. Nat Cell Biol 4:648–657

17. Chan SN, Tang BL (2013) Location and membrane sources for autophagosome formation from ER-mitochondria contact sites to Golgi-endosome-derived carriers. Mol Membr Biol 30:394–402
18. Taneike M, Yamaguchi O, Nakai A, Hikoso S, Takeda T, Mizote I et al (2010) Inhibition of autophagy in the heart induces age-related cardiomyopathy. Autophagy 6:600–606
19. Hsu HC, Chen CY, Lee BC, Chen MF (2016) High-fat diet induces cardiomyocyte apoptosis via the inhibition of autophagy. Eur J Nutr 55(7):2245–2254
20. Dimmeler S, Nicotera P (2013) MicroRNAs in age-related diseases. EMBO Mol Med 5:180–190
21. Wang JC, Bennett M (2012) Aging and atherosclerosis mechanisms, functional consequences, and potential therapeutics for cellular senescence. Circ Res 111:245–259
22. Leon LJ, Gustafsson AB (2016) Staying young at heart: autophagy and adaptation to cardiac aging. J Mol Cell Cardiol 95:78–85
23. Anisimov M, Zabezhinski A, Popovich IG, Piskunova TS, Semenchenko AV, Tyndyk ML et al (2011) Rapamycin increases lifespan and inhibits spontaneous tumorigenesis in inbred female mice. Cell Cycle 10:4230–4236
24. Harrison DE, Strong R, Sharp ZD, Nelson JF, Astle CM, Flurkey K et al (2009) Rapamycin fed late in life extends lifespan in genetically heterogeneous mice. Nature 460:392–395
25. Pyo JO, Yoo SM, Ahn HH, Nah J, Hong SH, Kam TI et al (2013) Overexpression of Atg5 in mice activates autophagy and extends lifespan. Nat Commun 4:2300
26. Lam YT (2016) Critical roles of reactive oxygen species in age-related impairment in ischemia-induced neovascularization by regulating stem and progenitor cell function. Hindawi Publishing Corporation Oxidative Medicine and Cellular Longevity, vol 2016, Article ID 7095901, 14 p. doi:10.1155/2016/7095901
27. Giannuzzi P, Temporelli PL, Corra U, Tavazzi L (2003) E-CS Group, antiremodeling effect of long-term exercise training in patients with stable chronic heart failure: results of the exercise in left ventricular dysfunction and chronic heart failure (ELVD-CHF) trial. Circulation 108:554–559
28. Wilson MG, Ellison GM, Cable NT (2015) Basic science behind the cardiovascular benefits of exercise. Heart 101:758–765
29. He C, Bassik MC, Moresi V, Sun K, Wei Y, Zou Z et al (2012) Exercise-induced BCL2-regulated autophagy is required for muscle glucose homeostasis. Nature 481:511–515
30. Blaha MJ, Hung RK, Dardari Z, Feldman DI, Whelton SP, Nasir K, Blumenthal RS, Brawner CA, Ehrman JK, Keteyian SJ, Al-Mallah MH (2016) Age-dependent prognostic value of exercise capacity and derivation of fitness-associated biologic age. Heart pii:heartjnl-2015-308537. doi:10.1136/heartjnl-2015-308537
31. Córdova C, Boullosa DA, Custódio MR, Quaglia LA, Santos SN, Freitas WM, Sposito AC, Nóbrega OT, Brazilian Study on Healthy Aging (2016) Atheroprotective properties of serum IGF-1 in the carotid and coronary territories and beneficial role on the physical fitness of the oldest old. J Gerontol A Biol Sci Med Sci 71(10):1281–1288
32. Wohlgemuth SE, Julian D, Akin DE, Fried J, Toscano K, Leeuwenburgh C et al (2007) Autophagy in the heart and liver during normal aging and calorie restriction. Rejuvenation Res 10:281–292
33. Han X, Turdi S, Hu N, Guo R, Zhang R, Ren J (2012) Influence of long-term caloric restriction on myocardial and cardiomyocyte contractile function and autophagy in mice. J Nutri Biochem 23:1592–1599
34. Gu XS, Wang ZB, Ye Z, Lei JP, Li L, Su DF et al (2014) Resveratrol, an activator of SIRT1, upregulates AMPK and improves cardiac function in heart failure. Genet Mol Res GMR 13:323–335
35. Sung MM, Das SK, Levasseur J, Byrne NJ, Fung D, Kim TT et al (2015) Resveratrol treatment of mice with pressure-overload-induced heart failure improves diastolic function and cardiac energy metabolism. Circ Heart Fail 8:128–137
36. Danz ED, Skramsted J, Henry N, Bennett JA, Keller RS (2009) Resveratrol prevents doxorubicin cardiotoxicity through mitochondrial stabilization and the Sirt1 pathway. Free Radic Biol Med 46:1589–1597
37. Gurusamy N, Lekli I, Mukherjee S, Ray D, Ahsan MK, Gherghiceanu M et al (2010) Cardioprotection by resveratrol: a novel mechanism via autophagy involving the mTORC2 pathway. Cardiovasc Res 86:103–112
38. Dinardo CL, Santos HC, Vaquero AR, Martelini AR, Dallan LAO, Alencar AM, Krieger JE, Pereira AC (2015) Smoking and female sex: independent predictors of human vascular smooth muscle cells stiffening. PLoS One 10(12):e0145062. doi:10.1371/journal.pone.0145062

Nutrition and Cardiac Health 10

Claudio Tomella, Veronica Di Nardo, and Massimo Fioranelli

Who would think that a calculator could promote cardiac health?

If we were to apply the principles of calculable efficiency and control used in fast-food restaurants to health, it would be unsuccessful in promoting healthy nutrition.

Mainstream nutrition is full of hoaxes, fads, and clichés that should be reviewed.

The dietary choices that people make on a daily basis are based on a complex combination of preference for flavor and smell; their beliefs, habits, culture, and relationships; in addition to marketing and economics. Nutritional approaches are numerous and differ from each other, and it is important to be clear that standard nutritional advice has limits.

The diet of most benefit to health will be one that is specifically designed to meet the various types of human constitution and individual biochemical needs. It is important to have a functional and tailored approach to nutrition in which the focus is on the "whole person."

Food is not only important for its calories or nutrients. There is a "harmonious whole" in the food we consume that interacts dynamically with each individual.

C. Tomella (✉) • V. Di Nardo
Guglielmo Marconi University, Rome, Italy
e-mail: claudio.tomella@gmail.com

M. Fioranelli
Department of Nuclear Physics, Sub-nuclear and Radiation, Guglielmo Marconi University, Rome, Italy

A modern approach to nutrition takes into consideration the succession of various meals that are consumed throughout the day. It takes into account how to choose, cook, and combine foods according to the functioning of organs and the specific needs of the subject.

Combining foods in the right way and using different methods of cooking to maximize their properties for different effects can influence the main functions of the body, such as the optimization of the liver, kidneys, and thyroid; insulin regulation; and the balance of hormones.

In particular, the human digestive system (liver, gut, pancreas, etc.) and the kidneys, which are primarily involved in food processing and in the elimination of waste products, are those that need to be evaluated most carefully. Regarding their diet, an individual should consider the succession of various meals that are consumed throughout the day, to support the liver detoxification process and drainage of the excretory organs and kidneys. The strength of the effects that toxins have on our health is dependent on our level of exposure and the level to which our detoxification systems are functioning. Nutrition is a matter of rhythm: just as the beat of the heart keeps its rhythm, nutrients are also able to influence the cellular processes, hormones, and stages of life. Moreover, nutrition influences key processes of the human body, such as inflammation, glycation, methylation, oxidative stress, and autophagy. It can also influence 5′ AMP-

M. Fioranelli (ed.), *Integrative Cardiology*, DOI 10.1007/978-3-319-40010-5_10

activated protein kinase (AMPK), mammalian target of rapamycin (mTOR), sirtuins, and mitochondrial function. A central role is played by molecules, which are essential to effecting key chemical reactions and are normally present in the body or introduced through the diet (micronutrients, vitamins, etc.). Presence at their optimal levels is critical for the heart and the prevention of cardiovascular disease.

Integrated medicine, which considers the person as a whole, takes into account all these aspects.

10.1 Body Types and Vulnerability Areas: More than Weight

Many people think that "body type" just describes the way someone looks. But how is "body type" perceived from a nutritionist's point of view? The body type can provide information about your hormonal and sympathetic nervous system characteristics and about how you respond to food intake.

In some subjects more than in others, certain foods cause an increase in bodily circumferences or selective accumulation in specific parts of the body.

Once someone establishes their body type, they can then adjust nutrient intake to maximize body composition and health-related goals. The functional assessment decodes the symptoms described by the patient based on their clinical significance [1]. In this way, the menu is created based on the characteristics of the subject and not on those of the food.

The definition of the body type is less obvious than it seems in the case of the human body. This is proved by the large number of terms and definitions that distinguish it.

Human constitution types have been studied since the early days of medicine.

The focus of these studies is to find similar characteristics among groups of people, as defined by their psycho-morpho-neuro-immuno-endocrine constitutions.

Hippocrates's humoral theory was based on the observation of natural phenomena to explain the onset of disease and different types of human temperament.

Physical and psychological characteristics and temperaments can be understood through the four humors. Ancient Chinese medicine has created more detailed and nuanced classifications of the human constitution types [2].

Each person has a constitution type that has corresponding areas of vulnerability in addition to physical and psychological features and nutritional guidelines.

The constitution types presented here are in five categories, allowing the reader to understand a framework of the prevailing characteristics connected with each element. In reality, many people have mixed constitution types, in which the characteristics of more than one element are observed.

10.1.1 Human Constitution Type 1: Liver

The liver constitution type manifests a particular psycho-emotional sensitivity owing to the prevalence of the sympathetic nervous system. The general shape of the body is gynoid and fat is localized mainly in the lower body (hips, thighs, and buttocks). The chest is tight, the breasts are small, the abdomen is flat, and the waist very evident (Fig. 10.1).

Those who have this liver constitution have a special vitality in their eyes. Their prominent physiological characteristic is rapidity and the ability to adapt quickly.

These subjects usually have a weak liver metabolism and biliary system.

They can develop spastic colitis, constipation, or hemorrhoids. They have a tendency toward muscle hypertonicity that lends itself to the phenomenon of contracture in addition to cramps and spasms. The rapidity in the reactions and the tendency to spasm expose them to possible heart attacks.

In this constitution type, it is suggested that subjects avoid food rich in xenoestrogens and cheese (their lipids worsen liver function), limiting foods that are too rich in iodine or excessively stimulating.

For optimal liver function, an adequate portion of energy deriving from easily assimilated

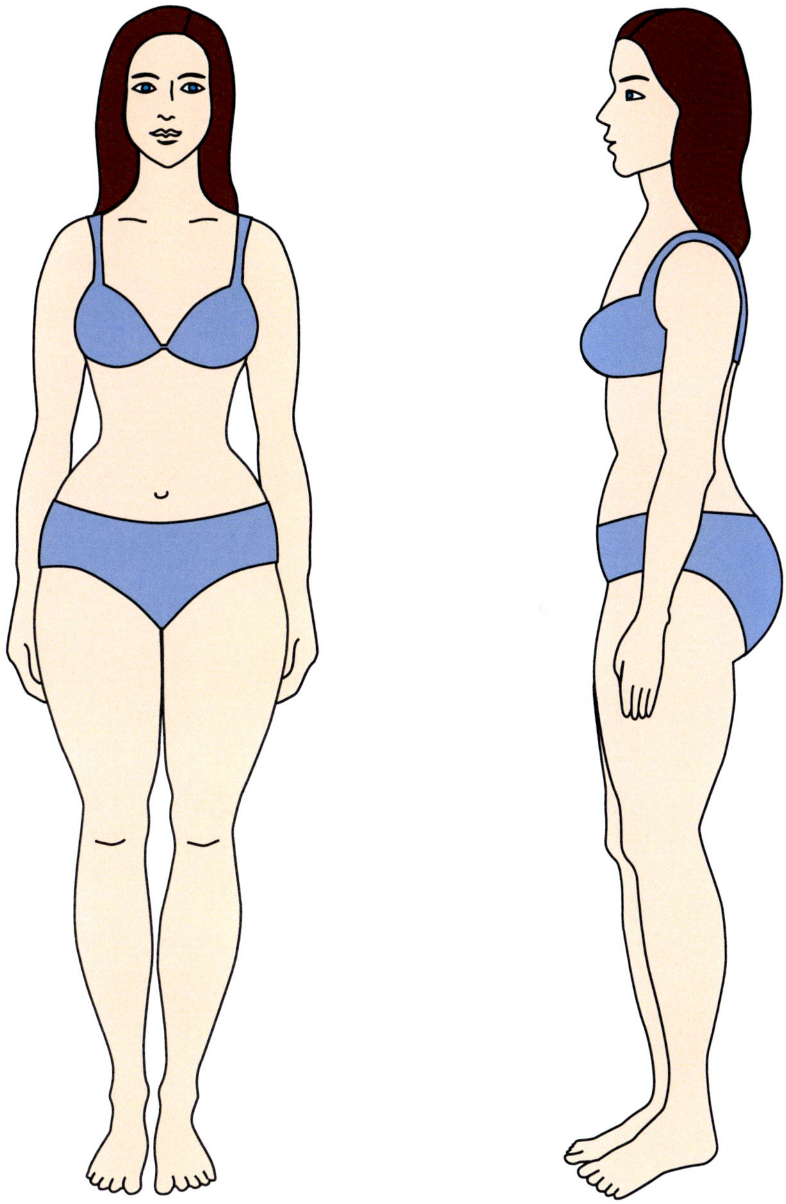

Fig. 10.1 Liver constitution type

carbohydrates and water content of fruits and vegetables, citric acid, vitamin C, and food rich in potassium can be very helpful.

10.1.2 Human Constitution Type 2: Heart–Adrenal

The distinguishing feature of these individuals is that they have very efficient adrenal gland activity. They can be compared with the blood–Hippocratic type. Fat deposition takes place in the areas most stressed by androgen hormones and cortisol. This form predominantly localizes fat in the upper area of the body (trunk, shoulders, and back of neck area) with barely evident waist line and remarkable development of the muscular system (Fig. 10.2).

From the psychological point of view, they are active and efficient, resolved, with good adaptability and capable of assuming positions. They are often persons of power. Areas of

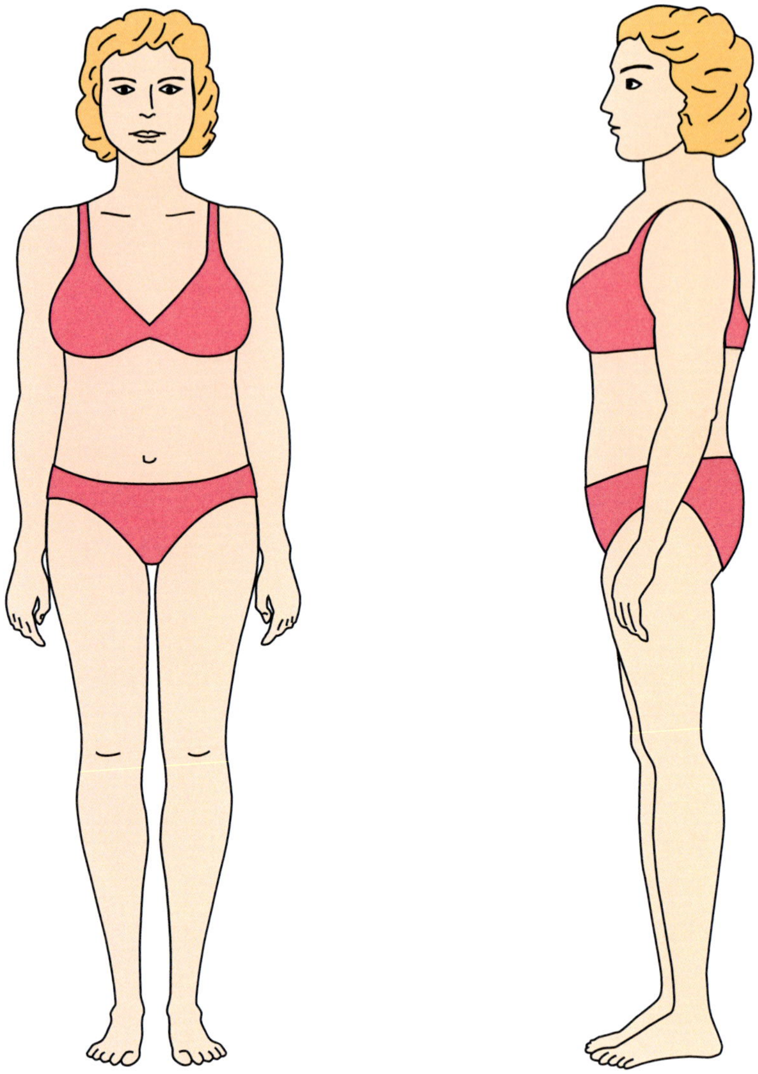

Fig. 10.2 Heart–adrenal constitution type

vulnerability are represented by cardiovascular disease, high blood pressure, dilated cardiomyopathy, hypercoagulable blood, headache, and facial flushing linked to high blood pressure. This is the constitution type that is most vulnerable to consequences related to excess of salt and oxalate.

The greatest risks for this type are associated with the kidneys and cardiac function, which are subjected to a blood pressure consistently above average, which produces frequent blood hypercoagulability, with the risk of thromboembolic phenomena. Glycemic imbalance or diabetes type II (related to hypercortisolemia) and imbibition tissues can be observed.

It is necessary to include in the diet foods that improve the function of the kidneys and also assist in the elimination of body fluids to counteract the imbibitions caused by increased cortisol.

Individuals with this constitution type must not use foods that promote the synthesis of androgens and the activities of the adrenal glands. They should also avoid anything that impairs the kidney function, such as red meat (which also stimulates the synthesis of androgens) and sometimes gluten. It may be useful to avoid excess minerals and antidiuretic food associations and limit all foods that stimulate anabolism.

10.1.3 Human Constitution Type 3: Pancreas

This type is comparable to the phlegmatic type of Hippocrates. The prevalence of the parasympathetic nervous system slows down overall metabolism easily with the accumulation of visceral fat located mainly around the waist and hips. The weak point is the metabolism of glucose and of insulin and thus the key is to promote their regulation.

The face is round, the mouth and lips are carnose, and the subcutaneous tissue is soft. Therefore, the keywords are: roundness and soft tissues (Fig. 10.3).

The appearance of subjects with this constitution type is calm and reassuring. They have great difficulty with adaptation. They show an increased risk for developing type II diabetes or insulin resistance and sometimes hypothyroidism.

As the endocrine and exocrine function of the pancreas often go hand in hand, subjects who belong to this constitution may suffer from digestive disorders: gastralgia, gastritis, ulcers, pancreatitis, hiatal hernia, fatty liver, and colitis, with a prevalence of diarrhea.

For this constitution type, it is more important to choose foods with low glycemic and insulin blood indexes, especially in the evening, and to use protein and fat to slow the peak of postprandial hyperglycemia. It is also recommended to boost the thyroid with iodine-rich foods, limiting the use of milk and derivatives and all foods that have sedative properties. Snacks are to be avoided, and are generally not required if the insulin is balanced.

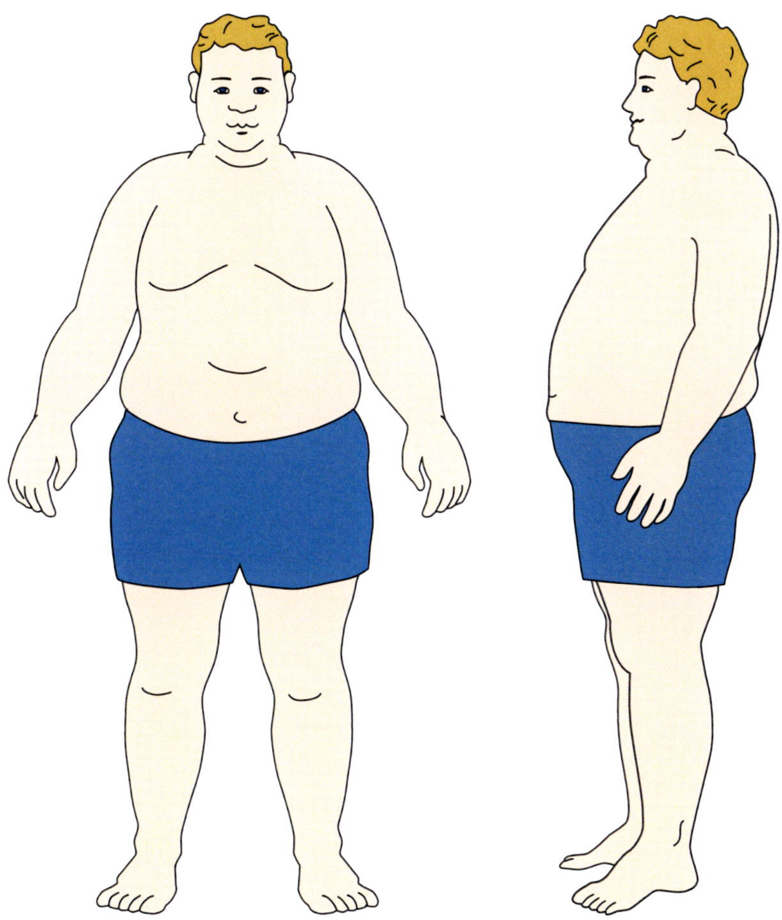

Fig. 10.3 Pancreas constitution type

10.1.4 Human Constitution Type 4: Lung

Classical pictures of the lung constitution type, which is comparable with Hippocrates's "melancholy" type, show individuals who are thin, pale, and with narrow shoulders.

Dryness and lack of elasticity that affect the skin and respiratory system are the main features (Fig. 10.4).

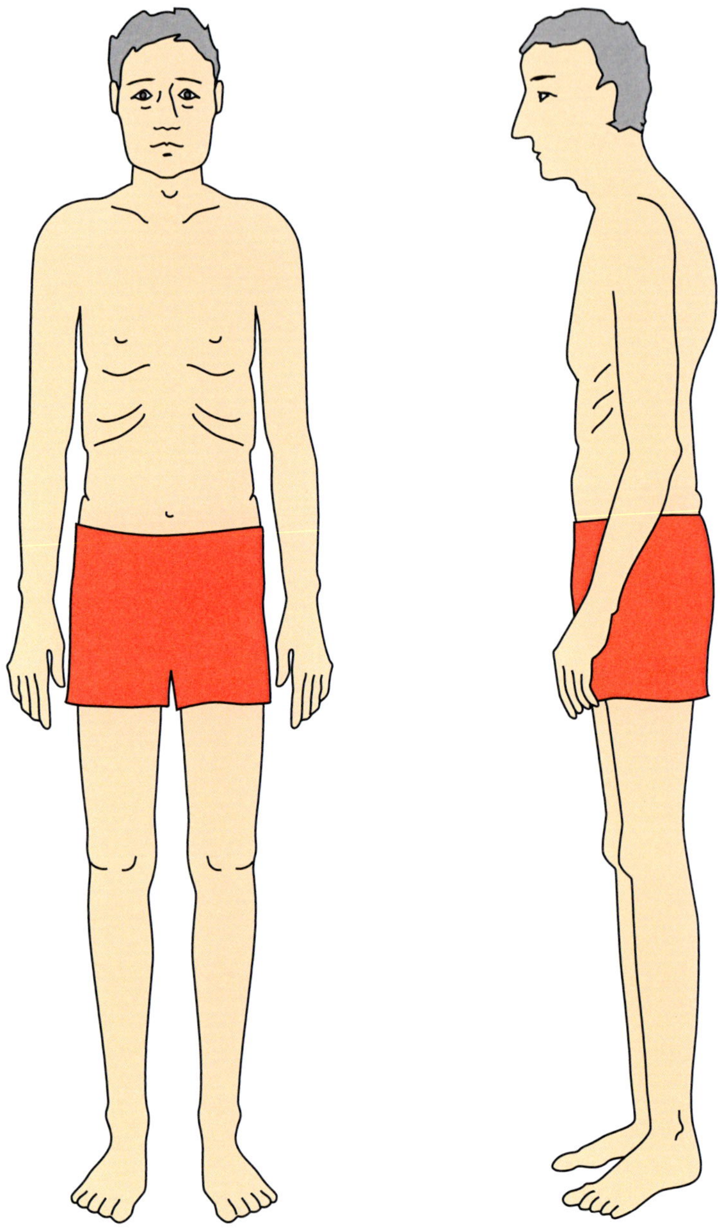

Fig. 10.4 Lung constitution type

This type often has insufficient vital energy, which is counterbalanced by considerable mental capacity.

Psychologically, they tend to reflect more than act. They tend to project their life experiences into the future leading to high levels of apprehension. They have a tendency to fall into pessimism or sadness and seem cold, cynical, and greedy.

They tend to have weak immune systems and are easily affected by bronchitis, pneumonia, laryngitis, chronic rhinitis, sinusitis, and in less favorable cases, asthma, chronic bronchitis, emphysema, and chronic pulmonary heart. They are at risk of thromboembolic events.

A curvature of the spine can be observed with aging leading to a predisposition for osteoporosis that is linked to vitamin D deficiency. In this constitution, the anabolism must be supported. It will be necessary to ensure adequate intake and absorption of iron, calcium, vitamins C and D, and protein of high biological value and carbohydrates.

From a nutritional perspective, lipids are essential in cases of dryness of the pulmonary pleura. They are substantial for the energy

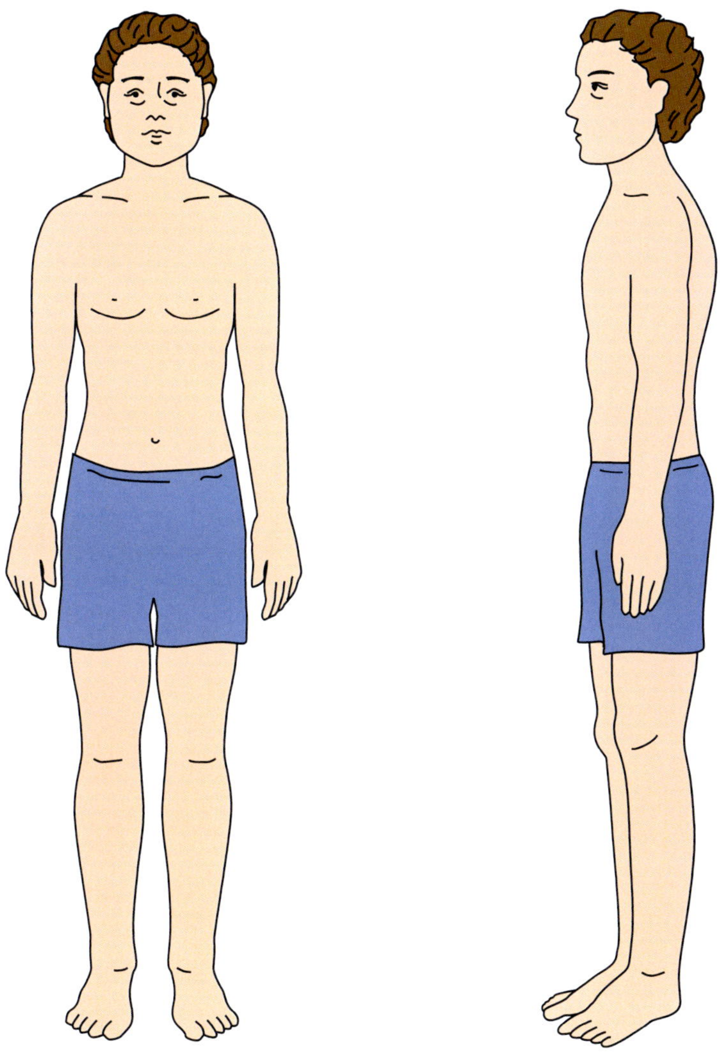

Fig. 10.5 Kidney constitution type

function as they compensate for the relative dryness and atrophy of the skin, of mucous membranes, and of all the structures of the respiratory system.

10.1.5 Human Constitution Type 5: Kidney

Not comparable to any Hippocratic type, the kidney constitution type has hypoadrenalism, which affects the body, psychology, and the behavior of a patient. Key signs are physical weakness and poor defenses (they easily get sick). For very thin people, it tends to be more embedded with a typical chillness that the patient often refers to as "cold to the bone" (Fig. 10.5).

This type is vulnerable from all points of view. They are continuously protecting themselves from attacks that originate outside and are felt internally. Not surprisingly, the basic emotion is fear. As it is a constitution that needs yang, it is usually known to absorb a great deal of energy from the doctor. From the psychobehavioral point of view, the kidney constitution type includes refined people, with a greater mental capacity. They are creative and lovers of beauty and of art in general. Individuals of this constitution type are subject to urogenital infections and kidney-related hypertension. As the kidney carries the essential energy, this type can develop chronic fatigue. Predominantly elderly people have degenerative osteoarticular systems. Nutritional guidelines for people with these characteristics are among the most difficult, because we must overload the kidney's metabolites, while at the same time managing the trend of the body's progressive decline of vital energy. Managing bodily fluids should be favored by avoiding antidiuretic foods and moderating the use of meat so as not to create nitrogenous waste. Excessive consumption of plant proteins, especially gluten, should be avoided. Eggs, milk, and dairy products form the best proteins.

√ **HOAX** FAD SECRET

If something tastes good it is harmful and what is not tasty is healthy, there are only two possibilities: a limitation diet in which cravings cannot be satisfied, or satisfaction, which leads to the uncontrolled use of food.

In reality, healthy food can and should be tasty.

HOAX √ **FAD** **SECRET**

Hydration is essential; therefore, one must drink a lot of water.

Drinking water is not always the best way. For effective hepatic detoxification water that comes from vegetables and fruit is essential, as it is used for biochemical reactions without fluid overload

HOAX **FAD** √ **SECRET**

The importance of cooking methods can influence the functional effects of foods.

10.2 Energy for the Heart

Choosing supplements and taking them can be an act of love toward oneself.

Diet is the essential starting point, but the correct number of nutrients cannot always be consumed through food. Studies have shown that several nutrients and functional foods play an important role in the prevention and progression of cardiovascular disease.

10.2.1 The Magic Organelle: The Mitochondria

There are many aspects to cardiovascular disease, with the central issues always being the loss of energy efficiency in the heart muscle and the coronary arteries that feed it (Fig. 10.6).

As the heart and blood vessels are rich with mitochondria, their tissues require a highly effective and efficient use of energy. Natural compounds can modulate mitochondrial functions by inhibiting organelle enzymes or metabolic pathways [3]. They alter the production of mitochondrial ROS and modulate the activity of transcription factors that regulate the expression of mitochondrial proteins. In the future, the importance of supporting energy production in the heart cells and preserving the mitochondria within them will be the focus of cardiovascular disease prevention.

The production of ATP requires coenzyme Q10 (CoQ10) as it is an essential component in the transfer of electrons from chemical bonds in food molecules to chemical bonds in the ATP molecules.

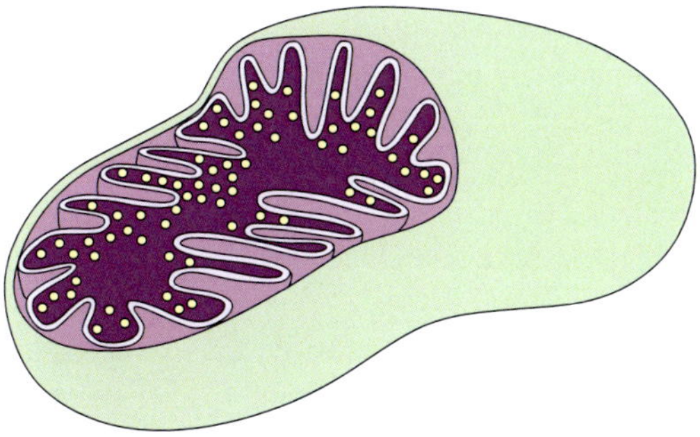

Fig. 10.6 Mitochondria

Coenzyme Q10 reduces inflammation, is a potent anti-oxidant, and is the first line of defense against low-density lipoprotein (LDL) oxidation. Statin therapy may lower plasma CoQ10 concentrations [4]. New data have shown that COQ10 as ubiquinol has a direct anti-aging effect as it assists the actions of the SIRT family of proteins that slow senescence through multiple biochemical mechanisms [5]. Significantly reduced cardiovascular mortality was observed in a 10-year follow-up of a group of healthy elderly participants, who were given 4 years of treatment with coenzyme Q10 and selenium.

The protective action continued beyond the intervention period into the follow-up period.

Carnosine has multi-targeted effects and is most prominent in the heart. It improves energy metabolism in the mitochondria, decreases ischemia, and enhances left ventricle function.

This protection derives from the anti-glycation, anti-oxidant, and anti-inflammatory actions of carnosine. It has the capacity to act on insulin resistance, and remove the accumulation of heavy metals and reduce damage to telomeres. A large systematic review published by researchers from the Mayo Clinic demonstrates strong evidence of carnitine's benefits for heart health [6].

Their publication shows that carnitine supplementation has been associated with a 27% reduction in all-cause mortality, a 65% reduction in ventricular arrhythmias, and a 40% reduction in angina symptoms in patients who have had heart attacks.

D-ribose, a naturally occurring pentose sugar that is a key component in the energy molecule ATP, may support energy generation and functional recovery for patients with ischemic heart disease and diastolic dysfunction [7]. Supplemental D-ribose is an excellent option for preventing and treating cardiovascular disease.

Selenium is essential for the proper functioning of the enzyme systems and heart. A decrease in selenium in the blood leads to decreased glutathione peroxidase activity. This in turn makes the heart tissue more vulnerable to damage, which can weaken its functioning.

A study was published of over 600 coronary artery disease patients in which it was found that the increased risk of cardiovascular events was independently associated with low activity levels of glutathione peroxidase in the red blood cells [8].

Selenium can be used when statins have significantly reduced the synthesis and activity of glutathione peroxidase.

High intake of dietary flavanols and flavones such as quercetin have been associated with a lowering of the risk of cardiovascular disease. In numerous studies, quercetin has been examined and found to be a powerful anti-oxidant and stimulator of nitric oxide and prompts reverse cholesterol transport. Intriguing new research on quercetin has suggested that this protection might be a result of the effects of quercetin on the preservation of mitochondria in the heart and sirtuins [9].

It has been shown that quercetin curbs oxLDL-induced endothelial oxidative injuries through the activation of SIRT1 and regulating the AMPK—NO synthase signaling pathway.

The benefits of resveratrol are well known. At the same time, its clinical efficacy and supplemental benefits in humans are controversial. Trans resveratrol offers various benefits to the cardiovascular system: it lowers the amount of inflammation and oxidation of LDL, supports a decrease in platelet aggregation, and promotes the relaxation of small blood vessels via nitrile oxide [10]. Additionally, resveratrol restricts ROS production in cardiomyocytes via SIRT1 and mitochondrial biogenesis signaling pathways [11].

Curcumin is well known for its anti-inflammatory and anti-oxidant properties. Curcumin has the ability to react directly with ROS and also to induce the expression of cytoprotective and anti-oxidant proteins through the transcription factor Nrf2. Recently, it has been suggested that mitochondrial function and metabolism are associated with Nrf2 and that curcumin activity decreases mitochondrial dysfunction [12].

Pomegranate also has multiple therapeutic functions beyond its anti-oxidant and anti-inflammatory properties, including improving mitochondrial function and increasing nitrile oxide.

Studies have demonstrated that pomegranate and its extracts work to decrease the accumulation of cellular cholesterol, protect LDL against oxidation and have the potential to significantly raise levels of activity of the enzyme paraoxonase-1 (PON-1) in the body, which protects high-density lipoprotein (HDL) from oxidation. These changes take place with an important decline in levels of vascular cell adhesion molecule-1 (VCAM-1), an important endothelial-produced inflammatory protein.

The active component in pomegranate, punicalagin, improves cardiac mitochondrial impairment in an experimental model via AMPK activation [13].

L-Arginine is known to serve as a precursor to nitric oxide in the endothelium.

New insights have been gained through recent data, which shows the role of L-arginine transport in mitochondrial biology and cardiovascular disease [14].

The increase in mitochondrial L-arginine is emerging as a new therapeutic strategy for myocardial disorders involving mitochondrial stress.

Lipoic acid is a unique anti-oxidant molecule that serves as a coenzyme in the energy metabolism of fats, carbohydrates, and proteins. It works at its best when combined with anti-oxidants, including vitamin E, CoQ10, carnitine, and selenomethionine.

Green tea extracts are abundant in natural anti-oxidant and antiplatelet agents and are commonly used in Asia to reduce high cholesterol and lower blood pressure [15].

Published research has shown that green tea could be beneficial as an anti-oxidant and to the reduction of hyperlipidemia and the incidence of atherosclerosis.

Vitamin C is a strong reducing agent that gives cytoprotection by scavenging ROS and therefore, defending DNA, protein, and lipids against peroxidation.

Vitamin C may have an impact on the bioavailability of nitrile oxide through the direct stimulation of the enzyme responsible for the synthesis of nitrile oxide synthase or tetrahydrobiopterin, an essential cofactor in nitrile oxide synthase activity [16].

Vitamin E is often known to work in conjunction with vitamin C for its potent anti-oxidant powers.

It has also been shown to have many other actions such as to lower lipid peroxidation and inhibit smooth muscle cell proliferation, platelet aggregation, and oxidized LDL uptake.

It acts on cytokine production, reducing blood levels of homocysteine and improving insulin sensitivity [16]. Physiological doses of gamma tocopherol are more effective than alpha tocopherol at enhancing the activity of superoxide dismutase and have more preventative effects on cardiovascular disease.

Vitamin D has protective effects for cardiovascular health that are carried out via several mechanisms. It affects systemic inflammation, insulin resistance, vascular endothelial function, and the hypertensive hormone angiotensin II, and lowers the risk of cardiovascular mortality [17].

Vitamin K2 is now emerging as an exciting long-acting vitamin in the prevention and potential regression of coronary atherosclerotic plaque because of its ability to lower vascular calcification and to help to prevent vascular disease [18]. Vitamin K2 can work together with vitamin D to slow arterial calcification, whereas statins can reduce vitamin K2, resulting in an increased risk for arterial calcification.

Anemia is increasingly recognized as an important factor in heart failure. In a recent study that included the analysis of more than 1,500 heart failure patients, 50% of subjects were found to have an iron deficiency [19].

Profound changes in how the heart, blood vessels, and other tissues function can be effected by moderate magnesium deficiency. It can be used therapeutically for a range of cardiac factors including arrhythmias, hypertension, atherosclerosis, and endothelial dysfunction.

This is a result of the vital role played by magnesium in tissues that have electrical or mechanical activity, such as nerves, muscles (including the heart), and blood vessels. Magnesium is critical to the way our body manages its energy and for maintaining normal metabolic function. It is an essential "cofactor" for more than 300 enzymes, and preliminary research has shown it to be an absolute requirement for maintaining and repairing telomeres [20].

Extra virgin olive oil is a kind of liquid gold. It has been shown to improve many cardiovascular risk factors, such as lipid profiles, blood pressure, postprandial hyperlipidemia, endothelial dysfunction, oxidative stress, and anti-thrombotic profiles.

The olive tree is a very old plant that can be traced back to Italy in the Neolithic Age (7000–3000 BC). It has been described as "the most genuine component of the Mediterranean diet" and is becoming known as a critical component of healthy nutrition. The beneficial effects of olive oil are due in part to the synergistic activity among various natural polyphenols, including reducing inflammation and decreasing oxidative stress. Investigators have concluded that polyphenols as opposed to solely monounsaturated fats are responsible for the multiple benefits of olive oil.

Extra virgin olive oil can be considered as a nutraceutical in the prevention of cardiovascular disease. Research also indicates that other enhanced benefits can be obtained by combining olive oil polyphenols with omega-3 fatty acids [21].

Many studies have demonstrated that omega-3 fatty acids reduce the risk of cardiovascular disease and improve the outcome of treatment [22].

It is currently unclear whether plant-derived omega-3 fatty acids (i.e., α-linoleic acid) or fish-derived omega-3 fatty acids (i.e., docosahexaenoic acid and eicosapentaenoic acid) are more important for the heart; thus, both can be considered beneficial to health. The favorable effects of omega-3 fatty acids on cardiovascular health are the result of several mechanisms. Omega-3 fatty acids increase HDL levels while lowering triglyceride levels. They may also reduce inflammatory stress in the body and decrease platelet aggregation. Omega-3 fatty acids are best consumed through food sources, although they can also be consumed in the form of capsules when the consumption of high-quality omega-3 is not feasible.

Garlic extract has long been known for its cardioprotective properties and ability to reduce inflammation, oxidative stress, high blood pressure and the damaging effects of cholesterol in the endothelium. It has recently been shown in an experimental animal model that garlic extract has cardioprotective effects, as it acts on mitochondrial dysfunction [23].

Pay attention to losses! There may be particular concern about micronutrient insufficiency among patients on certain heart failure medications. The use of diuretics is associated with the depletion of electrolytes (potassium and zinc) and may prevent the reabsorption of thiamine and increase its urinary excretion.

Magnesium, phosphate, and calcium excretion from the kidneys is increased with the use of loop diuretics.

It has been shown in numerous studies that low levels of testosterone can contribute to cardiovascular diseases. Glucose, insulin, and fat regulation in addition to other features of metabolism are all affected by testosterone levels. Additionally, testosterone is strongly involved in the reverse cholesterol transport process, which removes cholesterol from the arterial wall and improves endothelial function.

The situation can be of particular concern in men with chronic heart failure when in the presence of excess estradiol.

The careful replacement of testosterone with bio-identical hormones and the possible use of aromatase inhibitors are two new approaches in the management of cardiovascular disease [24].

Some evidence suggests that women with a history of heart failure might also benefit from testosterone replacement, possibly independently of other cardiovascular risk factors.

The level of free testosterone in men should range from 20 to 25 μg/mL and their estradiol levels between 20 and 30 pg/mL. For women, the range should be 8–15 pg/mL. Three of the most prominent risk factors for cardiovascular disease are atherosclerosis, endothelial dysfunction, and metabolic syndrome. New research has shown that dehydroepiandrosterone (DHEA), which is a precursor to testosterone and estrogen, directly attacks against these factors and its supplementation has been shown to improve cardiovascular health [25]. DHEA also modulates various pathways through direct actions, which promote the cell-signaling molecule nitric oxide through the activation of nitric oxide synthase and also restrains the inflammatory process in the endothelium.

After menopause, the risk of cardiovascular disease in women rises rapidly, showing the impact of decreased DHEA sulfate (DHEA-S) levels on the endothelial functions.

An ideal DHEA-S level for women is 280–400 and that for men is 350–500 μg/dL.

Many studies conducted on animals and humans have shown that a strategy for preventing cardiovascular disease in postmenopausal women is the use of bio-identical progesterone, which can inhibit the process of atherosclerosis [26].

New evidence suggests that other postmenopausal benefits to the cardiovascular system can also be gained via estriol [27].

It is necessary to carry out laboratory tests (blood, saliva, 24-h urine tests) to identify any specific deficiencies, and genetic tests focused on highlighting any areas of vulnerability.

CoQ10 as ubiquinol: 200–400 mg daily

Propionyl-L-carnitine: 1,000–2,000 mg daily

D-Ribose: 15–30 g in divided doses throughout the day

Selenium (SeMSc): 200 mcg daily

Quercetin: 500–1,000 mg daily

Trans-resveratrol: 250–500 mg daily

Standardized pomegranate extract: 500–1,500 mg daily

L-Arginine: 6,000–12,000 mg daily

R lipoic acid: 150–300 mg daily

Green tea, standardized extract: 725 mg daily

Curcumin: 400–800 mg daily

Vitamin C: 1,000–3,000 mg daily

Vitamin E: 400 IU daily (with 200 mg gamma tocopherol)

Vitamin B6 (as pyridoxal 50 phosphate): 100–300 mg daily

Vitamin B12: 1,000–2,000 mcg daily

Folate (as methyltetrahydrofolate): 1,000 mcg daily

Niacin: 1,000–3,000 mg daily

Vitamin D: 2,000–10,000 IU daily followed by vitamin D blood testing

(continued)

√ **HOAX** FAD SECRET

Carbohydrates at dinner make you fat.

Carbohydrates in the evening increase the levels of serotonin and melatonin and promote better sleep: studies shows that sleep is essential for the balance of neuroendocrine structure and cardiovascular health [28]. A low-calorie diet with carbohydrates eaten mostly at dinner changes diurnal hormone secretion and improves metabolic status.

HOAX √ **FAD** SECRET

To lose weight, eat only light food.

Eating light food is a gimmick. It does not satisfy the sense of hunger and only encourages you to eat more.

HOAX **FAD** √ **SECRET**

Nutrition is a matter of rhythm, just think about it: hormonal circadian rhythms, alternation between sleep and wakefulness, phases of the menstrual cycle, activities of the sympathetic and parasympathetic nervous systems, anabolism and catabolism, fasting and feeding are all matters of rhythm. Ancient traditional Chinese medicine has attributed value to everything and sees the different stages of life through an understanding of the theory of the five elements.

Vitamin K: 2,000 mcg daily; providing K1, MK-4, MK-7

Magnesium citrate: 160 mg, 1–6 times daily

Fish oil: 3,000–6,000 mg daily

Aged garlic extract: 1,200 mg daily

In addition, bio-identical hormone therapy may be necessary, depending on blood test results.

10.3 Tricks to Maintain Weight

Imagine you were in a situation where you knew you were making a bad mistake at the table, but you were not able to avoid it. Improving dysfunctional attitudes to food and providing strategies for changing behavior are essential for maintaining body weight.

10.3.1 Monitoring Diet, Physical Activity and Sleep

The food diary can have several advantages:

- Taking pictures helps to identify habits
- It creates a precise account of nutritional intake
- Instructions on how to prepare and cook food
- Determine the taste of the patient and psychological value of certain foods for the patient
- Highlights any ailments and symptoms of the patient
- Brings an awareness to the patient regarding their overall daily intake and the results obtained.

A diary of physical activity can provide information on the number of daily steps, the type, the strength, and duration of physical activity.

A sleep diary can provide information on the duration and quality of sleep.

10.3.2 If a Patient Needs to Lose Weight It Is Important to Set and Share Reasonable Weight Loss Goals with the Patient

In general, a loss of 5–10% of a patient's weight is sufficient to reduce cardiovascular risk and must be the primary objective. Once this has been obtained, a further evaluation should be completed regarding the need to decrease additional body weight.

It very important that the weight loss goal and the nutritional program are explained clearly because if there is a great cognitive dissonance between the goal of the patient and the result, the risk is that the patient could leave the new program and return to previous habits.

10.3.3 Maintaining Body Weight

The majority of patients overlook the need for active management of maintaining body weight and return to old habits, resulting in regaining weight lost [29].

Patients often tend to undervalue the improvements in health that are achieved.

The main obstacles to accepting the need for continued dietary maintenance should be addressed and clarified with patients:

- Having unrealistic goals for weight loss
- The tendency to maintain negative body images despite losing weight
- Having primary goals that are different than improving health (having better interpersonal relationships, finding a partner, improved self-esteem, etc.)

10.3.4 The Loss of Control over Food Can Result from Internal or External Stimuli

Internal stimuli that can lead to overeating are:

1. Negative emotions: boredom, loneliness, anxiety, depression, anger, etc.
2. Positive emotions: joy, celebrations, etc.

These emotions must be identified and a plan created to balance their effects with alternative activities. The patient may need the help of a psychologist.

External stimuli that lead to excess eating may occur:

a. Before eating
b. While eating
c. After eating (Tables 10.1, 10.2, and 10.3)

Table 10.1 Techniques for controlling external stimuli: before eating

Problem	Advice
Going shopping	1. Go shopping with a full stomach 2. Do the shopping based on a list so as not to buy food that is not needed 3. Buy foods that require preparation: prepared foods are often the least healthy 4. Avoid the junk food aisle
Food storage	1. Do not leave food in sight 2. Keep food stocks only in the kitchen 3. Place the tempting food in inaccessible places
Prepare food	1. Do not cook when you are hungry 2. Cook the exact amount of food that will be consumed (according to portion size). 3. Do not taste the food during preparation

Table 10.2 Techniques for controlling external stimuli: while eating

Problem	Advice
Eating quickly	1. Take small bites and chew slowly for a long time 2. Try to be the last person to finish the meal
Eating in different places and standing	1. Eat at the dinner table 2. Do not eat standing
Eating while doing other things (e.g., watching TV, reading, etc.)	1. While eating, do not do any other activity 2. Focus attention on what is being eaten 3. Focus on the flavor and taste of the food

Table 10.3 Techniques for controlling external stimuli: after having eaten

Problem	Advice
Remaining at the table for a long time after having eaten	1. Clear the table immediately after eating 2. If possible move from the kitchen to another room in the house when the food is finished
Storing leftovers	1. Cook only a single serving per person

Techniques for Controlling External Stimuli: Eating at Restaurants

- Try to choose a restaurant that has healthy cuisine and a wide selection of dishes
- Do not arrive at the restaurant too hungry
- Decide in advance what you want to eat
- Order first
- Eat slowly
- Look out for alcohol

Planning ahead: prepare properly for the event by increasing physical activity before the event and consider what dishes will be desired as well as the peer/social pressure of the occasion.

10.4 New Suggestions Behind Integrative Medicine

Give importance to your own space, time, and relationships regarding nutrition.

There are two important variables that are related, but should not be confused: what to eat and how to eat.

Nutritional pyramids have failed because they entrap people into the strict lines of a triangle, which does not allow any concessions for taste or the freedom of personal choice.

As a result, they have not been able to generate positive emotions in most people.

√ **HOAX** FAD SECRET

Saturated fats are always associated with an increased CHD.

Recently, it was shown that saturated fats were not associated with total CHD, even if there is a strong positive association between trans fats intake and CHD [30]. Fats in addition to having invaluable nutritional functions contribute to a sense of satiety.

HOAX √ **FAD** SECRET

Eating lots of fruit is always healthy.

Fruit is a priceless treasure of nature, rich in water and colorful vegetation with micronutrient anti-oxidants. Fructose has a lower glycemic index than glucose, but a high-fructose diet promotes insulin resistance, visceral obesity, and elevated serum triglycerides. Fructose has elevated glycation capacity [31] and elevates uric acid production.

HOAX FAD √ **SECRET**

It is useless to subtract and multiply the calories or use indexes: it is better to understand what happens when food meets the body and its metabolic pathways.

Nutrition in integrative medicine treats the "whole person" with a functional and tailored approach specifically designed to meet human constitution types and individual biochemical needs.

We suggest structuring the diet, taking into account these factors:

- The human constitution types should be considered.
- A variety of whole, natural, unprocessed foods should be eaten. This ensures a wide range of nutrients and reduces the chance of developing food addictions and sensitivities.
- Organic or wild foods should be eaten, where possible, to minimize exposure to pesticides, antibiotics, growth promoters, and other drugs.
- Genetically modified foods and commercially processed foods should be avoided as far as possible. Lack of time to shop and prepare food, stress, and the practice of eating commercial food can lead one off the path of healthy nutrition.
- A wide range of fruits, vegetables, herbs, and spices should be consumed, for their important phytochemicals.
- Protein and fat should be used to slow the peak of postprandial hyperglycemia.
- Foods with a low glycemic and insulin blood index should be chosen, particularly in the evening meal.
- Intake of sugars and refined carbohydrates should be limited, to control insulin resistance and glycation.
- Snacks are optional and should not be eaten unless necessary. They are permitted for the benefit of individuals who are doing more physical activity, children, and/or those who are vulnerable to hypoglycemic states between meals.
- Extra virgin olive oil, both raw and cooked, should be the main source of fats. Also, polyunsaturated fat from oily fish, nuts, seeds, and a small amount of saturated fatty acids (e.g., butter) should be added.
- Gastrointestinal function can be optimized by replacing dietary fiber and the factors necessary to optimize digestive secretions (e.g., capsaicinoids and zinc), prebiotic foods, and if necessary by supplementing probiotics.
- Cooking temperatures should be maintained below 200° C/400° F. Meat should be precooked in the microwave before conventional cooking and fibrous foods and fruit should be eaten at the same meal.
- The succession of the various meals that are consumed throughout the day should be taken into account, supporting the liver detoxification process and drainage of the excretory organs and kidneys. Eventually, detoxification should be optimized by the supply of vitamins and cofactor nutrients.

To complete the work:

- Laboratory and genetic tests should be carried out to identify any specific deficiencies and highlight any areas of vulnerability.
- Micronutrients (vitamins, cofactor, etc.) and functional foods should be introduced to meet individual biochemical needs and to improve mitochondrial function.
- Hoaxes and fads regarding nutrition should be considered.
- The tricks of behavior to maintain weight should be mastered.
- Importance should be attributed to stress management and regular sleep.
- An active lifestyle should be maintained every day and regular physical activity should be performed.

Centenarian diets (e.g., the Okinawa diet) are low in calories, yet nutritionally dense, particularly with regard to vitamins, minerals, and phytonutrients, several of which have potential nutraceutical properties.

Caloric restriction has been confirmed to provide a plethora of cardiovascular benefits including improvement of endothelial function, arterial stiffness, atherogenesis, myocardial interstitial fibrosis, cardiac autophagy, oxidative stress, inflammation, and ventricular diastolic function.

The last SECRET: SPACE, TIME and ... WOMEN

There are three key factors behind food and nutritional choices.
SPACE is the element where all cooking and eating take place. It starts with the fire around which people have gathered for years, looking for warmth, protection, and nourishment. Fire has developed the language of humans, as the family and social life revolved around it in the kitchen, the informal space of the house in which emotions, relationships, and food were formed.
TIME spent in the kitchen has led to the physical, mental, and social development of relationships with food and people. Not devoting space and time in the kitchen in the right balance is equivalent to not devoting space and time to the love of oneself and others.
WOMEN Multitasking and global vision are skills that women developed throughout the centuries; this allows them to play a fundamental role in the transmission of information, abilities, and rituals concerning food and feeding.

Although caloric restriction as such cannot be applied to humans, in the last few years scientists have tried to transfer its beneficial effects through caloric restriction mimetics and AMPK activators [32, 33].

Recently, they also assessed the possible positive effects of intermittent fasting on the same mechanisms and on the stimulation of the autophagy machinery [34].

References

1. Nicolle L, Bailey C (2013) The functional nutrition cook book: addressing biochemical imbalances through diet. Singing Dragon, London
2. Aufiero F, Pentassuglia M (2015) Il ruolo Nutrizionale e terapeutico degli alimenti. Vis Sanatrix Nauturae
3. Gibellini L, Bianchini E, De Biasi S, Nasi M, Cossarizza A, Pinti M (2015) Natural compounds modulating mitochondrial functions. Evid Based Complement Alternat Med 2015:527209. doi:10.1155/2015/527209
4. Banach M, Serban C, Ursoniu S, Rysz J, Muntner P, Toth P, Jones SR, Rizzo M, Glasser SP, Watts Gerald F, Blumenthal RS, Lip GYH, Mikhailidis DP (2015) Statin therapy and plasma coenzyme Q10 concentrations – a systematic review and meta-analysis of placebo-controlled trials. Pharmacol Res 99:329–336
5. Alehagen U, Aaseth J, Johansson P (2015) Reduced cardiovascular mortality 10 years after supplementation with selenium and coenzyme Q10 for four years: follow-up results of a prospective randomized double blind placebo-controlled trial in elderly citizens. PLoS One 10(12):e0141641
6. Di Nicolantonio JJ, Lavie CJ, Fares H, Menezes AR, O'Keefe JH (2013) L-carnitine in the secondary prevention of cardiovascular disease: systematic review and meta-analysis. Mayo Clin Proc 88(6):544–551
7. Shecterle LM, St Cyr JA (2014) A potential role of D-ribose for myocardial diastolic dysfunction. J Cardiol Ther 1(1):1–2
8. Pillai R, Uyehara-Lock JH, Bellinger FP (2014) Selenium and selenoprotein function in brain disorders. IUBMB Life 66(4):229–239
9. Hung CH, Chan SH, Chu PM, Tsai KL (2015) Quercetin is a potent anti-atherosclerotic compound by activation of SIRT1 signaling under oxLDL stimulation. Mol Nutr Food Res 59(10):1905–1917
10. Joshi MS, Williams D, Horlock D, Samarasinghe T, Andrews KL, Jefferis AM, Berger PJ, Chin-Dusting JP, Kaye DM (2015) Role of mitochondrial dysfunction in hyperglycaemia-induced coronary microvascular dysfunction: protective role of resveratrol. Diab Vasc Dis Res 2(3):208–216
11. Li YG, Zhu W, Tao JP, Xin P, Liu MY, Li JB, Wei M (2013) Resveratrol protects cardiomyocytes from oxidative stress through SIRT1 and mitochondrial biogenesis signaling pathways. Biochem Biophys Res Commun 438(2):270–276
12. Trujillo J, Granados-Castro LF, Zazueta C, Andérica-Romero AC, Chirino YI, Pedraza-Chaverrí J (2014)

Mitochondria as a target in the therapeutic properties of curcumin. Arch Pharm 347(12):873–884
13. Cao K, Xu J, Pu W, Dong Z, Sun L, Zang W, Gao F, Zhang Y, Feng Z, Liu J (2015) Punicalagin, an active component in pomegranate, ameliorates cardiac mitochondrial impairment in obese rats via AMPK activation. Sci Rep 5:14014
14. Parikh S, Saneto R, Falk MJ, Anselm I, Cohen BH, Haas R (2009) A modern approach to the treatment of mitochondrial disease. Curr Treat Opt Neurol 11(6): 414–430
15. Pang J, Zhang Z, Zheng T, Yang YJ, Li N, Bai M, Peng Y, Zhang J, Li Q, Zhang B (2015) Association of green tea consumption with risk of coronary heart disease in Chinese population. Int J Cardiol 179: 275–278
16. Goszcz K, Deakin SJ, Duthie GG, Stewart D, Leslie SJ, Megson IL (2015) Antioxidants in cardiovascular therapy: panacea or false hope? Front Cardiovasc Med 2:29
17. Wang TJ, Pencina MJ, Booth SL, Jacques PF, Ingelsson E, Lanier K, Benjamin EJ, D'Agostino RB, Wolf M, Vasan RS (2008) Vitamin D deficiency and risk of cardiovascular disease. Circulation 117:503–511
18. Juanola-Falgarona et al (2014) Dietary intake of vitamin K is inversely associated with mortality risk. J Nutr 144(5):743–750
19. Klip IT, Comin-Colet J, Voors AA, Ponikowski P, Enjuanes C, Banasiak W, Lok DJ, Rosentryt P, Torrens A, Polonski L, van Veldhuisen DJ, van der Meer P, Jankowska EA (2013) Iron deficiency in chronic heart failure: an international pooled analysis. Am Heart J 165(4):575–582
20. Rowe WJ (2012) Correcting magnesium deficiencies may prolong life. Clin Interv Aging 7:51–54
21. Venturini D, Simão AN, Urbano MR, Dichi I (2015) Effects of extra virgin olive oil and fish oil on lipid profile and oxidative stress in patients with metabolic syndrome. Nutrition 31(6):834–840
22. Chaddha A, Eagle Kim A (2015) Omega-3 fatty acids and heart health. Circulation 132:e350–e352
23. Supakul L, Pintana H, Apaijai N, Chattipakorn S, Shinlapawittayatorn K, Chattipakorn N (2014) Protective effects of garlic extract on cardiac function, heart rate variability and cardiac mitochondria in obese insulin-resistant rats. Eur J Nutr 53(3): 919–928
24. Arcopinto M, Salzano A, Isgaard J, Cittadini A (2015) Hormone replacement therapy in heart failure. Curr Opin Cardiol 30(3):277–284
25. Yoshida S et al (2010) Dehydroepiandrosterone sulfate is inversely associated with sex-dependent diverse carotid atherosclerosis regardless of endothelial function. Atherosclerosis 212(1):310–315
26. Prior JC (2015) Progesterone or progestin as menopausal ovarian hormone therapy: recent physiology-based clinical evidence. Curr Opin Endocrinol Diabetes Obes 22(6):495–501
27. Takahashi K, Manabe A, Okada M, Kurioka H, Kanasaki H, Miyazaki K (2000) Efficacy and safety of oral estriol for managing postmenopausal symptoms. Maturitas 34(2):169–177
28. Sofera S, Eliraza A, Madara Z, Froya O (2015) Concentrating carbohydrates before sleep improves feeding regulation and metabolic and inflammatory parameters in mice. Mol Cell Endocrinol 414:29–41
29. Dalle Grave R (2014) Terapia Cognitivo Comportamentale dell' Obesità. Positive Press
30. De Souza RJ, Mente A, Maroleanu A, Cozma AI, Ha V, Kishibe T, Uleryk E, Budylowski P, Schünemann H, Beyene J, Anand SS (2015) Intake of saturated and trans unsaturated fatty acids and risk of all cause mortality, cardiovascular disease, and type 2 diabetes: systematic review and meta-analysis of observational studies. BMJ 351:h3978. doi:10.1136/bmj.h3978
31. Polimeni A, Tomella C (2014) La Glicazione e le sue implicazioni sulla salute femminile. Bollettino Ginecol Endocrinol 8:15–22
32. Winnik S, Auwerx J, Sinclair DA, Matter CM (2015) Protective effects of sirtuins in cardiovascular diseases: from bench to bedside. Eur Heart J 36(48): 3404–3412
33. Qi D, Young LH (2015) AMPK: energy sensor and survival mechanism in the ischemic heart. Trends Endocrinol Metab 26(8):422–429
34. Godar RJ, Ma X, Liu H, Murphy JT, Weinheimer CJ, Kovacs A, Crosby SD, Saftig P, Diwan A (2015) Repetitive stimulation of autophagy-lysosome machinery by intermittent fasting preconditions the myocardium to ischemia-reperfusion injury. Autophagy 11(9):1537–1560

11 Psycho-neuro-endocrino-immunology Paradigm and Cardiovascular Diseases

Francesco Bottaccioli and Anna Giulia Bottaccioli

We are living through the end of a great illusion that has lasted more than 400 years: the illusion of being able to take the complexity of life, in health and disease, reduce it to simple determinants, and then order it into a system of incontrovertible knowledge [1, 2]. This illusion established the mechanistic and reductionist biomedical paradigm, which was nourished by the "mechanical philosophy" advocated by a vast movement of philosophers, physicists, and physicians from the seventeenth century onward [3].

The dominant paradigm, in its present state, no longer seems capable of producing significant advances in the knowledge and practice of care [4].

The paradigm of psycho-neuro-endocrino-immunology (PNEI) may offer an important answer to this crisis.

11.1 What Is Psycho-neuro-endocrino-immunology?

The discipline of PNEI studies the bidirectional relationships between the psyche and the biological systems [5–7]. After 1930, the accumulated knowledge of endocrinology, immunology, and the neurosciences converged to form a single model.

Hans Selye [8] demonstrated that stress response is independent of the nature of the stimulus. Further studies reinforced this concept, proving that stress can be activated by physical, infectious, and psychological factors. Independent of any type of stressor, a neuroendocrine and neurovegetative response is then activated, with the subsequent release of hormones and neurotransmitters from the adrenal glands. In the mid-1970s, the immunophysiologist Hugo Besedovsky et al. [9] proved that the immunosuppressive effect is caused by an increase in cortisol produced by the adrenal glands during a stress response. Thus, the first biological connection among the brain, stress, and the immune system was established. In the second half of the 1980s, the American physiologist Edween Blalock [10] showed how lymphocytes have receptors for the hormones and neurotransmitters produced by the brain, and at the same time produce hormones and neurotransmitters similar to the cerebral ones. Hence, the bidirectional communication between the brain and the immune system was proven (Figs. 11.1, 11.2, and 11.3). More recently, it has been demonstrated that the peripheral nerve fibers innervating the entire body release substances (neuropeptides) that activate or suppress the

F. Bottaccioli (✉)
University of L'Aquila, L'Aquila, Italy

Italian Society of Psycho-neuro-endocrino-immunology (SIPNEI), Via Trionfale 65, 00195 Rome, Italy
e-mail: bottac.fra@gmail.com

A.G. Bottaccioli
Sapienza University of Rome, Rome, Italy

M. Fioranelli (ed.), *Integrative Cardiology*, DOI 10.1007/978-3-319-40010-5_11

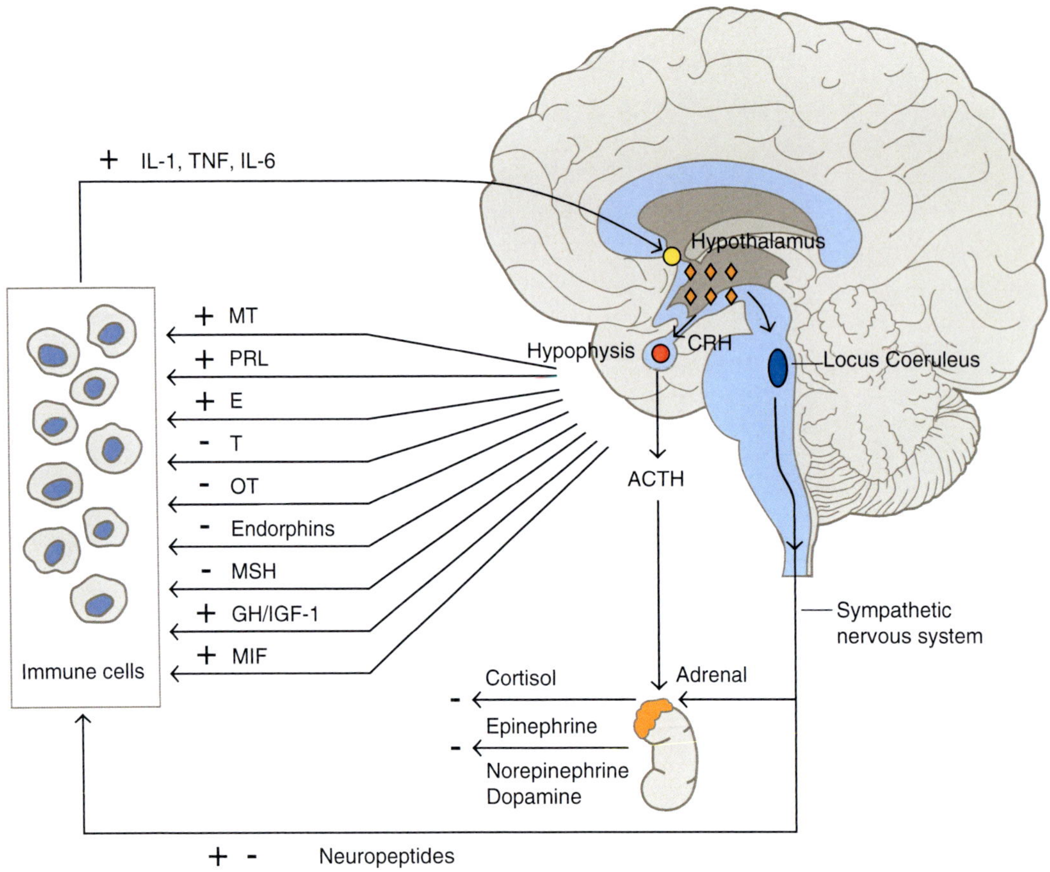

Fig. 11.1 The influence of the neuroendocrine system on the immune system. The symbols + and – indicate activation and inhibition, respectively. *MT* melatonin, *PRL* prolactin, *E* estrogen, *T* testosterone, *OT* oxytocin, *MSH* melanocyte stimulating hormone, *GH/iGF-1* growth hormone/insulin-like growth factor-1, *MIF* macrophage inhibitory factor

immune response. This discovery, for the first time, implies that inflammation may be of nervous origin (neurogenic inflammation).

At the same time, it has by now become clear how cytokines, which are released by the immune cells, pass through the blood or the large cranial nerves (such as the vagus nerve) and carry signals to the brain, thus influencing both biological (e.g., fever, hunger, satiety) and psychological activities (anxiety and depression) [11, 12].

During the 1990s, there was a significant boom in studies of the neurobiology of emotions. Emotions, traumas, and stressful events in general cause a dysregulation in the stress system that strongly alters the disposition and the functioning of the immune system. In the short-term, cortisol, epinephrine, and norepinephrine (NE) (catecholamines) also have a tonifying effect on the immune system. In the mid- to long-term, these substances place the immune response in an unsuitable position to fight viruses and tumors. Similarly, the dysregulation of the stress axis can favor the onset of different types of autoimmune diseases [13].

By the end of the twentieth century, the works of the American neuroscientist Robert Sapolsky and those of other scholars have proven that the alteration of the stress system and the overproduction of cortisol can result in atrophy of the hippocampus, the cerebral area responsible for long-term memory formation.

Studies of the first decade of the twenty-first century show that even diseases such as atherosclerosis and heart disease are usually

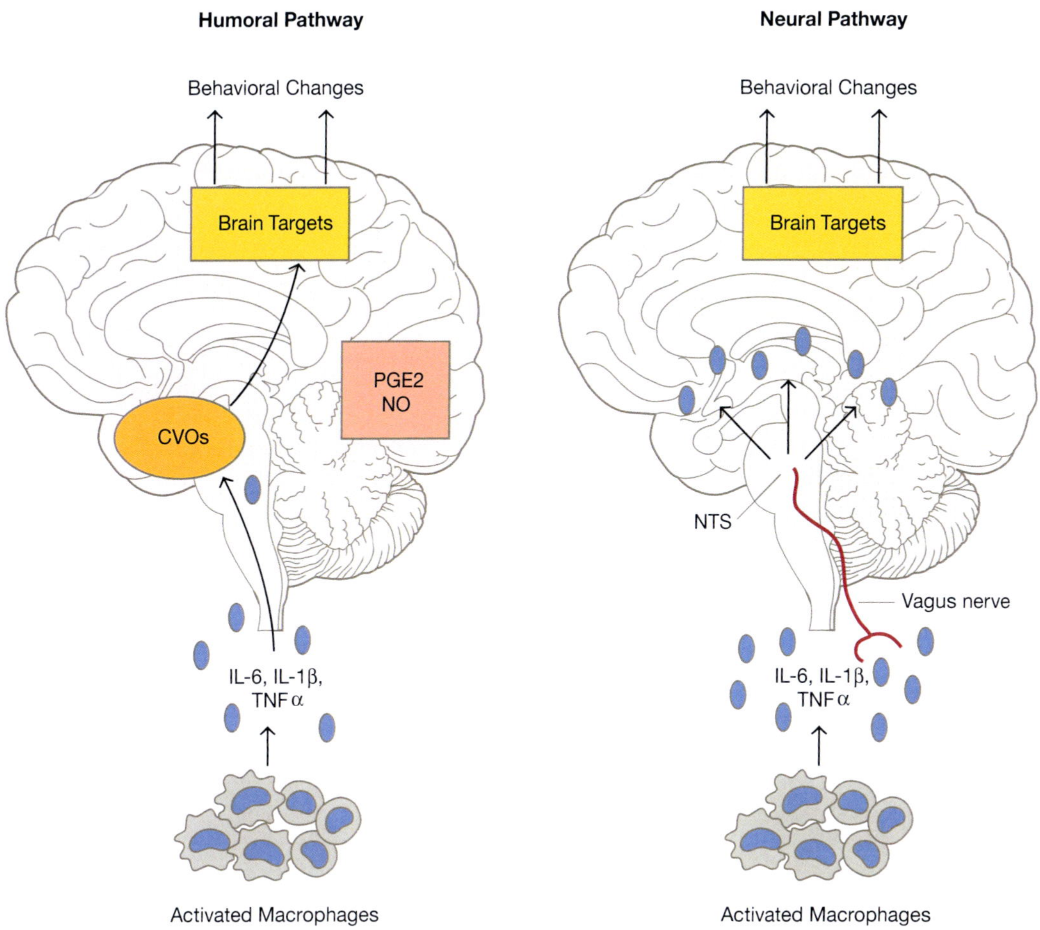

Fig. 11.2 Cytokines from immune cells activated (i.e., macrophage) reach the brain via the blood and the vagus nerve. Via the blood they reach the blood–brain barrier-free circumventricular organs (CVO) and elicit a second messenger (prostaglandins, nitric oxide) in blood–brain barrier too; via the vagus nerve they reach the nucleus tractus solitarius, the brain stem integration centre

strongly affected by mood. Depression, with the overproduction of cortisol and catecholamines, contributes to alterations in the inner vessel walls, favoring the formation of atherosclerotic lesions and worsening the prognosis of people who have suffered a heart attack [14]. Thus, the occurrence of some heart attacks or other acute cardiac failures tied to mood disorders, can be correlated with the presence of vascular alterations caused by an imbalance in serotonin levels, as suggested from animal research [15]. Serotonin has multiple physiological effects: in the brain the humor is regulated; in the gut, it is peristaltic activity; and in the blood it is coagulation that is regulated. Its decrement in the brain triggers depressive effects, whereas increment in the blood produces increased coagulation (prothrombotic effects).

To conclude, in the first decade of this century, research conducted mainly by the Belgian psychiatrist Michael Maes and the French neurobiologist Robert Dantzer proved that immune inflammatory dysregulation may be responsible for symptoms that are normally referred to as "somatization disorders" and "psychosomatic symptoms." All of these symptoms are tied to disorders that fall either within the purview of psychology and psychiatry (anxiety, depression, chronic fatigue syndrome) or to disorders belonging more specifically to the

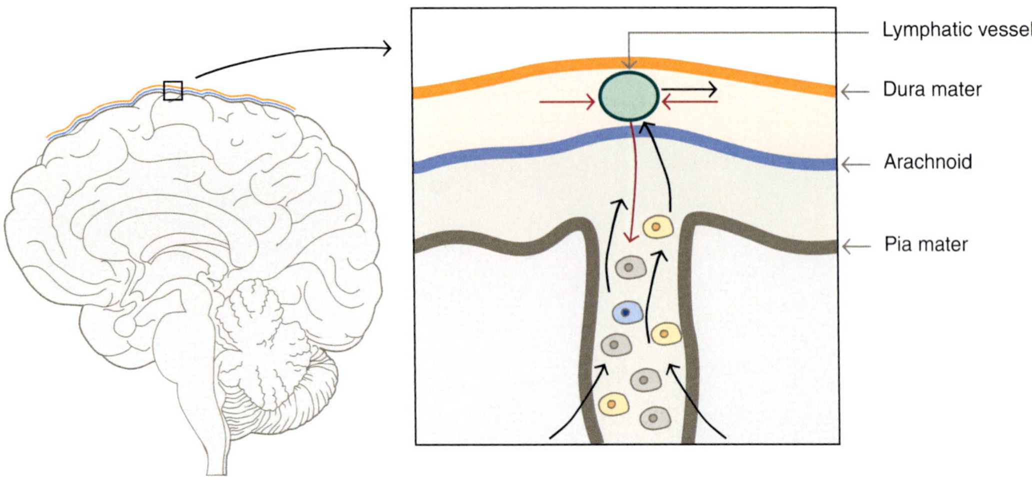

Fig. 11.3 The discovery of the lymphatic vessel [16] shows a new bidirectional pathway from the brain to the immune system

medical field (autoimmune diseases, cancer). For a recent general review, it is possible to consult the article by Irwin and Rothermund [17].

With PNEI, a model for research and for interpreting both health and disease has developed, one that considers the human body to be a structured and interconnected entity where the psychological and biological systems have a reciprocal influence. This provides the basis for new integrated approaches to the prevention and therapy of most common diseases, especially chronic ones. At the same time, it affords us the prospect of going beyond the old philosophical dichotomy between mind and body and the scientific dichotomy between medicine and psychology, by overcoming the respective reductionism that assigns the body (without the psyche) to the care of medicine, and the psyche (without the body) to that of psychology.

11.2 The Science of Stress

Research into PNEI has evolved out of the experimental pathological studies by Hungarian scientist Hans Selye, rightly considered the father of stress science.

From the 1930s until his death in 1982, Hans Selye focused his research on the adaptation of human and animal organisms in response to different kinds of stressors (physical, psychological, and toxic agents). Hence, the subject of Selye's investigations was the living organism as a whole. This approach to the unity of the organism was based on the experimental observation that the axis of stress in animals was activated independently of the nature of the stressor. The adrenal axis of an experimental mouse could be activated by a virus, a bath in icy water, or the animal's catching sight of a predator. This is now well documented. When bacteria or a virus get into the body, our immune system releases cytokines that reach the brain and activate the stress system. This same stress system can also be activated by an emotion. Today we know that this "nonspecificity" of stimuli is also present at the cellular level. Indeed, an immune cell can be activated by viral and bacterial products, inflammatory cytokines, oxidative derivatives in food, or by emotional stress: the cell has receptors for epinephrine and NE, which are the neurotransmitters of the stress response. Therefore, even if it seems inappropriate to presuppose a basic difference between psychological and biological stressors, there is undoubtedly a distinctiveness intrinsic to the psychological stressors.

Here is the fundamental question: how does the psyche work? What are the mechanisms by which an internal or external event activates the stress system?

11.3 The Psyche as a Product and Condition of the Life of the Organism

The psyche is an integral part of the meta-system. It is both the product of the biological organization and a fundamental source of its conditioning. It is necessary to fully understand that the biological and psychological levels are inextricably entwined. If we miss this point, we will be faced with two diverging philosophical trajectories: biologism and subjective idealism. The former considers the psyche nothing more than a synonym for the brain and the latter simply recycles the old metaphysical concept of Soul or Spirit. As a matter of fact, the psyche is an integral and vital part of the body.

A recent review lists the identified correlations between behaviors and brain plasticity (e.g., from navigation and hippocampus, from music and motor and auditory areas) and subsequently recalls humorously the famous conundrum: "what came first, the chicken or the egg?" [18].

Hand in hand with these correlations between brain structure and behaviors, a series of experiments has also hypothesized about the molecular paths that convert behaviors into a new cerebral asset, showing the increase in signals that are essential to the activation and growth of nerves such as *brain derived nervous factor* (BDNF), *nervous growth factor* (NGF), *n-methyl-D-aspartate* (NMDA).

Perspective-based parallel studies have been carried out. In these studies, researchers monitored people in the process of acquiring new knowledge and skills over a period of time.

In an experiment, they involved German medical students. At the end of their third academic year, students are required to pass an extremely demanding state medical examination, the so-called *Physicum*, a summary of all the main subjects studied in the previous years. This challenging examination requires on average a 2-month period of intense study. In this case, as in the other, the participants' brains were imaged three times, first before the study period, and then after, at the 2-month and 3-month marks. Neuroimages showed significant growth and an increase in grey matter in two crucial learning areas: the posterior parietal cortex and the hippocampus. Of particular relevance is the fact that after 3 months the hippocampus, especially the right side, continued to grow as if it were further processing the acquired information [19]. One may conclude from this that mental activity modifies brain morphology, regardless of whether it involves acquisition of abstract notions or acquisition of motor skills.

We can therefore make the following analogy: the software running on the brain machine modifies the machine itself.

For this reason, the psyche–brain system cannot be compared with the program computer system. In this latter case, if one changes the software, the hardware does not follow suit, whereas in the first case (the psyche–brain system), the software modifies the hardware.

11.4 Psycho-neuro-endocrino-immunology, the Science of Stress, and the Biopsychosocial Model

From the arguments and scientific data reported thus far, it can be deduced that it is now possible to unify the two great traditions (the biological and the psychological) of stress research, with the aim of reconstructing the health/disease balance and the mechanisms that concern the individual seen in his/her entirety. What is needed is a new unified science of stress.

Scholars of psychological sciences respond to this assertion by arguing that for some time there has been a systemic approach, called the "biopsychosocial model."

This proposal was published nearly 40 years ago in *Science* [20], where the author of the article, George Engel, did indeed present a very effective criticism of the dominant biomedical model by identifying its key elements: the reduction of complex phenomena to simple determinants (reductionism), the separation of the biological phenomena from the psychosocial ones (mind–body dichotomy), and the interpretation of vital phenomena in physical–chemical terms (physicalism).

Unfortunately, the course of history has not quite matched the vision set forth by Engel. Admittedly, the biopsychosocial model has trumpeted the idea, over the last few decades, that another vision of medicine and psychology is possible, but in all honesty, it has not advanced any research that explores the mechanisms contributing to the interdependence of the biological, the psychological, and the social. Thanks to PNEI we now have all the tools, as well as a rich and growing body of documentation, necessary for explaining and defining, in strictly scientific terms, the complex interaction between the different levels that determine human health and disease.

It is therefore no coincidence that distinguished researchers in psychological sciences, such as Shelley Taylor and Janice Kiecolt-Glaser, see PNEI as the forward path of choice for psychology. Kiecolt-Glaser writes that “Psychoneuroimmunology is psychology’s gateway to the biomedical future.” Indeed, it represents the principal contribution, she writes, that psychology can make in the effort to change the biomedical model and practice. It is her belief that to achieve this goal, an interdisciplinary framework for the training of health operators and researchers is necessary [21].

11.5 PNEI and Cardiovascular Diseases

Cardiovascular mortality and morbidity, and the problem of gender differences in cardiovascular diseases (CVDs) are relevant problems in world-wide disease epidemiology.

In the USA, the 2010 overall rate of death attributable to CVDs was 235.5 per 100,000. The rates were 278.4 per 100,000 for white males, 369.2 per 100,000 for black males, 192.2 per 100,000 for white females, and 260.5 per 100,000 for black females. From 2007 to 2010, 40.0% of men and 34.4% of women aged 40–59 suffered from CVD in the USA, and these percentages rise to 70.2 and 70.9% for ages 60–79 and 83.0% and 87.1% for ages 80 and above [22].

Working from a life-course perspective, Liu and Waite [23] have formulated hypotheses about age and gender differences in the link between marital quality and cardiovascular risk. They have tested these hypotheses using data from the first two waves of the National Social Life, Health, and Aging Project. The analysis sample includes 459 married women and 739 married men (aged 57–85 in the first series) who were interviewed in both periods. Results suggest that changes in marital quality and cardiovascular risk are more closely related for older married people than for their younger counterparts; and that the link between marital quality and cardiovascular risk is more pronounced among women than among men of older age. These findings fit with the gendered life-course perspective and the cumulative disadvantage framework.

In this disadvantage framework, depression and stress play an important role.

Recently, in the second wave of the Nord-Trøndelag Health Study in Norway (HUNT 2, 1995–1997), baseline data on symptoms of anxiety and depression, along with health status including cardiovascular risk factors, were registered for 62,567 adults, men and women, who were free for known indicators for heart failure. This group was monitored for incident heart failure (HF) from baseline throughout 2008. Symptoms of depression were associated with an increased risk for heart failure (HF) in a dose–response manner [24].

On 24 February 2014, the American Heart Association, with a scientific statement, determined that depression is a risk factor with a poor prognosis among patients with acute coronary syndrome [25]. With this report, we have for the first time unequivocal testimony of the negative influence that depression has on the progression of CVD. What are the possible biological mechanisms at work here?

11.6 Biological Mechanisms 1: Autonomic Cardiac System Dysregulation

Several forebrain areas form an interconnected network that initiates integrated autonomic, endocrine, and behavioral changes in response to emotionally relevant or homeostatically stressful stimuli [26]. This central stress network, including the insular cortex (IC), anterior cingulate cortex (ACC), amygdala (A), and several hypothalamic nuclei, projects to medullary and spinal nuclei controlling cardiac function by the vagus and sympathetic nerves.

This circuit appears essential to the regulation of autonomic responses to stressful stimuli. An imbalance in autonomic regulation may be linked to mental stress, resulting in a net shift toward increased sympathetic tone and/or withdrawal of parasympathetic tone. If chronic, this imbalance can increase the risk for cardiovascular disease by promoting arrhythmias, platelet aggregation, and vascular inflammation.

The sympathetic innervations of the heart originate in a group of neurons of the intermediolateral column (IML) of the spinal cord, which receives tonic excitatory glutamatergic inputs from neurons in rostral ventrolateral medulla (RVLM). The parasympathetic innervations of the heart are provided by the vagus nerve, by cardiovagal neurons primarily located in the nucleus ambiguus (NAmb) and in the minor extension in the dorsal motor nucleus of the vagus (DMN).

The autonomic cardiac system influences the intrinsic cardiac nervous system, a complex neural network composed of ganglia embedded in epicardial fat pads and the heart wall.

The sinoatrial (SA) node and atrioventricular (AV) node are two internal pacemakers that are responsible for initiating the heartbeat.

Sympathetic activation, via noradrenergic neurons, elicits an increase in the automatism of the SA node, with an increase in the heart rate (HR), and in AV conduction; in contrast, the main effects of the vagus, via cholinergic neurons, are the inhibition of the pacemaker activity of the SA node (decrease HR), and reduced AV conduction.

11.6.1 Arrhythmias and Autonomic Nervous System

It is well recognized that sympathetic inputs represent major neural triggers for both atrial and ventricular arrhythmias [27].

Atrial arrhythmia (atrial fibrillation and atrial flutter the most observed) is the most common rhythm disorder: the prevalence is increasing and accounts for nearly one quarter of ischemic strokes in the elderly population.

Ventricular arrhythmia is the leading cause of sudden death, a serious public health problem with 200,000–450,000 events in the USA annually [28]. About 50% of deaths in patients with heart failure are due to fatal arrhythmias.

Experimentally, sympathetic stimulation induces a change in ECG repolarization and reduces the fibrillation threshold, facilitating the initiation of ventricular fibrillation [29]. These effects are magnified in the presence of ischemic damage to the myocardial and conducting tissue.

Zhou et al. [30] demonstrated that ventricular fibrillation and sudden cardiac death, in ambulatory dogs, are immediately preceded by spontaneous sympathetic nerve discharge, indicating that sympathetic nerve discharge may serve as a trigger for arrhythmia.

A non-invasive marker of vulnerability to life-threatening arrhythmias in cardiovascular disease patients is heart rate variability (HRV); in general, reduced HRV indicates excessive cardiac sympathetic activity, reduced vagal modulation, and an increased risk of arrhythmic events.

Stress, through its impact on the autonomic cardiac system, can trigger both ventricular and atrial arrhythmias, as demonstrated by epidemiological, clinical, and laboratory studies.

Kop and collaborators [31] reported that mental stress can induce changes in T wave alternans (a sign of electrical instability) occurring at lower heart rates than with exercise in patients with implantable cardioverter defibrillators.

Other studies suggest that patients with heart failure experience alterations in autonomic nervous system function through increased sympathetic outflow to the heart and the peripheral vasculature and decreased parasympathetic activity, as documented by higher plasma NE concentrations and decreased clearance of NE from the circulation due to low cardiac output. Furthermore, increased plasma NE concentrations appear to predict negative outcomes in patients with congestive heart failure (CHF) [32].

In recent years, myocardial infarction with normal coronary arteries (MINCA) has been increasingly recognized and diagnosed. Recently, it was shown that MINCA occurs more frequently than previously thought, and data indicate that the prevalence ranges between 5 and 25% of all myocardial infarctions and approximately one-third of MINCA consists of Takotsubo stress cardiomyopathy.

Takotsubo cardiomyopathy (TTC) is characterized by transient systolic and diastolic left ventricular dysfunction with a variety of wall-motion abnormalities classified as apical, midventricular, basal or focal, in patients without coronary artery disease. It predominantly affects elderly women (except for Japan, where TTC is more prevalent among men) and is often preceded by an emotional trigger, although recent studies indicate that the disease may also occur with physical triggers or even without any evident preceding trigger.

Notably, 15.3% of patients with TTC have evidence of coexisting coronary artery disease on angiography.

The etiology of TTC is unknown, although indications point toward a strong relationship between TTC and acute physiological or mental stress with catecholamine excess and vasospasm.

Takotsubo cardiomyopathy is not an entirely benign and reversible condition. Data from the International Takotsubo Registry, a consortium of 26 centers in Europe and the USA, indicate that rates of severe in-hospital complications including shock and death are similar to acute coronary syndrome and younger patients with physical triggers and acute neurological or psychiatric diseases have a higher incidence of acute complications compared with elderly patients with emotional triggers. Ten-year follow-up combined end points of death and major adverse cardiac and cerebrovascular events reveal a rate of death from any cause of 5.6% per patient-year and a rate of major adverse cardiac and cerebrovascular events of 9.9% per patient-year among TTC patients. In both acute phase and long-term follow-up, men were at a higher risk for major adverse cardiac and cerebrovascular events than women [33].

11.6.2 The Role of the Vagus Nerve

In all the disorders mentioned above, the dysregulation of the autonomic cardiac system is characterized by sympathetic–vagal imbalance with parasympathetic withdrawal.

During the last decade, research has significantly advanced our understanding of the role of the vagus in the framework of neuroimmune communications.

The vagus nerve plays a prominent modulatory role in sympathetic effects. Moreover, the vagus nerve elicits a relevant cholinergic anti-inflammatory pathway named the "inflammatory reflex" [34].

Central nervous system efferent activity through the vagus nerve leads to acetylcholine (ACh) release in the organs of the reticuloendothelial system, including the liver, heart, spleen, and gastrointestinal tract. ACh interacts with nicotinic receptor (nAChr) on tissue macrophages, inhibiting the release of TNF-α, IL-1, and other pro-inflammatory cytokines. In 2000, Tracey and coworkers demonstrated that vagus nerve stimulation potently suppresses cytokine production in a rodent model of sepsis [35].

The observed withdrawal of parasympathetic activity during mental stress conversely results in the release of inflammatory cytokines by myocardial macrophages, leading to cardiac dysfunction and cardiomyocyte death.

Neuronal pathways, including the vagus nerve-based inflammatory reflex, are physiological regulators of immune function and inflammation. In parallel, neuronal function is altered in conditions characterized by immune dysregulation and inflammation [36].

11.7 Biological Mechanisms 2: Inflammation

The bidirectional association between stress, inflammation, and depression has been recognized for over two decades [37, 38].

Regarding inflammatory response triggered by mental stress, Kop and colleagues [39] reported that the mental arithmetic stress test causes transiently increased levels of the inflammatory markers, C-reactive protein (CRP), and interleukin-6 in patients with coronary artery disease. They also observed that patients with high catecholamine responses to mental stress also had an exaggerated increase in these inflammatory markers.

In depression, there are recorded elevations in the blood level of inflammatory cytokines (IL-1beta, IL-6, TNF-alpha) in addition to other markers of inflammation (CRP, ICAM-1).

In turn, inflammation increases depressive symptoms, as observed in a wide variety of clinical conditions: social context-related inflammation (e.g., impaired social relationships and loneliness), therapy-related inflammation (e.g., interferons (IFNs) for viral hepatic diseases, chemotherapy for cancer), and autoimmune disease-related inflammation (e.g., rheumatoid arthritis).

High rates of co-morbidity of depression and inflammatory diseases, such as diabetes, have been reported. The prevalence of depression, in a recent systematic review, was found to be more than three times higher in people with type 1 diabetes, and nearly twice as high in people with type 2 diabetes, compared with those without these conditions [40].

Affective disorders, including depression and anxiety, are common in patients with CHF. Studies suggest that depression occurs in approximately 40% and anxiety in 18–45% of patients with CHF. Depressive disorder worsens outcomes in patients with heart failure, reducing the quality of life, increasing the severity of cardiac symptoms, the rate of hospitalization, and death.

Many studies investigated the link between depression and cardiac disease, demonstrating that patients with depression exhibit autonomic nervous system changes comparable with those observed in patients with heart failure, such as increased circulating NO and decreased heart rate variability, and elevated levels of inflammatory markers (TNF-α and IL-1 cytokines, CRP, platelet hyperactivity, etc.) [32].

11.7.1 The Cardiac Immune System

The heart is receptive to inflammation, because, according to the most recent research, it is also an immune organ [41].

Innate and adaptive immunity cells reside in the heart: macrophages are the most abundant type, but dendritic cells, mast cells (MCs), and a small number of B cells and regulatory T cells also are located in the heart (Fig. 11.4).

Cardiac immune system plays a relevant role in myocardial infarction.

Resident cardiac immune cells are triggered by two distinct orders of "alarmins" [42]: pathogen-derived (PAMPs) and damage-derived (DAMPs) molecules, which are released by dying or injured myocardial cells and recognized by specific pattern recognition receptors (PRRs), such as toll-like receptors (TLRs). In mammals, 13 different TLRs have been identified. TLR2 and TLR4 are located on the surface of cardiac cells and are important mediators of inflammation following myocardial infarction and ischemia/reperfusion damage.

Damage-derived molecules also activate the complement system, another essential cascade in triggering inflammation and leukocyte infiltration in injured myocardium, as has been demonstrated with C3 cleavage in infarcted myocardial tissue (Fig. 11.4).

Damage-derived molecules can also be derived by mitochondria that are damaged because of hemodynamic stress, with the release of mitochondrial DNA and subsequent immune activation [43].

In acute myocardial infarction, due to prolonged ischemia, coagulative necrosis is the main mechanism of cell death, followed by cellular apoptosis.

Cellular death is characterized by oxidative stress. Following myocardial infarction, the antioxidant pool is overwhelmed, resulting in the net generation of a large amount of reactive oxygen

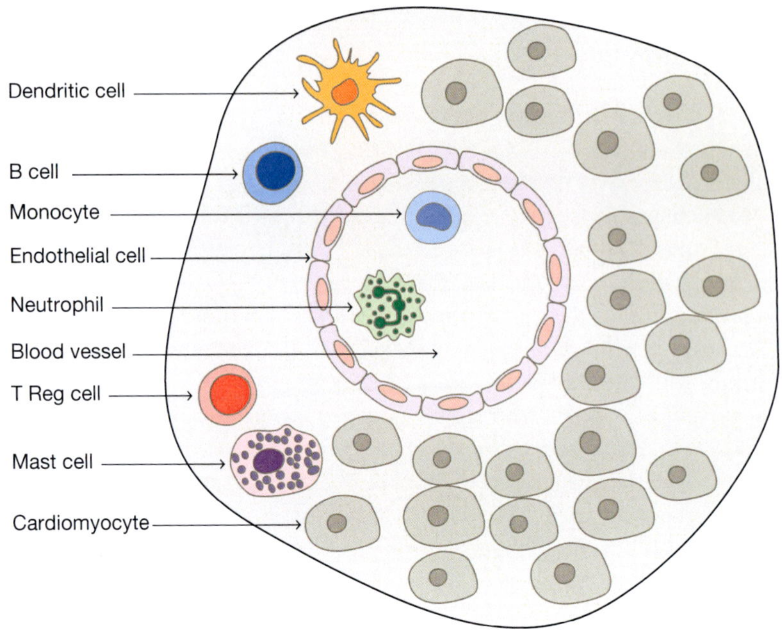

Fig. 11.4 Innate and adaptive immunity cells reside in the heart: macrophages are the most abundant type, but dendritic cells, mast cells, and a small number of B cells and regulatory T cells are also located in the heart

species (ROS) that may suppress myocardial function and activate leukocyte chemotaxis and inflammatory injury, causing loss of further cardiomyocytes through cell apoptosis and degradation of the extracellular matrix [44].

Toll-like receptors, complement, and ROS-related signal transduction activate the inflammatory transcription factors, including nuclear factor kB (NF-kB), which drives production of cytokines, interferons, and chemokines in the myocardial infarction zone.

As the prototypical pro-inflammatory cytokine, interleukin (IL)-1 mediates synthesis of chemotactic mediators and stimulates leukocyte recruitment in the infarct area, and plays an important role in inflammasome activation.

Tumor necrosis factor-alpha (TNF-α) is the other main pro-inflammatory cytokine released in the infarcted myocardium and may play a role in stimulating further cytokine synthesis in a vicious circle [45].

11.7.2 Mast Cells and Cardiac Events

Mast cells are important cells of the immune system of hematopoietic lineage, originating from pluripotent progenitor cells of the bone marrow. MCs are present throughout the body, mainly in mucosal and epithelial tissues.

Mast cells are also present in the heart and play a critical role, contributing to the development of the chemotactic gradient during acute coronary syndrome. MCs especially accumulate in the coronary artery during spasm, in the arterial adventitia, and in the shoulder region of the coronary atheromas and are involved in mechanisms of plaque erosion, and rupture. Coronary arteries of patients with ischemic heart disease contain more mast cells and histamine than normal vessels [46].

Oxidized low-density lipoprotein (LDL-ox), complement fragment 5a (C5a), IL-1, and ROS can activate MC degranulation. During hypoxic stress, MCs store and release TNF-α, IL-6, prostaglandins, and leukotrienes, metalloproteinases and renin, leading to increased local inflammation, vasoconstriction and rupture of the fibrous cap of the atherosclerotic plaque. Local renin, through the renin–angiotensin activation system, enhances the release of norepinephrine from cardiac nerve endings, triggering arrhythmias.

Mast cell-derived histamine, tryptase, and chymase are other proteases involved in plaque destabilization through collagen degradation and TLR-4 mediated smooth muscle cell apoptosis.

11.7.3 The Balance of the Inflammatory Response

The recruitment of neutrophils and other leukocytes from the blood into the area of myocardial infarction has the aim of removing dead cells, and releasing other cytokines and growth factors that lead to the formation of highly vascularized granulation tissue to maintain the integrity of the myocardial wall. The final phase is characterized by reparative myocardial fibrosis and angiogenesis.

Defects in the temporal and spatial regulation of the post-infarction inflammatory response may have catastrophic consequences. Excessive early inflammation may augment matrix degradation, leading to cardiac rupture. Prolongation of the inflammatory reaction may impair collagen deposition, producing a scar with reduced tensile strength, thus dilating the cardiac chambers.

Enhanced expression of pro-inflammatory mediators may activate pro-apoptotic pathways, inducing further loss of cardiomyocytes. Finally, defective containment of the inflammatory reaction may lead to extension of the inflammatory infiltrate into the non-infarcted myocardium, enhancing fibrosis and worsening diastolic function [45].

11.7.4 Mental Stress and Cardiovascular Damage

Mental stress can activate the sympathetic–adrenal–medullary (SAM) axis, eliciting the release of catecholamines (NE and EPI) resulting in the elevation of the heart rate (HR) and blood pressure (BP) with hemodynamic stress and DAMPs release. In turn, DAMPs can activate innate immune responses, leading to sterile inflammation, which in turn can result in myocarditis and dilated cardiomyopathy [41].

In an apolipoprotein E-deficient ($ApoE^{-}$) mice model, chronic intermittent mental stress resulted in a significant increase in the number of macrophages in atherosclerotic plaques of the proximal ascending aorta, where fibrous cap thickness was decreased. The coronary arteries showed larger plaques, more stenosis, and an increased degree of perivascular fibrosis. Moreover, myocardial infarctions occurred more frequently in the $ApoE^{-/-}$ mental stress group mice [47].

Acute mental or physical stress can activate cardiac MCs. Regulation of acute stress response activates neurohormonal pathways with hypothalamic release of a variety of hormones and neuropeptides, such as corticotropin-releasing hormone (CRH), CRH family peptide urocortin (Ucn), and neurotensin (NT), which act by binding CRH and NT receptors located both centrally and peripherally, including in the heart. Within the cardiovascular system, NT-containing neural fibers are found to be closed to cardiac myocytes, the cardiac conduction system, and coronary vessels. Stress-induced sympathetic hyperactivity also enhances neuropeptide synthesis outside the central nervous system, both in cardiomyocytes and in cardiac mast cells, leading to inflammatory cytokine release and mastocyte degranulation [48].

Pharmacological interventions moderating the inflammatory response to attenuate adverse remodeling and improve tissue repair may hold promise in patients with myocardial infarction [49].

Psychological stress has been shown to impair wound healing. In a randomized trial, it has been proven that a brief relaxation intervention, before surgery, reduces stress and improves surgical wound healing response. Patients in the intervention group had higher hydroxyproline deposition in the wound than did the control group patients [50].

11.8 Conclusions

What is needed for the prevention of CVD is a science that views the human organism as a whole. We also need care based on that science, and that focuses on increasing the self-adaptive capabilities of the individual, namely his or her ability to take care of him/herself. This endeavor can be aided by encouraging meditation and stress management techniques, which have a documented efficacy [51] and should be integrated into the mainstream prevention and care of CVD. This involves making important changes to the scientific and healthcare structures [52].

References

1. Bottaccioli F (2014) Epigenetica e psiconeuroendocrinoimmunologia. Edra-Lswr, Milan
2. Rose H, Rose S (2013) Genes, cells and brains. The promethean promises of the new biology. Verso Books, New York
3. Bottaccioli F (2014) La fine della grande illusione del riduzionismo in biologia e in medicina. Epistemologia Ital J Philos Sci XXXVII:5–21
4. Fani Marvasti F, Stafford RS (2012) From sick care to health care—reengineering prevention into the U.S. system. N Engl J Med 367(10):889–891
5. Kusnecov AW, Anisman H (eds) (2014) The Wiley-Blackwell handbook of psychoneuroimmunology. Wiley, Oxford
6. Ader R (2007) Psychoneuroimmunology, 4th edn. Academic Press-Elsevier, San Diego
7. Bottaccioli F (2005) Psiconeuroendocrinoimmunologia. Red, Milan
8. Selye H (1936) A syndrome produced by diverse nocuous agents. Nature 138:32
9. Besedovsky H, Del Rey A, Sorkin E, Da Prada M, Burri R, Honegger C (1983) The immune response evokes changes in brain noradrenergic neurons. Science 221:564–566
10. Blalock JE (1989) A molecular basis for bidirectional communication between the immune and neuroendocrine systems. Physiol Rev 69(1):1–32
11. Maier SF, Goehler LE, Fleshner M, Watkins LR (1998) The role of the vagus nerve in cytokine-to-brain communication. Ann NY Acad Sci 840:289–300
12. Pavlov VA, Tracey KJ (2012) The vagus nerve and the inflammatory reflex—linking immunity and metabolism. Nat Rev Endocrinol 8(12):743–754. doi:10.1038/nrendo.2012.189
13. Del Rey A, Besedovsky H (2014) The immune-neuroendocrine network in health and disease. In: Kusnecov AW, Anisman H (eds) The Wiley-Blackwell handbook of psychoneuroimmunology. Wiley-Blackwell, Oxford, pp 100–119
14. Lichtman JH, Froelicher ES, Blumenthal JA, Rm C, Doering LV, Frasure-Smith N, Freedland KE, Jaffe AS, Leifheit-Limson EC, Sheps DS, Vaccarino V, Wulsin L (2014) Depression as a risk factor for poor prognosis among patients with acute coronary syndrome: systematic review and recommendations. A scientific statement from the American Heart Association. Circulation 129 (12):1350–1369
15. Carnevali L, Mastorci F, Audero E, Graiani G, Rossi S, Macchi E, Callegari S, Bartolomucci A, Nalivaiko E, Quaini F, Gross C, Sgoifo A (2012) Stress-induced susceptibility to sudden cardiac death in mice with altered serotonin homeostasis. PLoS One 7:e41184. doi:10.1371/journal.pone.0041184
16. Louveau A, Smirnov I, Keyes TJ, Eccles JD, Rouhani SJ, Peske JD, Derecki NC, Castle D, Mandell JW, Lee KS, Harris TH, Kipnis J (2015) Structural and functional features of central nervous system lymphatics. Nature 523(7560):337–341. doi:10.1038/nature14432
17. Irwin MR, Rothermund M (2012) Clinical psychoneuroimmunology. In: Nemeroff CB, Schlaepfer TE (eds) Neurobiology of psychiatric disorders. Elsevier, Edinburgh, pp 211–225
18. May A (2011) Experience-dependent structural plasticity in the adult human brain. Trends Cogn Neurosci 15:475–482
19. Draganski B, Gaser C, Kempermann G, Kuhn HG, Winkler J, Büchel C, May A (2006) Temporal and spatial dynamics of brain structure changes during extensive learning. J Neurosci 26:6314–6317
20. Engel GL (1977) The need for a new medical model: a challenge for biomedicine. Science 196:129–136
21. Kiecolt-Glaser J (2009) Psychoneuroimmunology. Psychology's gateway to the biomedical future. Perspect Psychol Sci 4:367–369
22. Go AS, Mozaffarian D, Roger VL et al (2014) American Heart Association Statistics Committee and Stroke Statistics Subcommittee: AHA Statistical Update. Circulation 129(3):399–410
23. Liu H, Waite L (2014) Bad marriage, broken heart? Age and gender differences in the link between marital quality and cardiovascular risks among older adults. J Health Soc Behav 55(4):403–423. doi:10.1177/0022146514556893
24. Gustad LT, Laugsand LE, Janszky I, Dalen H, Bjerkeset O (2014) Symptoms of anxiety and depression and risk of heart failure: the HUNT Study. Eur J Heart Fail 16(8):861–870
25. Lichtman JH, Froelicher ES, Blumenthal JA, American Heart Association Statistics Committee of the Council on Epidemiology and Prevention and the Council on Cardiovascular and Stroke Nursing et al (2014) Depression as a risk factor for poor prognosis among patients with acute coronary syndrome: systematic review and recommendations: a scientific statement from the American Heart Association. Circulation 129(12):1350–1369. doi:10.1161/CIR.0000000000000019
26. Palma J-A, Benarroch EE (2014) Neural control of the heart. Neurology 83:261–271
27. Tan AY, Verrier RL (2013) The role of the autonomic nervous system in cardiac arrhythmias. In: Buijs RM, Swaab DF (eds) Autonomic nervous system. Elsevier, London, pp 134–145
28. Tomaselli GF (2015) Introduction to a compendium on sudden cardiac death. Epidemiology, mechanisms, and management. Circ Res 116:1883–1886

29. Shen MJ, Zipes DP (2014) Role of the autonomic nervous system in modulation cardiac arrhythmias. Circ Res 114:1004–1021
30. Zhou S, Jung BC, Tan AY et al (2008) Spontaneous stellate ganglion nerve activity and ventricular arrhythmia in a canine model of sudden death. Heart Rhythm 5:131–139
31. Kop W, Krantz D, Nearing B, Gottdiener J, Quigley J, O'Callahan M, Del Negro A, Friehling T, Karasik P, Suchday S, Levine J, Verrier R (2004) Effects of acute mental stress and exercise on T-wave alternans in patients with implantable cardioverter defibrillators and controls. Circulation 109:1864–1869
32. York KM, Hassan M, Sheps DS (2009) Psychobiology of depression/distress in congestive heart failure. Heart Fail Rev 14(1):35–50. doi:10.1007/s10741-008-9091-0
33. Templin C, Ghadri JR et al (2015) Clinical features and outcomes of Takotsubo (stress) cardiomyopathy. N Engl J Med 373:929–938. doi:10.1056/NEJMoa1406761
34. Soufer R, Jain H, Yoon AJ (2009) Heart-brain interactions in mental stress-induced myocardial ischemia. Curr Cardiol Rep 11(2):133–140
35. Borovikova LV, Ivanova S, Zhang M, Yang H, Botchkina GI, Watkins LR, Wang H, Abumrad N, Eaton JW, Tracey KJ (2000) Vagus nerve stimulation attenuates the systemic inflammatory response to endotoxin. Nature 405(6785):458–462
36. Pavlov VA, Tracey KJ (2015) Neural circuitry and immunity. Immunol Res 63(1–3):38–57. doi:10.1007/s12026-015-8718-1
37. Maes M (1999) Major depression and activation of the inflammatory response system. Adv Exp Med Biol 461:25–46
38. Dantzer R, O'Connor JC, Lawson MA, Kelley KW (2011) Inflammation-associated depression: from serotonin to kynurenine. Psychoneuroendocrinology 36(3):426–436. doi:10.1016/j.psyneuen.2010.09.012
39. Kop WJ, Weissman NJ, Zhu J, Bonsall RW, Doyle M, Stretch MR, Glaes SB, Krantz DS, Gottdiener JS, Tracy RP (2008) Effects of acute mental stress and exercise on inflammatory markers in patients with coronary artery disease and healthy controls. Am J Cardiol 101(6):767–773
40. Roy T, Ce L (2012) Epidemiology of depression and diabetes: a systematic review. J Affect Disord 142: S8–S21. doi:10.1016/S0165-0327(12)70004-6
41. Epelman S, Liu PP, Mann DL (2015) Role of innate and adaptive immune mechanisms in cardiac injury and repair. Nat Rev Immunol 15:117–129
42. Bianchi ME (2007) DAMPs, PAMPs and alarmins: all we need to know about danger. J Leukoc Biol 81:1–5
43. Oka T, Hikoso S, Yamaguchi O, Taneike M, Takeda T, Tamai T, Oyabu J, Murakawa T, Nakayama H, Nishida K, Akira S, Yamamoto A, Komuro I, Otsu K (2012) Mitochondrial DNA that escapes from autophagy causes inflammation and heart failure. Nature 485(7397):251–255. doi:10.1038/nature10992
44. Frangogiannis NG (2014) The immune system and the remodeling infarcted heart: cell biological insights and therapeutic opportunities. J Cardiovasc Pharmacol 63(3):185–195
45. Frangogiannis NG (2012) Regulation of the inflammatory response in cardiac repair. Circ Res 110(1): 159–173. doi:10.1161/CIRCRESAHA.111.243162
46. Krystel-Whittemore M, Dileepan KN, Wood JG (2016) Mast cell: a multi-functional master cell. Front Immunol 6:620. doi:10.3389/fimmu.2015.00620.eCollection.2015
47. Roth L, Rombouts M, Schrijvers DM, Lemmens K, De Keulenaer GW, Martinet W, De Meyer GR (2015) Chronic intermittent mental stress promotes atherosclerotic plaque vulnerability, myocardial infarction and sudden death in mice. Atherosclerosis 242(1): 288–294. doi:10.1016/j.atherosclerosis.2015.07.025
48. Alevizos M, Karagkouni A, Panagiotidou S, Vasiadi M, Theoharides TC (2014) Stress triggers coronary mast cells leading to cardiac events. Ann Allergy Asthma Immunol 112(4):309–316. doi:10.1016/j.anai.2013.09.017
49. Mann DL (2015) Innate immunity and the failing heart: the cytokine hypothesis revisited. Circ Res 116(7):1254–1268. doi:10.1161/CIRCRESAHA.116.302317
50. Broadbent E, Kahokehr A, Booth RJ et al (2012) A brief relaxation intervention reduces stress and improves surgical wound healing response: a randomized trial. Brain Behav Immun 26(2): 212–217. doi:10.1016/j.bbi.2011.06.014
51. Bottaccioli F, Carosella A, Cardone R, Mambelli M, Cemin M, D'Errico MM, Ponzio E, Bottaccioli AG, Minelli A (2014) Brief training of Psychoneuroendocrinoimmunology-based meditation (PNEIMED) reduces stress symptom ratings and improves control on salivary cortisol secretion under basal and stimulated conditions. Explore (NY) 10 (3):170–179. doi:10.1016/j.explore.2014.02.002
52. Bottaccioli F (2014) Stress science as a whole organism science. In: Rulli G (ed) Theories on stress. TAO Digital Library, Bologna, pp 5–17

12 The Role of Stress and Emotions in Cardiovascular Disease: Stress Management and Meditation Programs in the Prevention and Treatment of Cardiovascular Disease

Anna Giulia Bottaccioli

12.1 Introduction

There is growing evidence that psychosocial stress can influence the natural history of coronary heart disease (CHD). Established data from both population studies and an experimental animal model confirmed that adverse early life events, in particular during childhood and adolescence, predispose the individual to a greater rate of inflammatory-based diseases such as cardiovascular disease (CVD) in adulthood through epigenetic signature. Several epidemiological studies report that psychosocial factors such as acute and chronic stressors strongly increase the risk for cardiac events, worsening the prognosis in susceptible patients [1].

Since 1910, emotional triggers have been included in the pathogenesis of acute myocardial infarction by Obraztsov and Strazhesko [2]. Heterogeneous community-wide events, such as natural disasters, financial crashes, terrorist attacks, and wars, are associated with an increase in major cardiac events, in addition to positive emotionally charged events, such as sports matches and Christmas and New Year holidays [3].

Chronic stressors have also been linked to a worse prognosis in patients with existing CVD. Meta-analyses of prospective observational studies found that social isolation and loneliness were associated with a 50% increased risk of incident CVD events (pooled relative risk [RR] = 1.5, 95% confidence interval [CI]: 1.2–1.9). The increased risk associated with work-related stress (high work load, low reward) was similar at 40% (pooled RR = 1.4, 95% CI: 1.2–1.8) [4].

12.2 Emotions and CVD: Depression

Depression has been widely studied as an independent risk factor in patients with coronary artery disease (CAD) and heart failure, demonstrating a close relationship between highly depressive symptoms and a poor prognosis after an acute cardiac event, as established in the 2014 American Heart Association Scientific Statement [5].

Depression is also associated with incident CHD [6], with a pooled adjusted RR of 1.90 (95% CI: 1.49–2.42), and stroke [7], with a pooled adjusted hazard ratio (HR) of 1.45 (95% CI: 1.29–1.63).

A large number of epidemiological studies regarding racial differences in the incidence and mortality of CHD and racial disparities in depressive symptoms could be explained by biological (neuroendocrine stress pattern activation) and behavioral (smoking, physical inactivity, lower socioeconomic status) factors.

In REGARDS, 24,443 US blacks and whites without CHD at baseline were followed up to

A.G. Bottaccioli (✉)
M.D., Internal Medicine residency, Sapienza University, Rome, Italy
e-mail: annagiulia.bottaccioli@gmail.com; annagiulia.bottaccioli@uniroma1.it

M. Fioranelli (ed.), *Integrative Cardiology*, DOI 10.1007/978-3-319-40010-5_12

assess whether depressive symptoms are related to new cardiac events. Blacks who reported depressive symptoms were at a greater risk for the composite end point of CHD or revascularization (HR: 1.36; 95% CI: 1.01–1.81). Depressive symptoms were also associated with incident acute CHD or revascularization among blacks but not whites [8].

In another community-based cohort of blacks, the Jackson Heart Study, 3,309 participants showed, over a 10-year follow-up, that major depressive symptoms were associated with greater risks of incident stroke and CHD. Moreover, the authors found that the association between depressive symptoms and CHD risk was no longer significant after adjustment for coping strategies, demonstrating that coping strategies are particularly important for mitigating the increased CHD risk associated with depressive symptoms [9].

12.3 Emotions and CVD: Anxiety

The association between anxiety and onset of CVD is less significant. In a 2010 meta-analysis, great anxiety in healthy individuals is associated with an increased incidence of coronary disease. However, the meta-analytic estimate for the association of anxiety with CHD was not adjusted for depression, which is commonly comorbid with anxiety [10].

Sex differences were found about anxiety disorder and prevalence of CVD. Among 49,321 young military men, those who are diagnosed with anxiety are at an increased risk for experiencing CHD (adjusted HR: 2.17 [95% CI: 1.28–3.67]) and myocardial infarction (HR 2.51 [95% CI: 1.38–4.55]) [11]. A Finnish cohort showed an association between anxiety and an elevated risk of incident CHD over 7 years of follow-up only in women, with an HR of 1.24 (95% CI: 0.91–1.70) [12]. No clear association was found between anxiety and incidence of cardiac events and mortality among CHD patients.

12.4 Emotions and CVD: Post-Traumatic Stress Disorder

Evidence is better established for psychological trauma and post-traumatic stress disorder (PTSD) with incident CVD events and/or CVD death. Multiple prospective cohort studies have included general population subgroups and veterans. In a Danish study, associations were found between PTSD and CVD events, with limited evidence for gender differences [13]. The recently published Nurses' Health Study II investigated trauma exposure and PTSD symptoms in 49,978 women, finding that having elevated PTSD symptoms was associated with increased CVD risk, after adjusting for age, family history, and childhood factors (HR: 1.60; 95% CI: 1.20–2.13) [14].

A recently published analysis of active duty US military service members and veterans participating in the Millennium Cohort Study reported that combat deployment is associated with new-onset CHD by self-report or medical record diagnoses, demonstrating that experiences of recent combat exposure may increase the risk for CHD over a relatively short period of time (5.6-year follow-up) [15].

12.5 Positive Emotions and CVD

Some studies have focused on the importance of positive thoughts and emotions, along with social cohesion, on health outcome.

Prospective data from the Health and Retirement Study of older US adults included 6,808 participants who were followed for 4 years. Multiple logistic regression models are used to assess if optimism was independently associated with incident heart failure. Greater optimism was associated with a lower risk for incident heart failure over the follow-up period, adjusted for sociodemographic, behavioral, biological, and psychological covariates, with an odds ratio (OR) of 0.74 (95% CI: 0.63–0.85) [16].

Emerging ethnic differences between behavioral factors and the prognosis of CAD are also shown in a Japanese prospective study. Two hundred and one men enrolled in the Eastern Collaborative Group Study who have had CAD and undergone diagnostic coronary angiography were administered the Japanese Coronary-prone Behavior Scale (JCBS), a questionnaire that evaluates 10 psychological items. The authors have found that lower levels of impatience were associated with a 1.4-fold higher multivariable-adjusted risk of incidence of CHD and a 1.5-fold higher multivariable-adjusted risk for the incidence of myocardial infarction and nonfatal coronary disease. The fourth item of JCBS concerns the Japanese mentality, describing the Japanese "Spirit of Wa," transliterated as "harmonious groupism," a traditional attitude used to keep order in hierarchically organized social relationships in communities and groups. "Wa" represents a way of living that integrates a person into his or her community or group. Japanese Spirit of "Wa" was independently associated with coronary events (HR: 0.21) at the 7-year follow-up and thus is a preventive factor against coronary events for Japanese men with CAD [17].

Higher perceived neighborhood social cohesion may have a protective effect against myocardial infarction, as demonstrated in a cohort study of 5,276 American middle-aged adults with no history of heart disease, in which an increase in perceived neighborhood social cohesion was associated with a reduced likelihood of incident myocardial infarction (OR = 0.78, 95% CI: 0.63–0.94) over 4 years, even after further adjustments for behavioral, biological, and psychosocial factors [18].

12.6 Quantify Myocardial Stress: Mental Stress-Induced Myocardial Ischemia

An important method of assessing the effects of stress on cardiac function is Mental Stress-Induced Myocardial Ischemia (MSIMI) [19], a provocative test alternative to exercise and pharmacological stress-induced ischemia, in which the stimulus is psychological rather than physical. A wide range of stimuli were regarded as mental stressors, including mental arithmetic, simulated public speaking tasks, problem-solving tasks, cognitive tasks such as the Stroop color/word interference task, psychomotor challenges such as mirror tracing, and tasks involving the recall of a negative emotion.

Ischemic alterations in MSIMI are induced not by extreme emotional response to stress, but by behavioral challenges similar to those that might be experienced in everyday life. For this reason, anger, both as an emotional state and as a personality trait, is likewise associated with the propensity to develop myocardial ischemia during mental stress, but not during exercise/pharmacological stress [20].

Many different instrumental techniques have been used to assess reversible myocardial ischemic damage induced by psychological testing. Electrocardiogram (ECG) alone or in combination, echocardiography (ECHO), radionuclide ventriculogram, nuclear scintigraphy, positron emission tomography (PET), and quantitative coronary angiography show different characteristics of transient stress-induced ischemia: ST segment depression on ECG, wall motion abnormality on ECHO, left ventricular ejection fraction decrease on ventriculography, segmental hypoperfusion on scintigraphy, abnormal regional myocardial perfusion and reduced coronary flow reserve on PET, and finally coronary vasoconstriction on angiography.

Basing on recent evidence, myocardial perfusion imaging (e.g., with 99mTc-sestamibi SPECT) seems to be more accurate for the detection of MSIMI than methods based solely on electric changes and/or changes in the left ventricular function [21].

The main features of MSIMI are that it occurs more frequently among patients with CAD (about 50%) than in other groups, it is asymptomatic, and it occurs at a lower workload and oxygen demand than exercise-induced ischemia. Recent meta-analysis confirms a strong association between MSIMI and poor cardiovascular prognosis in terms of adverse outcome events in patients with CAD, with a pooled relative risk of 2.24 (95% CI: 1.59–3.15), although MSIMI is not directly related to the severity of coronary atherosclerosis [22].

In healthy controls, both mental and exercise/dipyridamole stress tests induce increased myocardial blood flow in normal coronary vessel, as a result of coronary microvascular dilation. In patients with CAD, coronary flow during mental stress was lower in regions without epicardial stenosis than in those with significant stenosis, suggesting microvascular constriction. In contrast, physical stress-induced ischemia occurred primarily by coronary steal when restricted vasodilation in a stenosed epicardial vessel causes selective hypoperfusion.

Moreover, subjects with exaggerated cardiovascular reactivity during mental stress have a greater likelihood of positive exercise/pharmacologic stress test [23].

Most significant hemodynamic features associated with MSIMI are the increase in systemic vascular resistance, vasoconstriction of normal coronary artery segments, impaired endothelial function, and increased heart rate and/or blood pressure, thereby resulting in myocardial oxygen supply–demand imbalance. Mental stress, through the activation of stress–response systems, increases levels of circulating catecholamines, also inducing cardiac electrical instability, as shown by ST segment and T-wave abnormalities [22].

It has been well established that among young post-myocardial infarction patients, higher levels of cognitive and somatic depressive symptoms are associated with a greater tendency to develop ischemia with MSIMI, but not with physical (exercise or pharmacologically)-induced stress. This association remains robust even after multivariate adjustments for other risk factors and disease severity, and applies to both somatic and cognitive depressive symptoms [24].

Recent research has investigated the role of baseline coping strategies and CVD outcomes, once again in a Japanese population cohort. Analyses of CVD incidence and mortality included 57,017 subjects aged 50–79 years without a history of CVD, who completed a coping behaviors and strategies questionnaire and were included in an approach-oriented behavior strategy or in an avoidance-oriented behavior strategy.

The authors have found that an approach-oriented coping strategy was associated with a significantly reduced incidence of stroke and reduced CVD mortality, in particular among hypertensive individuals. The specific fantasizing behavior avoidance-oriented strategy is only associated with CVD incidence and with increased CVD mortality among hypertensive subjects, whereas a positive reappraisal behavior approach-oriented strategy is associated with reduced CVD mortality [25].

12.7 Pharmacological Treatment of Depression in CVD and the Impact on Cardiovascular Outcomes: Current Evidence

Physiological derangements related to depression include autonomic and hypothalamic–pituitary–adrenal axis dysregulation, altered central and peripheral serotonin homeostasis, an increase in inflammatory signals, stress-related platelet activation [26, 27], and endothelial dysfunction. The results of these derangements may lead to cardiac events and cardiovascular death [28].

Pharmacology-based approaches to depression treatment have been shown to decrease platelet/endothelial activation markers (e.g., platelet factor 4 and β-thromboglobulin), reduce inflammatory markers (e.g., tumor necrosis factor-α and C-reactive protein), improve heart rate variability, and normalize brain serotonin turnover [29].

Among antidepressants, selective serotonin re-uptake inhibitors (SSRIs) are recommended as first-line therapy for the treatment of depression in CVD patients. TCA and IMAO use is discouraged because of the adverse cardiovascular effects [30]. Some SSRIs seem to exert a direct cardioprotective role during acute myocardial infarction, inhibiting myocardial apoptosis in a rat model [31].

The first randomized controlled trial of pharmacological therapy for depression in cardiovascular patients was the Sertraline Antidepressant Heart Attack Randomized Trial (SADHEART). This trial demonstrated that sertraline was safe in CAD patients and resulted in improvements in depressive symptoms and quality of life, without significant effects on cardiovascular outcomes [32]. Indeed, sertraline in depressed patients with congestive heart failure showed no statistical difference in the reduction of depressive symptoms and no difference in all-cause mortality [33].

The subsequent Myocardial Infarction and Depression–Intervention Trial (MIND–IT) involving depressed patients treated with mirtazapine depressed patients with acute myocardial infarction or with placebo, finding no difference in cardiac events rate [34].

The Improving Mood-Promoting Access to Collaborative Treatment (IMPACT) trial randomized 235 primary care patients with depression to a 12-month collaborative care program involving antidepressants and psychotherapy, finding a dramatic 48% lower risk of a CVD event over a 5-year follow-up only among patients without baseline cardiac disease, underlining the importance of integrated stress management in the primary prevention of CVD [35]. A recent randomized controlled trial (RCT) on 24-week escitalopram treatment in patients with depression and recent coronary events, confirmed the antidepressant effect of SSRI drugs without any harmful changes in cardiovascular safety measures. However, the study did not analyze cardiovascular outcomes [36]. Another recent randomized trial, named Responses of Mental Stress Induced Myocardial Ischemia to Escitalopram Treatment (REMIT), on the use of 6-week administration of escitalopram versus placebo among 127 patients with stable coronaropathy and evidence of MSIMI at baseline, resulted in a significantly lower prevalence of MSIMI in the treatment group, with no difference in exercise-induced ischemia [37].

12.8 Psychotherapy in CVD

The importance of managing stress to prevent and improve CVD is challenging.

This is particularly true for women. Although female coronary disease occurs later in life, those women who have clinical events at a younger age have a worse prognosis than men. Psychosocial factors have been hypothesized as relevant risk markers in this field. In the context of the Stockholm Female Coronary Risk study, 237 middle-aged women, who had experienced acute myocardial infarction and who underwent coronary artery bypass grafting or percutaneous coronary intervention, were randomized to a group-based psychosocial stress intervention program or usual care for 1 year. Over a mean period of 7 years, women in usual care had a mortality rate of 20%, whereas those in the psychosocial intervention group had a mortality rate of 7% [38].

Behavioral intervention has also been tested among patients with an implantable cardioverter defibrillator (ICD). A comprehensive review of cognitive-behavioral therapies coupled with relaxation strategies (e.g., diaphragmatic breathing, breath counting meditation, progressive muscle relaxation, visualization, self-hypnosis, and autogenic training) showed promising results with respect to reductions in psychological distress, whereas effects on cardiovascular endpoints (e.g., shocks and arrhythmias) remain elusive [39].

A cost-effectiveness analysis of the stress management program in secondary prevention in established CAD patients reveals lower medical costs than usual care in the first 2 years and lower cumulative costs over 5 years for stress management compared with usual care [40].

Psychotherapy also appears effective in treating the psychological symptoms of coronary disease patients, significantly improving quality of life [41].

The largest intervention trial of a non-pharmacology-based approach to depression in CVD is the Enhancing Recovery in Coronary Heart Disease Patients (ENRICHD) trial, in which 2,481 patients with an acute myocardial infarction and major depressive disorder, depressive symptoms, or dysthymia were randomized to cognitive-behavioral therapy (CBT) or usual treatment. If the score of the Hamilton scale was greater than 24, they also received an SSRI. CBT was found to significantly improve depression, social isolation, and the overall quality of life, with no effect on cardiac outcomes [42].

The safety and efficacy of CBT were confirmed in a recently published trial involving 158 heart failure patients with a major depressive disorder. At 6 months, depression and the anxiety score were significantly reduced, as along with the rate of hospitalization, but improvement of physical functioning was not observed [43]. Also, collaborative care interventions improve depression and quality of life and in some cases, relieve cardiac symptoms.

A dedicated Cochrane Review on psychological intervention for coronary disease established that psychological treatments are effective in treating the psychological symptoms of CHD patients. Uncertainty remains regarding the subgroups of patients who would benefit most from treatment (there is most evidence for "type A" behavior) and the characteristics of successful interventions [41]. A 2011 comprehensive Cochrane systematic review concluded that both pharmacological and psychological intervention for depression in CVD patients may have a small yet clinically meaningful effect on depression outcomes, without beneficial effects on the reduction of mortality rates and cardiac events, owing to the low number of high-quality trials [44].

12.9 Meditation Programs: State of the Art in Scientific Research

The physiology of meditation practices and their role in health and disease have been widely investigated in the last half century, with increased attention given to the effect of meditation on the cardiovascular system [45].

Meditation practice, by reducing the heart rate and respiratory rate (approximately 6 breaths per minute), positively affects autonomic balance, enhancing parasympathetic activity and improving heart rate variability and baroreflex sensitivity, in addition to inducing the vagal anti-inflammatory reflex [46]. Evidence from neurophysiological studies confirms the impact of mindful meditation on stress response in the brain through reduced amygdala activation, increased prefrontal cortex activation, and increased hippocampal gray matter density [47].

A review of RCTs demonstrates that mind–body practices produce encouraging results in patients with cardiac disease; however, the quality of the studies in this field remains low [48].

12.10 Transcendental Meditation

Transcendental meditation, introduced into the West in the second half of the nineteenth century by Yogi Maharishi Mahesh, is a technique that involves the use of a repeated sound (mantra) for 15–20 min twice per day to achieve a quiet state of awareness. It is estimated that there have been more than 600 studies published examining the impact of transcendental meditation on CVD, although, again, many studies have been criticized for their low quality and possible researcher bias.

A 2013 American Heart Association Statement described TM as a safe and effective alternative treatment to lowering high blood pressure, both in primary and in secondary prevention, with mean blood pressure reduction between 4.7 and 3.2 mmHg among young and older subjects [49]. It was found that a TM program also reduces left ventricular mass on echography, decreases the carotid intima-media thickness in African–American hypertensive adults, and reduces circulating levels of stress hormones norepinephrine and cortisol [50]. However, there are few trials with outcomes that are too limited to draw conclusions about the effectiveness of TM for the primary prevention of CVD [51].

A small group of 23 African–Americans with heart failure randomized to TM and usual care showed a significant increase in the 6-min walking distance in addition to improvement in depression scores and measures of quality of life in the TM group [52]. A more recent, large study involved 201 black patients with stable CAD who demonstrated a 48% risk reduction in the composite of mortality, nonfatal myocardial infarction, and nonfatal stroke, and a significant reduction in blood pressure during an average follow-up of 5.4 years and improvement in psychosocial distress, confirming that the TM program may be clinically useful in the secondary prevention of CVD [53].

12.11 Acem Meditation

Acem meditation is a systematic, nondirected, nonreligious approach to meditation theorized by physicians and psychologists and founded in Norway in 1966 by Are Holen. It subsequently spread worldwide. Acem meditation is based on the use of a simple combination of repeated sounds and release of the spontaneous activities of the mind, providing deep relaxation and free flow of thoughts and feelings. Also, Acem meditation may contribute toward a reduction in cardiovascular risk, as demonstrated in a study conducted recently among 27 middle-aged healthy participants of both genders practicing Acem meditation for 20 min: heart rate variability increased during meditation compared with rest, without a change in respiration and heart rates [54].

12.12 Mindfulness Meditation

Mindfulness is a modern Western movement, derived from the ancient Buddhist Vipassana meditation, founded by Jon Kabat-Zinn in the late 1970s. It is a nonjudgmental practice involving becoming aware moment to moment, improving emotion regulation, and cultivating the attention of mental events in the present moment with openness and acceptance. Mindfulness-based stress reduction (MBSR) is the most popular and validated mindfulness program, with a consistent number of scientific studies. MBSR provides 8 weeks of systematic training in formal mindfulness meditation practices, including a physical session with mindful yoga and a psychoeducational program.

The mindfulness stress reduction program improves psychological well-being through a reduction of distress, anxiety, and depression. In patients with mild-to-moderate depression, MBSR effect sizes for anxiety and depressive symptoms are comparable with the use of an antidepressant in a primary care population, without the associated toxicities [55].

There is currently limited evidence for the connection between mindfulness and CVD risk. Some small observational and not all randomized studies assess a global improvement in physical activity, smoking cessation, reducing caloric intake, and weight loss in high-risk and eating behavior patients, and show mixed and nonconclusive results in the reduction of blood pressure and limited evidence for glucose regulation in diabetic and nondiabetic subjects [56]. Meditation and mindfulness skills led to improved sleep, greater relaxation, and more accepting approaches to illness and illness experience among 40 patients with diabetes and CHD [57]. An interesting pilot study in a small sample of experienced and inexperienced meditators demonstrates an increased level of nitric oxide (arterial vasodilator), with the higher rate in experienced subjects and a more significant reduction of self-reported stress in the experienced group, after 20 min of loving kindness meditation [58].

The SAFE-LIFE randomized trial assesses the effects of a comprehensive lifestyle modification (to a Mediterranean diet) and stress reduction intervention on coronary stenosis progression, blood lipids, heart rate, blood pressure, angina symptoms, and quality of life. Stress reduction interventions included MBSR, guided imagery, yoga breathing techniques, and a body scan. Further elements included CBT (cognitive restructuring) and psychoeducational approaches (coping skills training). At 3 years, comprehensive lifestyle modification has no impact on coronary stenosis progression, but shows sustainable benefit for blood pressure, heart rate, the need for anti-ischemic medication, and overall quality of life [59].

12.13 Yoga

The practice of yoga began in India about 4,000 years ago, and has become increasingly common in Western countries since the beginning of 1960s. Ancient texts have described several types of yogic practices, including Dhyana Yoga (which emphasizes meditation), Mantra Yoga (which emphasizes the repetition of sacred words), and the most famous, Hatha Yoga (which emphasizes, through harmonic movements, the energy of the body). However, core components of Hatha yoga include stretching exercises and physical postures (*asanas*), breath control (*pranayama*), and concentration techniques (meditation).

Several controlled and uncontrolled studies have shown the short- and long-term usefulness of yoga in the treatment of hypertension [60].

Yoga-based programs also improve body weight and lipid profiles in healthy adults and in patients with diabetes, hypertension, and

CHD, estimating the reduction of total cholesterol to be between 5.8 and 25.2%, triglycerides between 22.0 and 28.5%, and low-density lipoprotein (LDL) cholesterol by 12.8–26% [61].

In a recent prospective study, short-term yoga-based lifestyle intervention involving 237 normal weight, overweight, and obese subjects significantly increased high-density lipoprotein (HDL) cholesterol levels. Moreover, there was a reduction in blood pressure, fasting blood glucose, and an improvement in global lipid profile [62]. Results of some small, nonrandomized studies provide evidence that yoga may reduce oxidative stress and circulating fibrinogen. Other trials have shown that 1 year of regular practice of yoga/meditation significantly reduced early atherosclerosis, as quantified by carotid intima media thickness, in individuals with metabolic syndrome [63].

12.14 Tai Chi Chuan

Tai Chi Chuan (TCC) is a mind–body intervention that derives from ancient Chinese martial arts and combines low- to moderate-intensity physical activity through flowing circular movements and balance and weight shifting, with meditation, body awareness, and breathing techniques. A typical session lasts 20–30 min and is safe and accessible for all types of patients. A recent meta-analysis confirmed that the traditional Chinese exercises, including TCC, significantly improves the quality of life and depression of patients with chronic diseases [64].

There are consistent findings for TCC and cardiac rehabilitation, showing greater exercise tolerance and an increase in functional capacity measured as peak oxygen consumption (VO_2 peak) in patients with recent myocardial infarction [65].

Among patients with congestive heart failure with preserved ejection fraction randomized to a TCC program or aerobic exercise, 12 weeks of TCC increases the 6-min walking distance through lower oxygen uptake, and a low respiratory rate and heart rate, compared with usual exercises [66].

In patients with severe heart failure (EF 29%), no significant differences in the change in the Six-Min Walk Test and peak oxygen uptake were observed in comparison with the education group, but patients in the tai chi group experienced an increase in daily activities, reporting improvements in their global quality of life [67].

12.15 Conclusion

The enormous amount of literature regarding the influence of emotions and daily stress in the pathogenesis and prognosis of CVD is well established. Emerging evidence for the beneficial effects of psychotherapies, stress reduction programs, and meditation techniques on symptom relief and outcomes in CHD needs further research and more rigorous experimental studies, to promote the large-scale application of stress management training in primary and secondary cardiovascular prevention.

References

1. Saban KL, Mathews HL, DeVon HA, Janusek LW (2014) Epigenetics and social context: implications for disparity in cardiovascular disease. Aging Dis 5(5):346–355. doi:10.14336/AD.2014.0500346
2. Obraztsov VP, Strazhesko ND (1910) The symptomatology and diagnosis of coronary thrombosis. In: Vorobeva VA, Konchalovski MP (eds) Works of the first Congress of Russian therapists. Comradeship Typography of A.E. Mamontov, Moscow, pp 26–43
3. Schwartz BG, French WJ, Mayeda GS, Burstein S, Economides C, Bhandari AK, Cannom DS, Kloner RA (2012) Emotional stressors trigger cardiovascular events. Int J Clin Pract 66(7):631–639. doi:10.1111/j.1742-1241.2012.02920.x
4. Steptoe A, Kivimäki M (2013) Stress and cardiovascular disease: an update on current knowledge. Annu Rev Public Health 34:337–354
5. Cohen BE, Edmondson D, Kronish IM (2015) State of the art review: depression, stress, anxiety, and cardiovascular disease. Am J Hypertens 28(11):1295–1302. doi:10.1093/ajh/hpv047
6. Nicholson A, Kuper H, Hemingway H (2006) Depression as an aetiologic and prognostic factor in coronary heart disease: a meta-analysis of 6362 events among 146 538 participants in 54 observational studies. Eur Heart J 27:2763–2774

7. Pan A, Sun Q, Okereke OI, Rexrode KM, Hu FB (2011) Depression and risk of stroke morbidity and mortality: a meta-analysis and systematic review. JAMA 306:1241–1249. doi:10.1001/jama.2011.128
8. Sims M, Redmond N, Khodneva Y, Durant RW, Halanych J, Safford MM (2015) Depressive symptoms are associated with incident coronary heart disease or revascularization among blacks but not among whites in the reasons for geographical and racial differences in stroke study. Ann Epidemiol 25 (6):426–432. doi:10.1016/j.annepidem.2015.03.014
9. O'Brien EC, Greiner MA, Sims M, Hardy NC, Wang W, Shahar E, Hernandez AF, Curtis LH (2015) Depressive symptoms and risk of cardiovascular events in blacks: findings from the Jackson heart study. Circ Cardiovasc Qual Outcomes 8(6):552–559. doi:10.1161/CIRCOUTCOMES.115.001800
10. Roest AM, Martens EJ, de Jonge P, Denollet J (2010) Anxiety and risk of incident coronary heart disease: a meta-analysis. J Am Coll Cardiol 56:38–46
11. Janszky I, Ahnve S, Lundberg I, Hemmingsson T (2010) Early-onset depression, anxiety and risk of subsequent coronary heart disease: 37-year follow-up of 49,321 young Swedish men. J Am Coll Cardiol 56:31–37
12. Nabi H, Hall M, Koskenvuo M, Singh-Manoux A, Oksanen T, Suominen S, Kivimäki M, Vahtera J (2010) Psychological and somatic symptoms of anxiety and risk of coronary heart disease: the health and social support prospective cohort study. Biol Psychiatry 67:378–385
13. Gradus JL, Farkas DK, Svensson E, Ehrenstein V, Lash TL, Milstein A, Adler N, Sørensen HT (2015) Associations between stress disorders and cardiovascular disease events in the Danish population. BMJ Open 5 (12):e009334. doi:10.1136/bmjopen-2015-009334
14. Sumner JA, Kubzansky LD, Elkind MS, Roberts AL, Agnew-Blais J, Chen Q, Cerdá M, Rexrode KM, Rich-Edwards JW, Spiegelman D, Suglia SF, Rimm EB, Koenen KC (2015) Trauma exposure and post-traumatic stress disorder symptoms predict onset of cardiovascular events in women. Circulation 132 (4):251–259. doi:10.1161/CIRCULATIONAHA.114.014492
15. Crum-Cianflone NF, Bagnell ME, Schaller E, Boyko EJ, Smith B, Maynard C, Ulmer CS, Vernalis M, Smith TC (2014) Impact of combat deployment and posttraumatic stress disorder on newly reported coronary heart disease among US active duty and reserve forces. Circulation 129:1813–1820
16. Kim ES, Smith J, Kubzansky LD (2014) Prospective study of the association between dispositional optimism and incident heart failure. Circ Heart Fail 7(3):394–400. doi:10.1161/CIRCHEARTFAILURE.113.000644
17. Hori R, Hayano J, Kimura K, Shibata N, Kobayashi F (2015) Psychosocial factors are preventive against coronary events in Japanese men with coronary artery disease: the Eastern Collaborative Group Study 7.7-year follow-up experience. Biopsychosoc Med 9(1):3. doi:10.1186/s13030-015-0030-8
18. Kim ES, Hawes AM, Smith J (2014) Perceived neighbourhood social cohesion and myocardial infarction. J Epidemiol Community Health 68 (11):1020–1026. doi:10.1136/jech-2014-204009
19. Strike PC, Steptoe A (2003) Systematic review of mental stress-induced myocardial ischaemia. Eur Heart J 24(8):690–703
20. Pimple P, Shah A, Rooks C, Bremner JD, Nye J, Ibeanu I, Murrah N, Shallenberger L, Kelley M, Raggi P, Vaccarino V (2015) Association between anger and mental stress-induced myocardial ischemia. Am Heart J 169(1):115–21.e2. doi:10.1016/j.ahj.2014.07.031
21. Krantz DS, Burg MM (2014) Current perspective on mental stress-induced myocardial ischemia. Psychosom Med 76:168–170
22. Wei J, Rooks C, Ramadan R, Shah AJ, Bremner JD, Quyyumi AA, Kutner M, Vaccarino V (2014) Meta-analysis of mental stress-induced myocardial ischemia and subsequent cardiac events in patients with coronary artery disease. Am J Cardiol 114 (2):187–192. doi:10.1016/j.amjcard.2014.04.022
23. Ramadan R, Sheps D, Esteves F, Zafari AM, Bremner JD, Vaccarino V, Quyyumi AA (2013) Myocardial ischemia during mental stress: role of coronary artery disease burden and vasomotion. J Am Heart Assoc 2 (5):e000321. doi:10.1161/JAHA.113.000321
24. Wei J, Pimple P, Shah AJ, Rooks C, Bremner JD, Nye JA, Ibeanu I, Murrah N, Shallenberger L, Raggi P, Vaccarino V (2014) Depressive symptoms are associated with mental stress-induced myocardial ischemia after acute myocardial infarction. PLoS One 9(7):e102986. doi:10.1371/journal.pone.0102986
25. Svensson T, Inoue M, Sawada N, Yamagishi K, Charvat H, Saito I, Kokubo Y, Iso H, Kawamura N, Shibuya K, Mimura M, Tsugane S, JPHC Study Group (2016) Coping strategies and risk of cardiovascular disease incidence and mortality: the Japan Public Health Center-based prospective Study. Eur Heart J. pii:ehv724
26. Jiang W, Boyle SH, Ortel TL, Samad Z, Velazquez EJ, Harrison RW, Wilson J, Kuhn C, Williams RB, O'Connor CM, Becker RC (2015) Platelet aggregation and mental stress induced myocardial ischemia: results from the responses of myocardial ischemia to escitalopram treatment (REMIT) study. Am Heart J 169(4):496–507.e1. doi:10.1016/j.ahj.2014.12.002
27. Mazereeuw G, Herrmann N, Bennett SA, Swardfager W, Xu H, Valenzuela N, Fai S, Lanctôt KL (2013) Platelet activating factors in depression and coronary artery disease: a potential biomarker related to inflammatory mechanisms and neurodegeneration. Neurosci Biobehav Rev 37(8):1611–1621. doi:10.1016/j.neubiorev.2013.06.010
28. Carnevali L, Mastorci F, Audero E, Graiani G, Rossi S, Macchi E, Callegari S, Bartolomucci A, Nalivaiko E, Quaini F, Gross C, Sgoifo A (2012) Stress-induced susceptibility to sudden cardiac death

in mice with altered serotonin homeostasis. PLoS One 7(7):e41184. doi:10.1371/journal.pone.0041184
29. Bradley SM, Rumsfeld JS (2015) Depression and cardiovascular disease. Trends Cardiovasc Med 25 (7):614–622. doi:10.1016/j.tcm.2015.02.002
30. Mavrides N, Nemeroff CB (2015) Treatment of affective disorders in cardiac disease. Dialogues Clin Neurosci 17(2):127–140
31. Wang Y, Zhang H, Chai F, Liu X, Berk M (2014) The effects of escitalopram on myocardial apoptosis and the expression of Bax and Bcl-2 during myocardial ischemia/reperfusion in a model of rats with depression. BMC Psychiatry 14:349. doi:10.1186/s12888-014-0349-x
32. Glassman AH, O'Connor CM, Califf RM, Swedberg K, Schwartz P, Bigger JT, Krishnan KR, van Zy LT, Swenson JR, Finkcl MS, Landau C, Shapiro PA, Pepine CJ, Mardekian J, Harrison WM, Barton D, Mclvor M, Sertraline Antidepressant Heart Attack Randomized Trial (SADHEART) Group (2002) Sertraline treatment of major depression in patients with acute MI or unstable angina. J Am Med Assoc 288:701–709
33. O'Connor CM, Jiang W, Kuchibhatla M, Silva SG, Cuffe MS, Callwood DD, Zakhary B, Stough WG, Arias RM, Rivelli SK, Krishnan R, SADHART-CHF Investigators (2010) Safety and efficacy of sertraline for depression in patients with heart failure. Results of the SADHART-CHF (Sertraline Against Depression and Heart Disease in Chronic Heart Failure) Trial. J Am Coll Cardiol 56(9):692–699
34. van Melle JP, de Jonge P, Honig A, Schene AH, Kuyper AM, Crijns HJ, Schins A, Tulner D, van den Berg MP, Ormel J, MIND-IT Investigators (2007) Effects of antidepressant treatment following myocardial infarction. Br J Psychiatry 190:460–466
35. Stewart JC, Perkins AJ, Callahan CM (2013) Effect of collaborative care for depression on risk of cardiovascular events: data from the IMPACT randomized controlled trial. Psychosom Med 76(1):29–37. doi:10.1097/PSY.0000000000000022
36. Kim JM, Bae KY, Stewart R, Jung BO, Kang HJ, Kim SW, Shin IS, Hong YJ, Kim JH, Shin HY, Kang G, Ahn Y, Kim JK, Jeong MH, Yoon JS (2015) Escitalopram treatment for depressive disorder following acute coronary syndrome: a 24-week double-blind, placebo-controlled trial. J Clin Psychiatry 76 (1):62–68. doi:10.4088/JCP.14m09281
37. Jiang W, Velazquez EJ, Kuchibhatla M, Samad Z, Boyle SH, Kuhn C, Becker RC, Ortel TL, Williams RB, Rogers JG, O'Connor C (2013) Effect of escitalopram on mental stress-induced myocardial ischemia: results of the REMIT trial. JAMA 309 (20):2139–2149. doi:10.1001/jama.2013.5566
38. Orth-Gomér K, Schneiderman N, Wang HX, Walldin C, Blom M, Jernberg T (2009) Stress reduction prolongs life in women with coronary disease: the Stockholm Women's Intervention Trial for Coronary Heart Disease (SWITCHD). Circ Cardiovasc Qual Outcomes 2(1): 25–32. doi:10.1161/CIRCOUTCOMES.108.812859
39. Habibović M, Burg MM, Pedersen SS (2013) Behavioral interventions in patients with an implantable cardioverter defibrillator: lessons learned and where to go from here? Pacing Clin Electrophysiol 36(5):578–590. doi:10.1111/pace.12108
40. Blumenthal JA, Babyak M, Wei J, O'Connor C, Waugh R, Eisenstein E, Mark D, Sherwood A, Woodley PS, Irwin RJ, Reed G (2002) Usefulness of psychosocial treatment of mental stress-induced myocardial ischemia in men. Am J Cardiol 89 (2):164–168
41. Whalley B, Rees K, Davies P, Bennett P, Ebrahim S, Liu Z, West R, Moxham T, Thompson DR, Taylor RS (2011) Psychological interventions for coronary heart disease. Cochrane Database Syst Rev 8:CD002902. doi:10.1002/14651858.CD002902.pub3
42. Bekke-Hansern S, Trockel M, Burg MM, Taylor CB (2012) Depressive symptom dimensions and cardiac prognosis following myocardial infarction: results from the ENRICHD clinical trial. Psychol Med 42:51–60
43. Freedland KE, Carney RM, Rich MW, Steinmeyer BC, Rubin EH (2015) Cognitive behavior therapy for depression and self-care in heart failure patients: a randomized clinical trial. JAMA Intern Med 175 (11):1773–1782. doi:10.1001/jamainternmed.2015.5220
44. Baumeister H, Hutter N, Bengel J (2011) Psychological and pharmacological interventions for depression in patients with coronary artery disease. Cochrane Database Syst Rev 9:CD008012. doi:10.1002/14651858.CD008012.pub3
45. Emani S, Binkley PF (2010) Mind-body medicine in chronic heart failure: a translational science challenge. Circ Heart Fail 3(6):715–725. doi:10.1161/CIRCHEARTFAILURE.110.951509
46. Olex S, Newberg A, Figueredo VM (2013) Meditation: should a cardiologist care? Int J Cardiol 168 (3):1805–1810. doi:10.1016/j.ijcard.2013.06.086
47. Marchand WR (2014) Neural mechanisms of mindfulness and meditation: evidence from neuroimaging studies. World J Radiol 6(7):471–479. doi:10.4329/wjr.v6.i7.471
48. Younge JO, Gotink RA, Baena CP, Roos-Hesselink JW, Hunink MM (2015) Mind-body practices for patients with cardiac disease: a systematic review and meta-analysis. Eur J Prev Cardiol 22 (11):1385–1398. doi:10.1177/2047487314549927
49. Brook RD, Appel LJ, Rubenfire M, Ogedegbe G, Bisognano JD, Elliott WJ, Fuchs FD, Hughes JW, Lackland DT, Staffileno BA, Townsend RR, Rajagopalan S (2013) Beyond medications and diet: alternative approaches to lowering blood pressure: a scientific statement from the American Heart Association. Hypertension 61:1360–1383. doi:10.1161/HYP.0b013e318293645f
50. Barnes VA, Orme-Johnson DW (2012) Prevention and treatment of cardiovascular disease in adolescents and adults through the transcendental meditation(®) program: a research review update. Curr Hypertens Rev 8(3):227–242

51. Hartley L, Mavrodaris A, Flowers N, Ernst E, Rees K (2014) Transcendental meditation for the primary prevention of cardiovascular disease. Cochrane Database Syst Rev 12:CD010359. doi:10.1002/14651858.CD010359.pub2
52. Jayadevappa R, Johnson JC, Bloom BS, Nidich S, Desai S, Chhatre S, Raziano DB, Schneider R (2007) Effectiveness of transcendental meditation on functional capacity and quality of life of African Americans with congestive heart failure: a randomized control study. Ethnic Dis 17:72–77
53. Schneider RH, Grim CE, Rainforth MV, Kotchen T, Nidich SI, Gaylord-King C, Salerno JW, Kotchen JM, Alexander CN (2012) Stress reduction in the secondary prevention of cardiovascular disease: randomized, controlled trial of transcendental meditation and health education in Blacks. Circ Cardiovasc Qual Outcomes 5(6):750–758. doi:10.1161/CIRCOUTCOMES.112.967406
54. Nesvold A, Fagerland MW, Davanger S, Ellingsen Ø, Solberg EE, Holen A, Sevre K, Atar D (2012) Increased heart rate variability during nondirective meditation. Eur J Prev Cardiol 19(4):773–780. doi:10.1177/1741826711414625
55. Goyal M, Singh S, Sibinga EM, Gould NF, Rowland-Seymour A, Sharma R, Berger Z, Sleicher D, Maron DD, Shihab HM, Ranasinghe PD, Linn S, Saha S, Bass EB, Haythornthwaite JA (2014) Meditation programs for psychological stress and well-being: a systematic review and meta-analysis. JAMA Intern Med 174 (3):357–368. doi:10.1001/jamainternmed.2013.13018
56. Loucks EB, Schuman-Olivier Z, Britton WB, Fresco DM, Desbordes G, Brewer JA, Fulwiler C (2015) Mindfulness and cardiovascular disease risk: state of the evidence, plausible mechanisms, and theoretical framework. Curr Cardiol Rep 17(12):112. doi:10.1007/s11886-015-0668-7
57. Keyworth C, Knopp J, Roughley K, Dickens C, Bold S, Coventry P (2014) A mixed-methods pilot study of the acceptability and effectiveness of a brief meditation and mindfulness intervention for people with diabetes and coronary heart disease. Behav Med 40(2):53–64. doi:10.1080/08964289.2013.834865
58. Kemper KJ, Powell D, Helms CC, Kim-Shapiro DB (2015) Loving-kindness meditation's effects on nitric oxide and perceived well-being: a pilot study in experienced and inexperienced meditators. Explore (NY) 11(1):32–39. doi:10.1016/j.explore.2014.10.002
59. Lehmann N, Paul A, Moebus S, Budde T, Dobos GJ, Michalsen A (2011) Effects of lifestyle modification on coronary artery calcium progression and prognostic factors in coronary patients – 3-year results of the randomized SAFE-LIFE trial. Atherosclerosis 219 (2):630–636. doi:10.1016/j.atherosclerosis.2011.08.050
60. Hagins M, States R, Selfe T, Innes K (2013) Effectiveness of yoga for hypertension: systematic review and meta-analysis. Evid Based Complement Alternat Med 2013:649836. doi:10.1155/2013/649836
61. Chu P, Gotink RA, Yeh GY, Goldie SJ, Hunink MM (2014) The effectiveness of yoga in modifying risk factors for cardiovascular disease and metabolic syndrome: a systematic review and meta-analysis of randomized controlled trials. Eur J Prev Cardiol. pii:2047487314562741
62. Yadav RK, Magan D, Yadav R, Sarvottam K, Netam R (2014) High-density lipoprotein cholesterol increases following a short-term yoga-based lifestyle intervention: a non-pharmacological modulation. Acta Cardiol 69(5):543–549
63. Manchanda SC, Madan K (2014) Yoga and meditation in cardiovascular disease. Clin Res Cardiol 103 (9):675–680. doi:10.1007/s00392-014-0663-9
64. Wang X, Pi Y, Chen B, Chen P, Liu Y, Wang R, Li X, Zhu Y, Yang Y, Niu Z (2015) Effect of traditional Chinese exercise on the quality of life and depression for chronic diseases: a meta-analysis of randomised trials. Sci Rep 5:15913. doi:10.1038/srep15913
65. Nery RM, Zanini M, de Lima JB, Bühler RP, da Silveira AD, Stein R (2015) Tai Chi Chuan improves functional capacity after myocardial infarction: a randomized clinical trial. Am Heart J 169 (6):854–860. doi:10.1016/j.ahj.2015.01.017
66. Yeh GY, Wood MJ, Wayne PM, Quilty MT, Stevenson LW, Davis RB, Phillips RS, Forman DE (2013) Tai chi in patients with heart failure with preserved ejection fraction. Congest Heart Fail 19 (2):77–84. doi:10.1111/chf.12005
67. Yeh GY, McCarthy EP, Wayne PM, Stevenson LW, Wood MJ, Forman D, Davis RB, Phillips RS (2011) Tai chi exercise in patients with chronic heart failure: a randomized clinical trial. Arch Intern Med 171 (8):750–757. doi:10.1001/archinternmed.2011.150

13 Ozone Therapy as a Complementary Treatment in Cardiovascular Diseases

N. Dardes, V. Covi, and G. Tabaracci

13.1 The Therapeutic Effect of Ozone

Ozone is a metastable gas, made up of three oxygen atoms, is faintly blue, and owes its name to the characteristic pungent odor (from the Greek *ozein*: smell). It is known for the layer existing 22 km from the Earth, which is necessary to largely protect us from ultraviolet radiation, and for its toxicity to the airways, as a result of air pollution.

Soon the stigma of ozone toxicity was overcome, thereby encouraging its use as a therapeutic agent. Many other gaseous and nongaseous molecules are harmful if used in excessive doses and concentrations, but if they are used within the correct range of values, and via appropriate routes of administration, they have a useful and important therapeutic effect in many fields of medicine [1].

Ozone has been used for therapeutic purposes since the end of the eighteenth century. The history of the therapeutic use of ozone is shown in the box.

History of ozone as a therapeutic agent
1785: ozone was mentioned for the first time in the scientific literature: it was described in an experiment by Martin van Marum, a Dutch physicist
1840: Professor C.F. Schonbein perceived a distinctive smell while studying the slow oxidation of white phosphorus and water electrolysis. This smell was similar to that smelled during a storm; thus he coined the term "ozone" from the Greek *ozein* (smelling)
1850: first scientific publications in journals such as *The Lancet* and the *British Medical Journal*
1896: first ozone generator was patented by Tesla
1897: Major G. Stoker established the Oxygen Hospital in London, for the treatment of ulcers and wounds by oxygen
1932: the Swiss dentist E.A. Fisch understood the enormous advantages of using ozone in local therapies. He treated the surgeon E. Payr for his gangrenous pulpitis using gas injections and ozonated water
1957: H. Wolff and J. Hänsler began to use major autohemotherapy
1980: The advent of ozone therapy in Italy is due to C. Verga: he noticed that myalgic pain disappeared after local injection, and in 1989 he published "New therapeutic approach to lumbar herniations and protrusions"
Recent years: many scientific works written by Cuban, Spanish, German, Russian, Italian, American physicians (and those from other many countries) have been published

The current applications of ozone therapy include many fields of medicine, such as orthopedics (e.g., herniated discs, arthritis, spinal stenosis, tendinitis, peripheral neuropathy from compression), internal medicine (hepatitis, diabetes), cardiology (outcomes of ischemia and

N. Dardes (✉)
Guglielmo Marconi University, Rome, Italy
e-mail: nicoladardes@hotmail.com

V. Covi • G. Tabaracci
San Rocco Clinic Center, Montichiari, Brescia, Italy

M. Fioranelli (ed.), *Integrative Cardiology*, DOI 10.1007/978-3-319-40010-5_13

infarction, atherosclerosis), bronchopneumology (chronic obstructive pulmonary disease, pulmonary fibrosis, emphysema), rheumatology (rheumatoid arthritis, systemic lupus erythematosus, Sjögren's syndrome), neurology (vasomotor and cluster headaches, multiple sclerosis, dementia of various causes), gastroenterology (Crohn's disease, ulcerative colitis), ophthalmology (retinal arterial disease, dry eye syndrome), gynecology (vaginitis, dysmenorrhea), surgery (vascular ulcers, diabetic foot, infected wounds), aesthetic medicine (cellulitis, visible capillaries, wrinkles, dystrophic scars).

13.2 Biochemical and Pathophysiological Basis of the Therapeutical Effect of Ozone

13.2.1 Biochemistry

Ozone is detectable at concentrations between 98.16 and 19.63 μg/m^3 (0.002 ppm). It is composed of three atoms of oxygen (allotropic form) and is formed by an endothermic process: $3O_2$ + 68,400 cal → $2O_3$; it has a PM of 48 and a rate of decomposition of 105–106 mol/s.

In water, ozone is 1.6 times denser and 10 times more soluble than oxygen (49 ml/100 ml of water at 0 °C). Although it is not a radical, it is the third largest oxidant, after fluoride and persulfate.

Ozone is produced from three sources of energy: chemical electrolysis, electric discharge and UV radiation, through a reversible reaction. Ozone half-life depends inversely proportional to the ambient temperature and the salinity of the water, and directly proportional to the pressure, the capacity of the syringe and the concentration of the mixture. For medical purposes, therefore, it can't be stored, but it must be prepared at the moment of use.

Ozone has the ability to react with the majority of organic and inorganic substances until it reaches complete oxidation. It presents a preferable selectivity for the double and triple bonds present in the cells, fluids or tissues, such as amino acids and unsaturated fatty acids, part of lipoprotein complexes of the plasma and of the double layer of cell membranes, DNA molecules and cysteine residues of the protein. When the gas mixture comes into contact with biological fluids, it dissolve within a few seconds in water. The effectiveness of administration is closely linked to the reaction with phospholipid membranes, determining, after partial initial consumption, the formation of ozonides, aldehydes, reactive oxygen species (ROS), including hydrogen peroxide (H_2O_2), and lipoperoxides (LOPs), in controlled amounts.

Formation of ROS in plasma is very rapid (less than 1 min), and it is accompanied by a transient decrease in antioxidant capacity (5–25%), returning it to a normal value within 15–20 min. Hydrogen peroxide and other mediators spread within the cells, triggering more pathways into erythrocytes, leukocytes, and platelets.

Considering the small amount of ozone used in the blood, compared with the various systemic actions, a direct action of such products on all the membranes is not possible, but there is a mechanism of induction of the synthesis and activation of various biologically active components. The obtainable effects on the organism determine an improvement in many metabolic processes.

13.2.2 Effects on Oxygen Metabolism and Rheology

Peroxides produced by the interaction of ozone with the phospholipid bilayer enter into erythrocytes, producing controlled oxidative stress. Thus, glycolysis is stimulated in the red blood cells, through the activation of the pentose phosphate pathway, resulting in:

- Increased production of adenosine triphosphate (ATP), which stabilizes the membrane potential and improves the mechanical strength
- A slow decrease in intracellular pH (Bohr effect)

- Increased 2,3-DPG, a direct inhibitor of the affinity of hemoglobin for oxygen

The newly generated red blood cells have an increased G-6PD activity (super gifted erythrocytes), and very gradually they replace only those that have completed their life cycle, without affecting the patient's hematocrit.

There are also several rheological effects, such as the activation of the nitric oxide (NO) synthase, with subsequent NO production, induction of carbon monoxide (CO) production, and the activity of enzymes such as trypsin, some proteases, and elastase, in a controlled manner. In addition, an increasing negative charge on the membrane surface of red blood cells is induced, improving the elasticity and deformability of these cells. From these biochemical processes a greater oxygen supply for the tissues, a controlled anticoagulant effect, a reduced stacking of erythrocytes, a reduced blood viscosity and platelet aggregation, an increased oxygen partial pressure in arterial blood, and a decrease in oxygen pressure in venous blood, with a consequent decrease in venous and capillary stasis, can be achieved.

13.2.3 Modulation of Oxidative Stress

Ozone is consumed within minutes after administration, because of its high reactivity and solubility. As previously mentioned, hydrogen peroxide and LOPs are formed from it at doses not exceeding the anti-oxidant capacity of the organism. The oxidation products effectively determine a transient increase in oxidative processes, and they induce the activation of anti-oxidant systems after a few minutes, such as superoxide dismutase (SOD), catalase, and glutathione peroxidase, leading to a rebalancing of the redox components.

Hydrogen peroxide is rapidly converted into water, LOP 4-hydroxynonenal (4-HNE) enhances anti-oxidant enzymes, acting as a trigger: it forms a compound with Cys 34 of albumin and with glutathione, and it induces adaptive responses through the increase in NO and bilirubin, acting as direct anti-oxidants.

4-HNE reacts with the cytosolic Nrf2-Keap1 system, forming a complex that releases Nrf-2, a protein present in all body cells, activated by controlled oxidative stress, and a key compound in the defense against oxidative stress.

This repeated oxidative stress causes a "preconditioning effect," balancing the redox system, altered by pathogenic stimuli. At ozone concentrations usually employed in medicine, these are transient and controlled processes, compatible with the anti-oxidant capacity in the blood. The redox imbalance is correlated with many diseases, from inflammatory processes to autoimmune diseases. All of these pathological conditions can be treated with ozone, with remarkable results. However, it is very important to know the correct ozone concentration and doses that are effective against a specific pathological condition to be treated and do not exceed the anti-oxidant capacity of the organism [2].

13.2.4 Reactivation of Innate Defense System

After its release, Nrf2 translocates to the nucleus and binds to DNA at the site of the antioxidant response element anti-oxidant response element (ARE; or hARE: human) regulator of the entire antioxidant system.

The activation of Nrf2/ARE causes:

- An increase in anti-oxidant enzymes direct (GSH, CO, and bilirubin) and detoxification (catalase, SOD, GPx, GSTR, NADPH-quinone oxidoreductase [NQO1], HO-1, HSP70)
- An increase in phase II enzymes (glutathione *S*-transferase, UDP-glucuronosyltransferase, *N*-acetyltransferase, and sulfotransferase)
- Inhibition of the production of inflammatory cytokines, induction of leukotriene B4 reductase
- A reduction of serum iron, and the resulting oxidative stress from high ferritin

- Recognition, repair, and removal of damaged proteins
- Protection from apoptosis due to oxidative stress
- Increased activity of DNA repair
- Increase of adrenocorticotropic hormone, cortisol, and corticotropin-releasing hormone

13.2.5 Immunomodulation

Ozone induces in balanced amounts the synthesis of cytokines by monocytes, macrophages, and lymphocytes, the release of cytokines and immunosuppressive immunostimulants (TGF-β1, IFNβ, γ, and δ, TNF, IL-1β, 2, 4, 6, 8, 10), and activation of nonspecific defense systems, humoral and cellular immunity.

Therefore, considering the induced modulation, ozone can be used both in autoimmune diseases and in immune deficiencies.

13.2.6 Bactericidal, Virus Static, and Antifungal Action

According to the literature data, ozone acts against any Gram-positive and Gram-negative bacterium known, including *Pseudomonas aeruginosa* and *Escherichia coli*, all lipophilic and hydrophilic viruses, and each fungal spore and protozoa.

Ozone alters plasma membrane permeability and homeostasis within the cell. During lipid peroxidation, new bonds are formed between proteins and lipids, causing ultrastructural damage in the cytoplasm leading to the destruction of the cellular organelles within 10–20 min.

These direct actions occur if the mixture is used at high concentrations. Unlike most antiseptics, ozone does not irritate or affect the healthy tissue surrounding the area of administration.

Furthermore, ozone can be generated in vivo in activated neutrophils; for this reason, it is not only a bactericidal agent, but also a component of the physiological mechanisms of inflammation, probably related to a reaction catalyzed by antibodies. It acts on a nonspecific immune system (activation of phagocytosis, increased synthesis of cytokines and interferon, interleukins, and TNF), and cellular and humoral immunity.

The use of ozone against infection can be systemic, local, or combined, because it acts either through the rupture of cell membranes by local action or via the stimulation of the immune system, increasing the defense capacity of the organism.

13.2.7 Metabolic Activation of Carbohydrates and Lipids

Low doses of ozone promote the oxidation of carbohydrates, lipids, and proteins, forming ATP, and activating the Krebs cycle and the beta-oxidation of fatty acids, determined by the displacement of equilibrium toward the oxidized form of NAD; the acetyl coenzyme A formed is incorporated into the Krebs cycle.

Ozone enhances the use of glucose, and decreases partially oxidized metabolites in the blood and the respiratory rate.

13.2.8 Anti-Inflammatory and Analgesic Action

Ozone has the ability to oxidize compounds in a double layer, such as arachidonic acid and prostaglandins, inducing and maintaining inflammation.

Furthermore, ozone is capable of inactivating metabolic mediators of pain. Therefore, it acts as a painkiller and as an anti-inflammatory agent, and induces an improvement in the microcirculation, with an increase in the transport of oxygen to tissues.

13.2.9 Action on the Endothelium

Hydrogen peroxide induces the synthesis of NO and the trans-endothelial migration of leukocytes, increasing the number of fibroblasts and remodeling of endothelial cells.

13.2.10 Detoxifying Action

In liver cells, ozone administration determines the system of cytochrome p450 enzyme accumulation, increasing the amount of glycogen and of antioxidants, and inducing the production of ATP.

The detoxifying effect manifests as the optimization of liver microsomes and filtering liver. The use of glucose is increased at a systemic level, in addition to enzymes such as lactate and pyruvate, and gluconeogenesis.

13.2.11 Effect on Well-Being

Administered ozone induces a complex release of hormones such as CRH, ACTH, cortisol, DHEA, GH, and endorphins, with an increase in serotonin and dopamine, resulting in the patient reporting a feeling of well-being.

13.2.12 Action on the Intervertebral Nucleus Pulposus

The action of ozone on the intervertebral disk takes place on several levels:

- Inhibition of PLA2 and PGE2 and other pro-inflammatory cytokines (IL-1, -2, -8, -12, -15, and IFN)
- Increased release of immunosuppressive cytokines (IL-10, factor B1), with analgesic and anti-inflammatory effect
- An increase in local microcirculation, reducing venous stasis, with an analgesic effect as the nerve root is very sensitive to hypoxia
- Direct effect on mucopolysaccharides and proteoglycans in the nucleus pulposus, with dehydration and production of chemical lysis
- Matrix degeneration, replaced by collagen fibers, and the formation of new blood cells, reducing the volume of the disk

There is therefore a combination of vascular and biochemical effects of ozone on the disk and nerve root compression, leading to an improvement in the symptoms and, in many cases, to the complete resolution of the syndrome.

13.3 Oxygen–Ozone Therapy in Cardiovascular Disease

Literature data indicate that supportive treatment with ozone administered by major autohemotherapy may be useful in patients suffering from ischemic heart disease, in patients with chronic heart failure due to cardiomyopathy or cardiac valve defects, and in subjects with peripheral arterial circulatory disorders.

13.3.1 Ischemic Heart Disease

As far as ischemic heart disease is concerned, it has been demonstrated that oxygen radicals play a role in the pathogenesis of myocardial ischemia and that peroxidation of arachidonic acid increases platelet aggregation. Moreover, the in vivo activation of macrophages causes a reduction of intracellular glutathione peroxidase activity, which is associated with the increased capacity of the cells to generate ROS, including hydroperoxides. This macrophage activation occurs both in inflammatory processes and in atherosclerotic disease. Effectively, a decrease in glutathione peroxidase and superoxide dismutase activity has been observed in patients with myocardial infarction. These data suggest the usefulness of scavenger agents in the therapy of infarction. Hernandez and colleagues reported that ozone autohemotherapy induces a significant increase in glutathione peroxidase activity, whereas a reduction in blood cholesterol levels has been reported by Rilling and co-workers.

Twenty-two patients who had myocardial infarction between 3 months and 1 year before the study were treated with ozone by autohemotherapy carried out in 15 sessions in the Ozone Research Center of Havana, Cuba, by Hernandez and colleagues. The authors reported a significant decrease in plasma total cholesterol and low-density lipoprotein (LDL). Erythrocyte glutathione peroxidase and glucose 6 phosphate dehydrogenase activity increased significantly, whereas no changes in plasma lipid peroxidation were found. The results indicated a significant activation of the anti-oxidant protection system in patients with myocardial infarction. These observations suggest that complementary therapy with ozone might play a relevant role in ischemic cardiac patients; nonetheless, further controlled clinical trials are necessary to evaluate the impact of the treatment on long-term survival, quality of life, and recurrence of acute episodes [3–7].

13.3.2 Chronic Cardio-Respiratory Insufficiency

One of the most striking features of the intravenous administration of ozone via autohemotherapy concerns the changes in the metabolic and rheological properties of the red blood cells. As mentioned above, owing to the specific intervention of ozone in the metabolism of red blood cells, glycolysis and the pentose phosphate shunt are activated to such an extent that new 2,3-DPG is produced and the oxygen affinity of the hemoglobin is reduced. This action on the red blood cells causes a shift in the O_2 bonding curve of hemoglobin to the right, increasing oxygen delivery to the peripheral tissues.

In healthy professional sportsmen, there was as a rule a 2,3-DPG increase of approximately 10% after a series of systemic ozone applications. In pathophysiological conditions, such as chronic respiratory failure due to either cardiac or pulmonary diseases, a similar effect could be achieved by treatment with ozone [8, 9].

In our personal experience, 40 patients suffering from chronic respiratory failure due to chronic obstructive pulmonary disease and 30 patients with cardiac insufficiency due to ischemic coronary disease and/or valvular disorders have been treated with complementary therapy with ozone administered by major autohemotherapy according to a standard procedure in 12 sessions of treatment. A significant reduction in the dyspnea score, measured by the Analogic Scale, the Borg Scale and the MMRC scale, was recorded in both groups. The Six-Minute Walk Test improved in most patients in both groups. We concluded that the observed improvement in the exercise tolerance could be due to the increased peripheral delivery of oxygen.

13.3.3 Peripheral Circulatory Disorders

Peculiar pathophysiological conditions may result in reduced or high fluctuating 2,3-DPG levels in diabetics, contributing to causing a reduction in oxygen supply to peripheral tissues.

In a group of patients with stage III and IV arterial circulatory disorders, according to Fontaine, the effect of ozone therapy on 2,3-DPG levels was evaluated and compared using Student's *t* test versus placebo. A significant increase in 2,3-DPG was found in treated patients who showed signs of improved peripheral oxygenation [10].

13.4 Guidelines

Vieban-Hansler and a group of members of the International Ozone Association recently proposed Guidelines for Ozone Therapy. In fact, medical ozone produces the same therapeutic effects in each specific disease and condition if properly applied. Improper application for erratic methods and doses is the most frequent cause of ineffectiveness and adverse effects. The basis of the guidelines for the medical use of ozone can be summarized as follows:

1. The pharmacological effect of medical ozone follows the principle of hormesis: low doses show a high efficacy, which decreases with increasing doses or concentrations, finally reversing into a questionable or toxic effect. On this basis, according to the literature reports, the dose/effect or concentration/effect relationship for the systemic use of ozone (autohemotherapy or rectal insufflations) has been standardized as follows:
   a. Oxygen–ozone mixture of 10–40 μg ozone/ml is physiologically effective and recommended for systemic application.

b. Within the high concentration range of 60–100 μg/ml the application of ozone has an antibiotic effect with a wide range of applications completely restricted to the topical forms of application.

2. Ozone is applied complementary to a corresponding basic therapy. Diabetes, cardiovascular diseases, chronic inflammatory diseases, diabetic angiopathy, and macular disease represent the classical indications for low-dose systemic ozone treatment.

In the field of cardiovascular disease, the complementary treatment with ozone is carried out exclusively by major autohemotherapy. The indications as a complementary treatment are:

1. Peripheral arterial circulatory disorders
2. Cerebral and ocular circulatory disorders
3. Inner ear circulatory diseases (acute hearing loss, tinnitus)
4. Diabetic angiopathy
5. Cardio-respiratory insufficiency
6. Coronary disease

The treatment is contraindicated in glucose-6-phosphate dehydrogenase deficiency, uncontrolled hyperthyroidism, pregnancy (first 3 months).

Treatment with ozone is not indicated in leukemia [11–13].

13.5 Medical Ozone: Production, Devices, and Methods of Administration

13.5.1 Generation of Medical Ozone

Medical ozone is a mixture of ozone in oxygen, under normal therapeutic indications it must be used within a concentration range between 0.5 and 5% (7–50 μg ozone/ml of oxygen).

The total dose is equivalent to the volume of gas (mL) multiplied by the ozone concentration (mg/mL). The equipment generating ozone induces the passage of an electrical discharge through a flow of pure oxygen for medical use. It must produce the mixture in a reliable manner, i.e., at accurate and reproducible concentrations, which must remain constant against the resistance of the syringe (spectrophotometric control), and all the materials in contact with ozone are inert to it.

In the European Union, ozone generators are considered to be health products and are registered with qualification II-b, and they will be reviewed in due course. Cylinders containing pure oxygen must be certified by a full license, and require a pressure reducer, which allows an emission at 0.8 bar.

The gas in the syringe should be aspirated through a bacterial filter that is resistant to ozone and made of hydrophobic Teflon with a pore size of 0.2 μm, to prevent contamination.

When a continuous flow of gas is required, for example, in bagging, an adequate connection, silicone, PVC, or polyethylene can be incorporated, to the valve output of the ozone generator.

Ozone must be prepared at the time of use, because of its decay to oxygen in relatively short times.

For various medical applications, physicians must know the optimal ozone doses and concentrations required to achieve a specific therapeutic effect, avoiding any toxicity, and in accordance with the guidelines.

13.5.2 Administration Modalities

Depending on the pathological condition to be treated, in addition to the doses and appropriate concentrations, the choice of the correct method of administration is crucial. The route of administration can be local or systemic:

a. Local administration
   - Injections: intramuscular, intra- and periarticular, intraforaminal and intradiscal, myofascial, perinervous and peritendinous, subcutaneous, intralesional

- Insufflation: nasal or vaginal
- Bagging: this method consists in using a bag which raises the part to be treated; after creating the vacuum, it fills the bag with the ozone concentration required in order (disinfection or regeneration), leaving everything for 20 min
- Ozonated oil
- Ozonated water

b. Systemic administration
- Major autohemotherapy: this procedure consists in the withdrawal in a special container (soft plastic bag or glass, inert to ozone) of a specific amount of blood (100–200 ml) from a peripheral vein; this blood is then placed in contact with the same amount of ozone (ratio = 1:1) inside the kit employed, reinfusing all via the same route (closed circuit).
- Minor autohemotherapy: cycle treatment includes 10–12 sessions twice a week, and subsequent references, at intervals to be determined based on the patient and condition being treated. Changing the method of administration and the concentration of the mixture of oxygen and ozone we can obtain different biological effects.
- Rectal insufflation: this procedure consists in the administration of ozone at the concentration of 10–50 μg ozone/ml of oxygen. The volume administered ranges between 150 and 300 ml. Administration is carried out using a rectal catheter connected to a 50-ml silicon-coated disposable syringe. This is one of the earliest forms of application in ozone therapy and is considered an alternative to major autohemotherapy.

References

1. Viebahn-Hansler R (2007) The use of ozone in medicine. ODREI, Iffezheim
2. Leon Fernandez OS (2014) Ozone therapy, oxidative conditioning, basis for its clinical effectiveness. ODREI, Iffezhheim
3. Hernandez F, Menendez S, Wong R (1995) Decrease of blood cholesterol and stimulation of the antioxidative response in cardiopathy patients treated with endovenous ozone therapy. Free Rad Biol Med 19:1115–1119
4. O'Neil W, Timmis G, Bourdillon P, Lai P et al (1986) A prospective randomized clinical trial of intracoronary Streptokinase versus coronary angioplastic therapy of acute myocardial infarction. N Engl J Med 314:812–828
5. Ellis SG, Wynne J, Braunwald E, Henschke CI, Sandor T, Kloner RA (1984) Response to reperfusion salvaged stunned myocardium to inotropic stimulation. Am Heart J 107:13–19
6. Hernandez F, Menendez S, Gomez M, Eng L (1989) Efecto de la ozonoterapia intravascular sobre el sistema de la glutation peroxidasa. Rev CENIC Ciencias Biol 20:37–40
7. Rilling S (1985) The basic clinical application of ozone therapy. Sci Eng 7:259–274
8. Parnham MJ et al (1987) Selenium hydroperoxides and atherosclerosis. Agent Actions 22:353–354
9. Ambrosio G, Becker LC et al (1986) Reduction in experimental infarct size by recombinant human superoxide dismutase: insights into the pathophysiology of reperfusion injury. Circulation 74:1424–1433
10. Dardes N, Covi V, Vaccaro MF, Tabaracci G (2015) Oxygen-ozone therapy in patients with chronic respiratory failure. In: Proceeding of CHEST national congress. CHEST Delegation Italy. Rome
11. Bocci V, Zanardi I, Travagli V (2011) Oxygen/ozone as a medical gas mixture. A critical evaluation. Med Gas Res 1:6
12. European Communities. Directives 2008/50/EC. Offi J Eur Union. L152:1–44
13. Viebahn-Hansler R, Leon Fernandez OS, Fahmy Z (2012) Ozone in medicine: the low-dose ozone concept. Guidelines and treatment strategies. Ozone 34: 408–424

Part II

Integrated Approach to Cardiovascular Disease

Integrated Approach to Dyslipidemia 14

Mara Piccoli, Massimo Fioranelli, Maria Grazia Roccia, Veronica Di Nardo, Claudio Tomella, and Carlo Dal Lin

14.1 Introduction

Life expectancy has lengthened in the past century in Italy: the average age for men is 79.21 years and for women, 84.59 years. The current aging population is affected by chronic diseases. People can live longer and healthier if they become aware of preventive medicine and if they change their lifestyle and nutrition. Despite the availability of numerous therapies for the treatment of cardiovascular diseases, these are still the leading cause of mortality and morbidity in the industrialized world (Circulation, 2008).

M. Piccoli (✉)
UO Cardiologia, Policlinico L.di Liegro, Rome, Italy
e-mail: mandimara@libero.it

M. Fioranelli, MD
Department of nuclear physics, Sub-nuclear and Radiation, Guglielmo Marconi University, Rome, Italy

M.G. Roccia, PhD
University B.I.S. Group of Institutions, Punjab Technical University, Punjab, India

V. Di Nardo, PhD • C. Tomella, MD
Guglielmo Marconi University, Rome, Italy

C. Dal Lin, MD
Department of Cardiological, Thoracic and Vascular Sciences, Padua University Medical School, Padova, Italy

14.2 Nutrition

The relationship between diet and cardiovascular risk is very complex and more detailed knowledge on the subject has recently been developed. It has become increasingly evident how important are the quality and the amount of carbohydrate ingested, and the quantity and quality of fatty acids consumptions. The action of a single nutrient is not decisive, nor is the effect of a single risk factor, but comprehensive assessment of the impact of all the risk factors involved is needed, integrating information relating to the direct effect of a nutrient or of "examined food" on clinical events.

In the first half of 1900, Angel Keys, physiologist at the University of Minnesota, began what is known as the Seven Countries Study of Cardiovascular Diseases. In addition to being the prototype of epidemiological studies concerning cardiovascular diseases; it showed the benefits of a high consumption of plant foods, with plenty of unrefined grains, vegetables, fruits, legumes, fish, olive oil, and moderate amounts of wine. A reduction of 25% of foods of animal origin, and an increase of 25% of foods of plant origin, would be associated with a 32% reduction in cardiovascular mortality to 25 years [1].

The Mediterranean diet has proven to be a successful model in cardiovascular prevention, based simply on the availability of raw material that could be accessed, and it is not designed with

M. Fioranelli (ed.), *Integrative Cardiology*, DOI 10.1007/978-3-319-40010-5_14

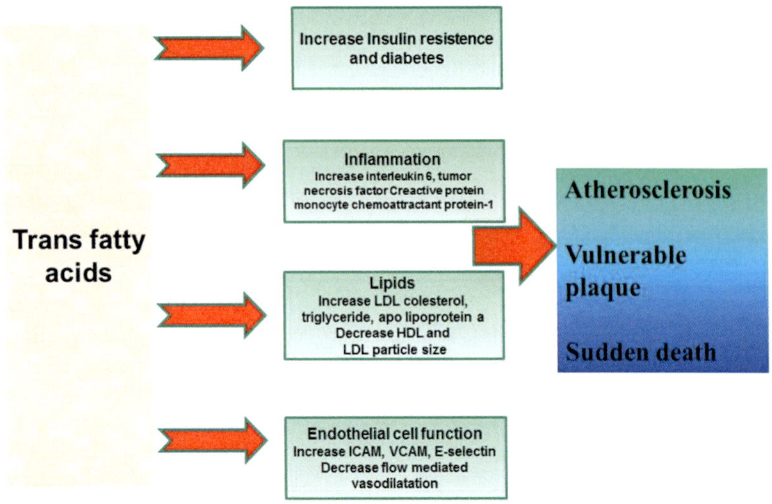

Fig. 14.1 Trans-fatty acids and atherosclerotic effects

a role of cardioprotection. Therefore, it can be improved based on current scientific knowledge.

One of the bases of the Mediterranean diet is olive oil, whose beneficial properties (improved lipid profile, improving the oxidation of low-density lipoprotein [LDL], insulin resistance, and inflammation) have been the subject of numerous studies. These benefits were initially attributed to the high concentration of monounsaturated fatty acids, but other active compounds exist, including polyphenols.

In fact, olive oil is made up of 99% fat, 85% of which consists of unsaturated fatty acids (70–80% monounsaturated oleic acid, 4–12% linoleic acid, a polyunsaturated fatty acid) and in smaller amounts from palmitic and stearic acid, both saturated fatty acids. In addition to fats, squalene and β-carotene, sterols (β-sitosterol), colored pigments (chlorophyll and carotenoid), fat-soluble vitamins (A and D), and phenolic compounds (simple secoiridoids, phenols, lignans, and flavonoids) are found. Just the phenolic compounds bind to the LDLs by increasing the resistance to oxidation of these lipoproteins, which are highly atherogenic [2]. In the Lyon Diet Heart Study of a post-infarcted population, a Mediterranean diet with the addition of 1 g linoleic acid was compared with a "conservative" diet. In the 27-month follow-up, a 73% reduction of coronary events was shown [3].

As already reported, the quality of fatty acids seems to make a difference. The data agree on excluding trans fatty acids from the diet (Fig. 14.1). Moreover, the amount of saturated fatty acids should be kept below 10%.

Increasing evidence in the literature shows that adequate dietary intake (between 4 and 8% of total calories) of omega 6, in particular, linoleic acid, is useful in reducing cardiovascular risk. Increasing intake of omega 6 is associated with decreased concentrations of plasma LDLs and triglycerides and increased concentrations of high-density lipoproteins (HDLs) without unfavorable evidence for arterial inflammation markers and arterial pressure and hemostasis parameters. Simple replacement of 5% of the calories from saturated fat with omega 6 causes a reduction of serum cholesterol greater than is obtained by drastically reducing dietary cholesterol (Fig. 14.2). A recent study [4] showed that the substitution of saturated fats with polyunsaturated fats entails a reduction in coronary risk; replacement with simple carbohydrates is associated with an increased risk, whereas with complex carbohydrates this risk is reduced. We cannot merely rely on a single risk marker because, if we consider the effect on

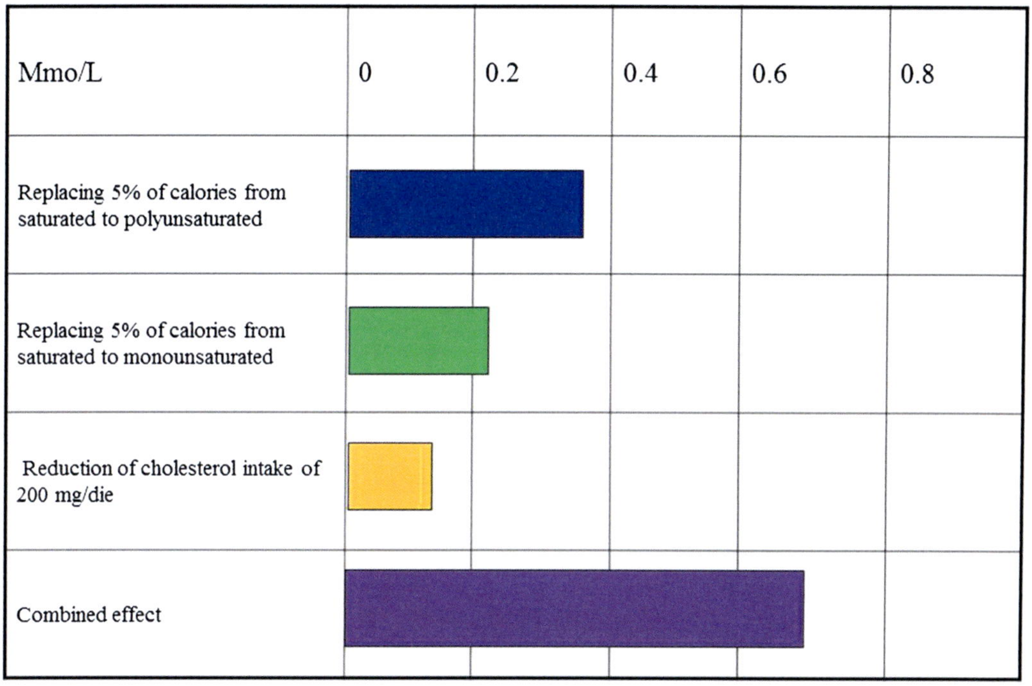

Fig. 14.2 Reduction in serum cholesterol due to substitution of saturated intake with polyunsaturated or monounsaturated or intake of dietary cholesterol reduction. Source: Clarke R, Frost C, Collins R et al. Dietary lipids and blood cholesterol: quantitative meta-analysis of metabolic ward studies. BMJ 1997;314:112–117

HDL cholesterol, all fatty acids increase this protective parameter, especially saturated fats.

Omega-3s have a known cardioprotective effect. In 1975, Sinclair observed a low incidence of heart attack and consumption of foods high in omega 3 consumption in the population of Greenland. The protective effect appears to be due to reduced synthesis and secretion of VLDL and increased clearance of plasma triglycerides and an anti-arrhythmic effect. They also have a positive effect on blood pressure, platelet aggregation, endothelial dysfunction, and systemic inflammation [5]. Omega-3s have a dose-dependent effect on the level of triglycerides, and the recommended dose is 2–3 g/day. Studies have shown a 25–52% reduction in plasma triglyceride levels.

14.2.1 Phythosterols

Phythosterols are substances naturally present in many foods, including nuts, almonds, dried fruit, cereals, vegetables (pulses), and olive oil.

Of the phytosterols identified (at least 40 types), those most frequently present in food are beta-sitosterol (50%), campesterol (33%), and stigmasterol (4%).

Phytosterols are structurally similar to human cholesterol and present poor intestinal absorption. They cannot be synthesized endogenously and are derived exclusively from the diet or are added to foods such as yogurt, margarine, sauces, and cream cheeses. Two grams per day of phytosterols have been shown to reduce LDL by about 7–10%.

Three grams per day should not be exceeded, in combination with a diet rich in vegetables and fruits, to balance the reduced blood levels of beta-carotene.

Phythosterols should not be used in:

- Pregnant and lactating women
- Children under the age of 5 years

There are limited data about the effect on risk factors for atherosclerosis and no major randomized cardiovascular outcomes data [6].

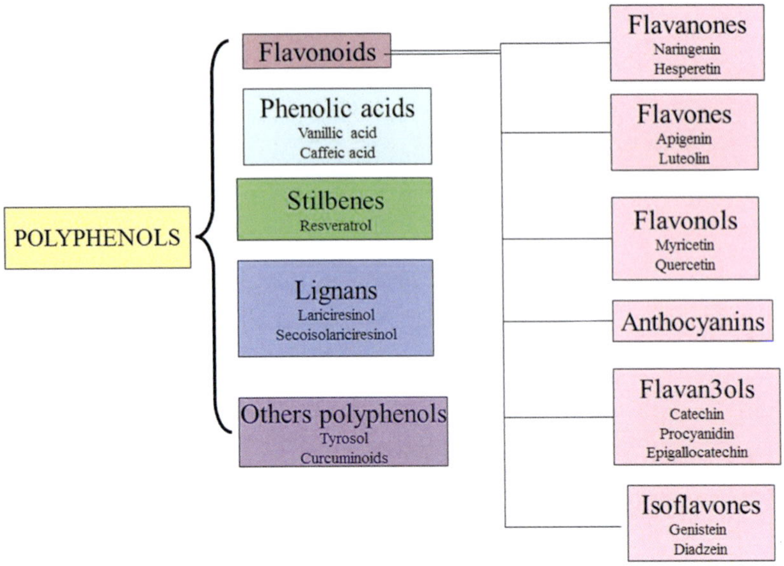

Fig. 14.3 Polyphenol classification

14.2.2 Polyphenols and Flavonoids

The term polyphenols refers to many classes of compounds with a common chemical structure, derived from benzene with one or more hydroxyl groups associated with the benzene ring. This makes these materials excellent scavengers. The high intake by diet of these compounds leads to the high reduction (50%) in cardiovascular mortality [7].

Figure 14.3 shows polyphenol classification. The beneficial effects are principally linked to the anti-oxidant capacity of these compounds and their metabolites [8, 9].

14.3 Resveratrol

Resveratrol is a polyphenol that belongs to the class of stilbenes present in small quantities in blackberries, grapes, peanuts, and red wine. Its mechanism of action seems to be the activation of SIRT1 deacetylase (silent mating type information regulation 2 homolog 1), a protein involved in the modulation of glucose and lipid metabolism and cell survival mechanisms. Studies are increasingly highlighting the power to reduce the chronic inflammation that predisposes to many diseases. Testing, whether with a low dose (8 mg) or a high dose (5 g) did not reveal any significant adverse events. Timmers et al. [10], in a study of obese individuals showed an improvement in the metabolic profile, the inflammatory status, blood pressure, and initial liver damage. Benefits for secondary cardiovascular prevention have also been shown [11].

14.4 Soy

From the botanical terms, the soy plant (*Glycine max* L. Merr.) belongs to the legume family with a high protein content (high biological value proteins), and rich in lipids and minerals (potassium calcium, phosphorus).

In the group of lipids, phosphatidylcholine is known as soy lecithin, which is the raw material of cell structures and contributes in part to reducing the levels of serum cholesterol to synergistic action with all the other constituents of the legume, such as protein, isoflavones (which behave as phytoestrogens), fibers, and saponins [12, 13].

Soybeans, because of the presence of phytoestrogens (genistein), interact with warfarin and tamoxifen and should be contraindicated in patients with estrogen-dependent tumors. Absolute caution must be applied when in constant use during childhood and adolescence because they may lead to the disorders of sexual development and somatic interference in the hypothalamic–pituitary–gonadal axis, with alterations to the sexual cycle. Furthermore, genistein inhibits the activity of cytochrome CYP3A4.

14.5 Bergamot and Bergamot Polyphenolic Fraction

Bergamot is a citrus fruit of the genus Citrus (*Citrus bergamia* Risso), belonging to the family Rutaceae, with a high content of flavonoids and flavonoid glycosides, especially naringenin and hesperetin. These compounds are absorbed by the small intestine and are hydrolyzed at the level of colon microflora in aglycones and aromatic acids. The bergamot polyphenols can activate AMP kinase (a regulator of glucose metabolism and fatty acids) or inhibit hydroxymethyl-coenzyme A (HMG-CoA) reductase (statin-like action). In popular tradition, bergamot was used as a neuro-sedative, antiseptic, and clinical bacteriostatic. Several studies have shown that the polyphenol fraction of bergamot (BPF) is effective at reducing total cholesterol, LDL, triglycerides, and glucose [14] and potentiates the effect of rosuvastatin in improving the lipid profile [15].

14.6 *Curcuma longa* L. (Zingiberaceae)

Turmeric is a herbaceous, rhizomatous, perennial native to the Far East and Australia, and *Curcuma longa* L. (also known by the name of *Curcuma domestica* Val.) is the most common species from which, after boiling and drying, the spice obtained is used, especially in Indian cooking. The rhizome, in addition to food use, is prescribed for its choleretic and cholagogue effects in functional disorders of the digestive processes attributable to the liver.

The main elements are the curcuminoids (which account for 3–5% of the drug), a mixture among which curcumin is the most abundant.

The main biological effects attributed to turmeric and curcumin are anti-oxidant, anti-inflammatory, anti-tumor, hepatoprotective, and hypolipidemic [16]. These effects are enhanced in combination with a substance of natural origin, piperine, which represents the main constituent of pepper. Serum levels of curcumin, when taken alone, are usually very low or undetectable; however, by means of a clinical study, carried out in eight healthy subjects, an increase in the curcumin bioavailability following joint administration of curcumin (2 g) and piperine (20 mg) was observed. This suggests that piperine might be beneficial to both the absorption and, consequently, its biological effects, also found in rats, in which it was shown that the concomitant use of these two substances enhances the cholesterol-lowering activity of curcumin itself. It is reasonable to hypothesize that cholesterol reduction is attributable to an increase in the bioavailability of curcumin; therefore, such a combination could represent a valuable contribution in the treatment of hyperlipidemia [17].

14.6.1 Phytotherapy

Until the advent of new drugs of plant origin acting like statins (*Monascus ruber*) and rebalancing the lipemic state (policosanol from sugarcane), herbal medicine benefitted from therapeutic agents that are still effective, even if they have been replaced with new protocols. In fact, in addition to excessive lipid intake, this condition can also be due to increased endogenous triglyceride synthesis in the liver or to insufficient exogenous elimination. In that case, we use hepatoprotective and choleretic–cholagogue function and balance hepatobiliary and intestinal functionality.

- *Cynara scolymus*
- *Taraxacum officinale*
- *Silybum marianum*
- *Peumus boldus*
- *Rosmarinus officinalis*

Other herbal remedies are used, resources still valid, even if they have been superseded by new protocols:

- *Olea europae*: the glycerin macerate Olivo, traditionally used as a hypolipidemic remedy.
- *Cynara scolymus*: artichoke, for its action as a cholagogue and laxative, is useful in hypercholesterolemia because it helps to remove bile salts via the bile and stimulating peristalsis, and their elimination through feces, resulting in decreased hepatic cholesterol. Also, it has recently been awarded a statin-like bland, formulation-titrated cynaroside.
- *Silybum marianum*: acts in dyslipidemia with a cholagogue–choleretic and liver tonic mechanism, balancing the metabolism of the hepatocytes.
- *Garcinia cambogia*: its mechanism of action is to inhibit the enzyme HMG-CoA reductase, and endogenous hepatic cholesterol production, with discrete hypolipidemic activities in overweight patients who do not follow the diet.
- *Commiphora mukul*: this Ayurvedic resin shows activity with a lipid-lowering mechanism peripheral receptor sequestrant and is therefore rationally associated with the other statin remedies above.

14.6.2 Policosanols

The alcoholic extract of sugar cane (*Saccharum officinarum*), present in significant quantities in the integuments of this plant, containing a mixture of mono-hydroxy long chain aliphatic alcohols, high molecular weight, the main representative of "1-octacosanol," which alone represents 64% of the total:

- Tetracosanol, 0.7%
- Heptacosanol, 0.7%
- Monacosanol, 0.8%
- Triacontanol, 0.9%
- Dotriacontanol, 5.4%
- Triacontanol, 12.8%
- Octacosanol, 64.5%

Although the exact mechanism of policosanol action is not yet known, it seems clear that the inhibitory activity on the enzyme HMG-COA reductase is not the only action, although it is the most relevant. They advanced various other assumptions to be verified:

- Mechanisms that directly involve the intestinal mucosa
- Intracellular carrier of fatty acid and cholesterol
- Donors h + ions to the respiratory chain
- Increased catabolism of LDL

In the literature, many data collections show very interesting results, with percentage lipid reduction similar to or even better for those obtained using synthesis statins by Cuban groups (Menendez R et al Biol Res, 1994; Menendez R et al Biol Res, 1996; Menendez R et al Arch Med Res, 2001). Ten milligrams per day of policosanol administration for at least 6 weeks reduces total cholesterol (17–21%), LDL cholesterol (21–29%), and triglycerides (13%) and increases HDL cholesterol (8–15%) [18]; however, randomized controlled trials in hyperlipemic Caucasian subjects do not confirm these data [19]. In 2015, the attenuated effects of atorvastatin on PCSK9 are obtained thanks to policosanol used in combination. The recommended dose is 10 mg per day in a single dose.

In the most challenging cases, it is possible to begin with a double dose and then decrease in function to clinical results. Useful associations are:

Monascus purpureus
Olea europaea
Garcinia cambogia
Cynara scolymus
Commiphora mukul Hook

14.7 Prebiotics

They have mechanical and physical actions and produce an acceleration of intestinal transit with more frequent evacuations and consequent elimination of some of the nutrients in the diet that are not yet absorbed, including a some of the lipids. Therefore, a portion of dietary fat is incorporated in the mucilage, once imbibed in water in the intestine, and are excreted in the feces.

This leads to lower fat absorption and a lowering of the blood lipid levels in general and triglycerides in particular:

- *Plantago ovata*
- Glucomannan

14.7.1 Monascus Ruber

The *Monascus ruber* is a mushroom traditionally used in the fermentation of red rice: the process used for centuries in China for the preparation of so-called "rice wine."

The term *Monascus ruber* indicates at least seven strains of this fungi.

- *Monascus albidus* Sato
- *Monascus pilosus* Sato
- *Monascus pubigereus* Sato
- *Monascus ruber* van Tieghem
- *Monascus paxii* Linge
- *Monascus fuliginosus* Sato
- *Monascus purpureus* Went

These mushrooms contain many active substances:

- Polyunsaturated fatty acids
- Phytosterols (b-sitosterol, campesterol, stigmasterol)
- Isoflavones and their glycosides
- Saponins
- Various red pigments
- Monacolin (at least 10: k, j, l, x etc.)

The monacolin substances derived from terpene, are certainly the most important active ingredients of the plant complex, in particular, monacolin K.

Currently, there are certain natural strains of *Monascus* at a maximum concentration of 0.4 and 0.8% of monakoline. The action at higher concentrations implies an artificial manipulation of the active principles. All clinical work from the USA cite compounds titrated to 0.4% monacolin K; Chinese studies have made use of compounds titrated to 0.8%.

All results indicate that the compound title to 0.8% does not guarantee superior results to that at 0.4%; the use of higher concentrations does not currently offer any clinical evidence.

Monascus ruber acts exactly like statin synthesis, inhibiting the enzyme HMG-CoA reductase, which, in the liver, is responsible for cholesterol synthesis. The first synthetic statin, incidentally, was developed and patented by Professor Endo, from Japan, who analyzed the chemical products in this mushroom rice [20].

The recommended dose is 400 mg (standardized to 0.4% of monacolin K), one capsule, twice a day (equivalent to 3.2 mg of monacolin K).

14.7.2 Berberine

Berberine is a plant preparation extract from the bark of *Berberis aristata*, a thorny shrub native to the Himalayas and Nepal (Berberidaceae family), still widely used in traditional local medicine. Intestinal absorption is very low (<5%), but presents a good tolerance and low side effects. Berberine has been shown to inhibit the biosynthesis of triglycerides through the activation of protein kinase activated by AMP (AMPK) enzyme that activates the (acetyl-CoA carboxylase (ACC), responsible for the transformation of acetyl-CoA in malonyl-CoA. Besides, berberine increases the expression of LDL receptor and LDL uptake in hepatic cells. In addition, berberine shows a reduction in PCSK9 protein expression, and this plays a positive role if associated with statin therapy, because statins increase PCSK9 expression. Numerous studies show benefits produced by berberine therapy used in combination with policosanols and red yeast rice (Fig. 14.4): reduction of cholesterol and glucose levels, increase in HDL and endothelial function, and a decrease in the body mass index without

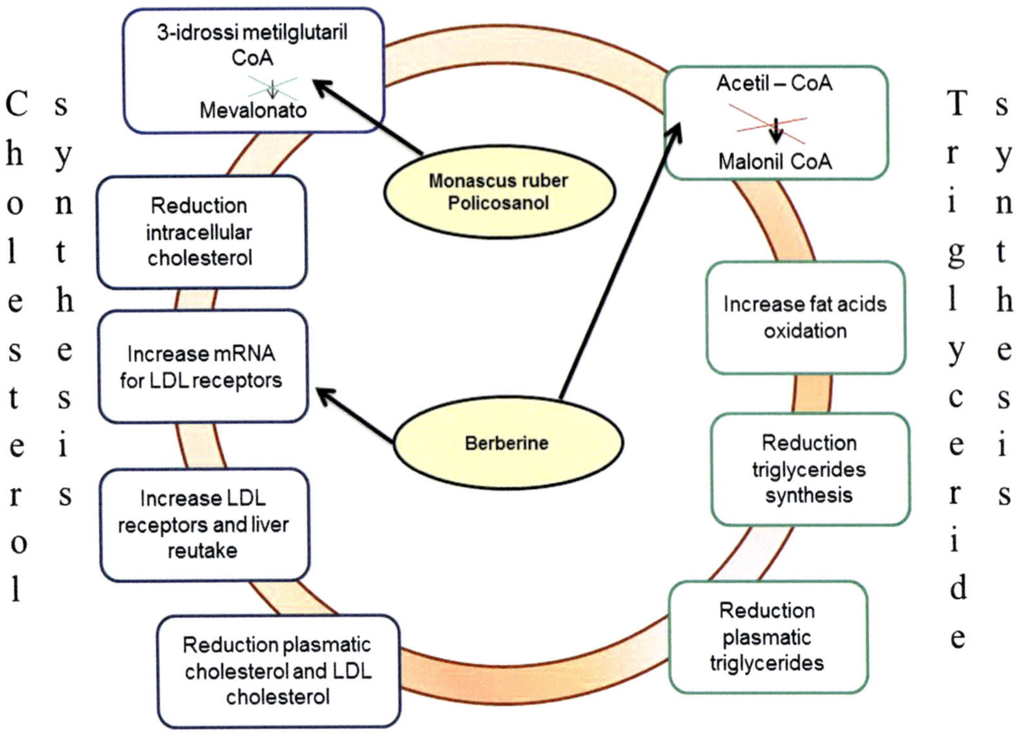

Fig. 14.4 Mechanisms of berberine activity

major adverse effects [21]. Recently, berberine use has been considered a safe potential therapeutic approach in hypercholesterolemia and diabetes treatment, especially in patients who not do tolerate statins or do not attain target LDL. Also, in association with ezetimibe, berberine is safe and efficacious and improves the lipid profile [22].

14.8 Coenzyme Q10

Coenzyme Q10 plays a key role in cell bioenergetics, both mitochondrial (respiratory chain) and at the level of ATP production, and plays an anti-oxidant role in relation to LDL. Being a lipophilic substance in the gastrointestinal tract, it is incorporated into chylomicrons, then passes into the lymphatic vessels, and ends in the bloodstream. The degree of absorption per se is very poor, because of its insolubility in water and the high molecular weight, and it is very important to the choice of pharmaceutical formulation, which allows a high solubility [23]. Statin therapy reduces the plasma concentrations of coenzyme Q10, and this could be the reason for muscle pain. Increasingly important is the supplementation of coenzyme Q10 in patients with muscle pain induced by statins, also with varying degrees of success [24, 25].

14.9 Medicinal Mushrooms

Medicinal mushrooms are active molecules in cardiovascular diseases in general and in dyslipidemia (see Chap. 6).

14.10 Acupuncture

Preliminary data, performed only in a Chinese population, are reported in the literature on the treatment of obesity and associated dyslipidemia

Table 14.1 Daily doses recommended based on the data presented in the literature

Berberine	500 mg
Bergamot	500 mg
Fiber	25–30 g
Phytosterols	1.6–2 g
Omega 3	3 g
Policosanol	10 mg
Soy protein	25 g
Red yeast rice	200 mg
Green tea	150 mg

Reducing cholesterol is estimated at between 10 and 20%

Table 14.2 Patients' target

Patients' target
• Primary prevention, hypercholesterolemic subjects who have a mile cardiovascular risk
• Patients' intolerant to statins
• High-risk patients who do not tolerate high doses of statins
• High-risk patients that even with the maximum tolerated dose of stains do not attain the target of LDL: security association with stains, ezetimibe, and phenols
• To enhance the treatment of adults and children (>6AA) with familial hypercholesterolemia

combining statin (atorvastatin) and acupuncture, and show a favorable synergistic effect [26].

Recently, a randomized clinical trial was designed that will provide additional information about using this method [27].

14.11 Conclusion

Epidemiological and clinical studies have shown that lifestyle modifications, such as nutrition and exercise, are the most important measures for reducing cardiovascular risk. Plant-derived food and nutraceutical products have been recognized to be primary preventive factors (Table 14.1).

Statins are the most important drug for reducing high cholesterol and cardiovascular risk, and their use has increased over the past few decades.

Along with this increased utilization of statins, we have observed an increase in therapy discontinuation and the presence of statin intolerance (Table 14.2). Combined therapy must be a potential positive strategy for treating these patients.

References

1. Keys A, Aravanis C, Blackburn H et al (eds) (1980) Seven countries study. A multivariate analysis of death and coronary artery disease. Harvard University Press, Cambridge, pp 1–381
2. Gimeno E, Torre-Carbot K, Lamuela-Raventos RM et al (2007) Changes in the phenolic content of low density lipoprotein after olive oil consumption in men. A randomized crossover controlled trial. Br J Nutr 98(6):1243–1250
3. De Lorgeril M, Salen P, Martin JL et al (1999) Mediterranean diet, traditional risk factors, and rate of cardiovascular complications after myocardial infarction: final report of the Lyon Diet Heart Study. Circulation 99:779–785
4. Li Y, Hruby A, Bernstein AM et al (2015) Saturated fats compared with unsaturated fats and sources of carbohydrates in relation to risk of coronary artery disease: a prospective cohort study. J Am Coll Cardiol 66:1538–1548
5. Mozzafarian D, Wu JH (2011) Omega-3 fatty acids and cardiovascular disease: effects on risk factors, molecular pathway and clinical events. J Am Coll Cardiol 58:2047–2067
6. Gylling H, Simonen P (2015) Phytosterols, phytostanols and lipoprotein metabolism. Nutrients 7: 7965–7977
7. Hertog MGL, Feskens EJM, Hollman PCH et al (1993) Dietary antioxidant flavonoids and risk of coronary artery disease: the Zutphen Elderly Study. Lancet 342:1007–1011
8. Tangney C, Rasmussen HE (2013) Polyphenols, inflammation and cardiovascular disease. Curr Atheroscler Rep 15:324
9. Prasad C, Imrhan V, Juma S et al (2015) Bioactive plant metabolites in the management of non-communicable metabolic diseases: looking at opportunities beyond the horizon. Metabolites 5:733–765
10. Timmers S, Konings E, Bilet L et al (2011) Calorie restriction-like effects of 30 days of resveratrol supplementation on energy metabolism and metabolic profile in obese humans. Cell Metab 14:612–622
11. Magyar K, Halmosi R, Palfi A et al (2012) Cardioprotection by resveratrol: a human clinical trial in patients with stable coronary artery disease. Clin Hemorheol Microcirc 50:179–187
12. Hertog MGL, Kromhout D, Aravanis C et al (1995) Flavonoid intake and long-term risk of coronary artery disease and cancer in the seven countries study. Arch Intern Med 155:381–386
13. Hooper L, Kroon PA, Rimm EB et al (2008) Flavonoids, flavonoid-rich foods, and cardiovascular risk:

a meta-analysis of randomized controlled trials. Am J Clin Nutr 88:38–50
14. Jung UJ, Kim HJ, Lee JS et al (2003) Naringin supplementation lowers plasma lipids and enhances erythrocyte antioxidant enzyme activities in hypercholesterolemic subjects. Clin Nutr 22:561–568
15. Gliozzi M, Walker R, Muscoli S (2013) Bergamot polyphenolic fraction enhances rosuvastatin-induced effect on LDL-cholesterol, LOX-1 expression and protein kinase B phosphorylation in patients with hyperlipidemia. Int J Cardiol 170(2):140–145
16. Epstein J, Sanderson IR, MacDonald TT (2010) Curcumin as a therapeutic agent: the evidence from in vitro, animal and human studies. Br J Nutr 103(11): 1545–1557
17. Tu Y, Sun D, Zeng X et al (2014) Piperine potentiates the hypocholesterolemic effect of curcumin in rats fed on a high fat diet. Exp Ther Med 8(1):260–266
18. Goumi-Berthold I, Berthold HK (2002) Policosanol: clinical pharmacology and therapeutic significance of a new lipid-lowering. Am Heart J 143:356–365
19. Cubeddu LX, Cubeddu RJ, Heimowitz T (2006) Comparative lipid lowering effects of policosanol and atorvastatin: a randomized, parallel, double-blind, placebo-controlled trial. Am Heart J 152:982
20. Endo TO, Kuroda M, Tanzawa K (1976) Competitive inhibition of 3-hydroxy-3-methyl-glutaryl coenzyme a reductase by ml-236a and ml -236b, fungal metabolites having cholesterolemic hypoactivity. FEBS Lett 72:323–326
21. Pirillo A, Catapano AL (2015) Berberine, a plant alkaloid with lipid and glucose-lowering properties: from in vitro evidence to clinical studies. Atherosclerosis 243:449–461
22. Marazzi G, Pelliccia F, Campolongo G et al (2015) Usefulness of nutraceuticals versus ezetimibe and combination in statin-intolerant patients with dyslipidemia with coronary artery disease. Am J Cardiol 116:1798–1801
23. Bhagavan HN, Chopra RK (2006) Coenzyme Q10: absorption, tissue uptake, metabolism and pharmacokinetics. Free Radic Res 40(5):445–453
24. Littelfield N, Beckstrand RL, Luthy KE (2014) Statins' effect on plasma levels of coenzyme Q10 and improvement in myopathy with supplementation. J Am Assoc Nurs Pract 26:85–90
25. Marcoff L, Thompson PD (2007) The role of coenzyme Q10 in statin associated myopathy: a systematic review. JACC 49:2231–2237
26. Sun YZ, Song J (2015) Clinical trials for treatment of primary hyperlipidemia by using acupuncture in combination with Lipitor. Zhen Ci Yan Jiu 40(1):61–64
27. Gao Z, Yu Z, Song ZX et al (2015) Comparative effectiveness of electro-acupuncture plus lifestyle modification treatment for patients with simple obesity and overweight: study protocol for a randomized controlled trial. Trials 16:525. doi:10.1186/s13063-015-1046

Integrated Approach to Hypertension 15

Carlo Dal Lin, Marco Silvestro, Raffaele Migliorini, Francesco Tona, and Massimo Fioranelli

15.1 Introduction

Hypertension, usually defined as persistent blood pressure (BP) at 140/90 mmHg or higher, affects about a quarter of the adult population in many countries, particularly in industrialized societies. Hypertension is a risk factor for most, if not all, cardiovascular diseases (coronary artery disease, myocardial infarction, thoracic and abdominal aneurysms, heart failure, and stroke) and renal failure. Hypertension is also associated with cognitive dysfunction, erectile dysfunction, and loss of vision. The higher the pressure, the greater the risk of complications [1].

Normal BP is defined as less than 120 mmHg systolic and less than 80 mmHg diastolic [2].

The status of hypertension breaks down into three grades (Table 15.1): grade 1, 140–159 mmHg systolic and 90–99 mmHg diastolic; grade 2, 160–179 mmHg systolic and 100–109 mmHg diastolic; and grade 3, 180 mmHg or higher systolic and 110 mmHg diastolic [1]. Between normal and grade 1 values is a category termed "prehypertension," a condition characterized by systolic blood pressure of 120–139 mmHg and diastolic blood pressure of 80–89 mmHg. We talk about "isolated systolic hypertension" in the presence of a systolic pressure greater than 140 mmHg with normal diastolic values. Isolated systolic hypertension should be graded (1, 2, 3) according to systolic blood pressure values within the ranges indicated, provided that diastolic values are <90 mmHg. For persons with diabetes or renal disease and hypertension, the BP treatment goal is less than 130/80 mmHg [2].

This classification is very important because it heightens awareness of both risk and opportunities for prevention, adopting therapeutic management based on lifestyle changes, and adding incremental drug therapy if necessary.

Hypertension has both modifiable and nonmodifiable risk factors. Gender and genetic heritage are nonmodifiable factors, although the latter is uncertain. As we discussed in a recent review [3], epigenetic inheritance plays a key role in determining the activation of the genome and the axis of stress. This type of information is a stable genetic trace, transmitted from generation to generation, but can gradually be changed and modulated by lifestyle and the surrounding environment (for details, see the section "Allostatic load and the building of cardiovascular diseases" in the aforementioned review, part B).

Systolic blood pressure rises throughout the adult age range, whereas diastolic blood pressure

C. Dal Lin, M.D. (✉) • M. Silvestro, N.D. • R. Migliorini, M.D. • F. Tona, M.D., Ph.D.
Department of Cardiological, Thoracic and Vascular Sciences, Padua University Medical School, Padova, Italy
e-mail: carlodallin@libero.it

M. Fioranelli, M.D.
Department of Nuclear Physics, Sub-Nuclear and Radiation, Guglielmo Marconi University, Rome, Italy

M. Fioranelli (ed.), *Integrative Cardiology*, DOI 10.1007/978-3-319-40010-5_15

Table 15.1 Definitions and classification of blood pressure levels (mmHg). Modified from Camm et al. [1]

Category	Systolic		Diastolic
Optimal	<120	And	<80
Normal	120–129	And/or	80–84
High normal	130–139	And/or	85–89
Grade 1 hypertension	140–159	And/or	90–99
Grade 2 hypertension	160–179	And/or	100–109
Grade 3 hypertension	≥180	And/or	≥110
Isolated systolic hypertension	≥140	And	<90

peaks at about age 60 years in men and 70 years in women and falls gradually thereafter [1]. Even if both systolic and diastolic blood pressures are independently predictive of stroke and coronary mortality, in the elderly, a wide pulse pressure (systolic blood pressure minus diastolic blood pressure) has been shown in some observational studies to be a better predictor of adverse cardiovascular outcomes than either systolic or diastolic pressures individually [1]. Thus, hypertension has always been considered a condition of aging: more than 65% of persons 65 years old or older are hypertensive, but, surprisingly, a person who is normotensive at age 55 years still has a 90% lifetime risk of developing hypertension [4]. This seems to strongly suggest that hypertension might be the result of an integrated and multifaceted individual adaptation to the environment and dramatically emphasizes the importance of environmental factors together with individual psychosocial and emotional factors in dealing with this issue [3].

Rather than focusing on chronological aging, the emphasis should be on physiological aging, which can be changed.

As we will see, lifestyle modifications demonstrably reduce BP: losing weight and certain diets, sodium intake reduction, moderate physical exercise, alcohol consumption reduction, smoking cessation, and stress and pain management.

This is very important because there is a considerable gap between what has been shown in pharmaceutical trials and what happens in daily clinical practice in terms of achievable BP reductions. Although pharmaceutical therapy has been demonstrated to be effective in reducing heart attacks and stroke, outside of clinical trials, only approximately one-third of patients achieve optimal BP control using drug therapy [2]. This efficacy gap in hypertension treatment represents an ideal opportunity to codevelop with a patient a customized action plan that addresses logical options for diet, exercise, supplementation, smoking cessation, and mind–body skills development [5]. Additional insights may also come from both Ayurvedic and traditional East Asian medicine.

In this chapter, several examples regarding the anti-hypertensive effectiveness of each individual factor previously listed are reviewed. Each of them can then be associated with obtaining a synergistic effect [5]. This can be very important because a reduction of just 5 mmHg in systolic BP is associated with a 7% reduction in all-cause mortality [6].

Hypertension is often dubbed the "silent killer" because it is frequently asymptomatic; the pressure value remains as an abstract number devoid of real significance for the patient. If no pain is felt, no disease is present. Thus, it is problematic to arrange a treatment for a condition that is not perceived by the subject and, in addition, a chronic therapy, of long duration.

It is essential that the doctor can find the time to go on a therapeutic journey with the patient, picking up and respecting the patient's beliefs, meanings, and interpretations of personal experience of hypertension and all that accompanies it.

Another key aspect in the management of the hypertensive patient is awareness of the problem and the fact that the condition persists even at home, in everyday life, and that it is not just a clinical quirk. Home BP monitoring with records in a diary or 24-h BP digital monitoring are simple means of raising awareness and compliance [1]. The data collected from the patient can be employed by the physician to educate the patient to take care of his health. They can be used to fill with him his individual cardiovascular risk score monitoring how it can improve over time (to this end, an electronic calculator can be used, such as: http://my.clevelandclinic.org/services/heart/prevention/risk-factors/Heart_Center_Risk_Tool).

More and more people ask not strictly pharmacological and symptomatic therapies for their health problems [7]. They seek integrative clinicians who can counsel from an evidence base on the logical options available to them (Fig. 15.1). Prehypertension is an early warning to modify lifestyle and probably is the ideal scenario to get the best results from an integrative approach. In addition, the change of lifestyle

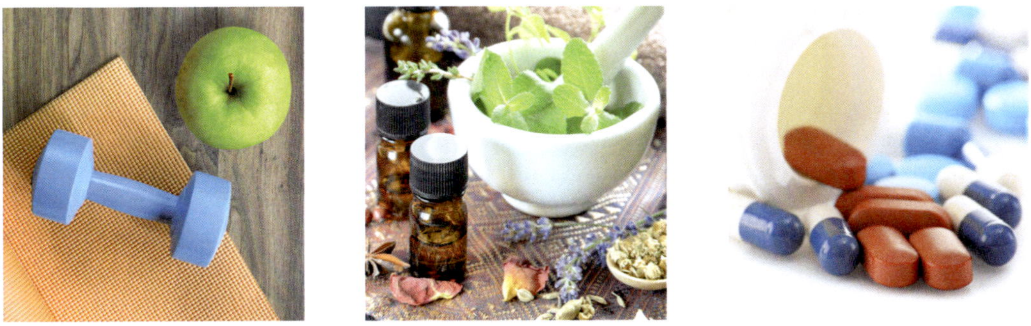

Minimize obstacles to healing ⟶

- Obesity: weight management program to achieve ideal body weight.

- Eliminate lifestyle factors contributing to hypertension: avoid coffee, alcohol, smoking and salt.

- Modify sedentary lifestyle: tailored exercise program (30 min aerobic exercise per day al least 4 days a week).

- Stress management: relaxation techniques.

- Diet: K, fibers, low sugar, Ca, Mg, vitamin C, dark chocholate, increase whole plant foods, celery, garlic, onions, cold-water ocean fish, nuts and seeds, green vegetables, grains, legumes, broccoli.

Tailor natural interventions to patient needs ⟶

- Mild hypertension: high potency vitamin-mineral; vitamin C and E, magnesium, garlic, flaxseed oil.

- Moderate hypertension: All of mesures indicated above; CoQ10; Crataegus.

Determine need for conventional therapy

- Mild/Moderate hypertension unresponsive to natural approach: refer to antihypertensive drugs (start with a single drug treatment).

- Severe hypertension: refer to antihypertensive drugs (strat with two-drug regimen).

Fig. 15.1 In summary: staged integrative approach to hypertension. Eat food, not too much and mostly plants. Exercise 30 min per day for at least 4 days per week. Limit alcohol. Don't smoke. Breathe: incorporate mind–body practices into your daily routine. Build an organized system of regular follow-up and review with self-monitoring and appointment reminders

is a fundamental step, which is boosted at any degree of hypertension (Table 15.2). The physician should try to increase his/her knowledge about nonpharmacological interventions that can be adopted in the treatment of hypertension, moving beyond the basic and often vague recommendations on lifestyle modifications that can be found in guidelines [2] or traditional books [1].

15.2 The Role of Oxidative Stress

Oxidative stress (an imbalance of harmful oxygen species and the anti-oxidant defense mechanism) represents an etiological factor of human hypertension [8–10], hypertensive patients have a higher level of oxygen free radicals [11] and an impaired anti-oxidant defense mechanism [12]. This, together with an imbalance in vasodilators (nitric oxide) and vasoconstrictors (angiotensin), contributes to the initiation and perpetuation of hypertension [13]. This is particularly important because oxidative stress depends on external factors (alimentation, pollution, etc.), but also on inner factors such as individual psychological profile [3, 14, 15]. Thus, it is of paramount importance to act at both these levels.

15.3 Lifestyle Modification

15.3.1 Smoking Cessation

Smoking (tobacco addiction) is the most significant of the modifiable cardiovascular risk factors [16]. At least 1 billion adults worldwide are smokers and at least 700 million children are passive smokers at home [17]. Many people mistakenly describe their tobacco addiction as a "habit" or "behavioral choice," and the onset of this state quickly follows the acquisition of an ability to inhale cigarette smoke, leading to a transformation of neurophysiological function and nicotine-receptor density [16]. To maintain

Table 15.2 Initiation of antihypertensive treatment

Other risk factors, OD, or disease	Normal SBP 120–129 or DBP 80–84	High normal SBP 130–139 or DBP 85–89	Grade 1 HT SBP 140–159 or DBP 90–99	Grade 2 HT SBP 160–179 or DBP 100–109	Grade 3 HT SBP ≥180 or DBP ≥110
No other risk factors	No BP intervention	No BP intervention	Lifestyle changes for several months then drug treatment if BP uncontrolled	Lifestyle changes for several weeks then drug treatment if BP uncontrolled	Lifestyle changes +immediate drug treatment
1–2 risk factors	Lifestyle changes	Lifestyle changes	Lifestyle changes for several weeks then drug treatment if BP uncontrolled	Lifestyle changes for several weeks then drug treatment if BP uncontrolled	Lifestyle changes +immediate drug treatment
3 or more risk factors, MS, or OD	Lifestyle changes	Lifestyle changes and consider drug treatment	Lifestyle changes+ drug treatment	Lifestyle changes+ drug treatment	Lifestyle changes +immediate drug treatment
Diabetes	Lifestyle changes				
Established CV or renal disease	Lifestyle changes +immediate drug treatment	Lifestyle changes +immediate drug treatment	Lifestyle changes +immediate drug treatment	Lifestyle changes +immediate drug treatment	Lifestyle changes +immediate drug treatment

CV cardiovascular, *MS* metabolic syndrome, *OD* subclinical organ damage, *SBP* systolic blood pressure, *DBP* diastolic blood pressure, *HT* hypertension
Modified from Camm et al. [1]

the personal "comfort," the patient becomes addicted to nicotine [3]. Smokers inhale thousands of other chemicals, many of which play critical roles in the initiation and accentuation of atherosclerosis by influencing vasomotor activity, vascular dysfunction, oxidation of lipids, atheroma development, and thrombosis [1].

Smoking cessation, of course, should be part of every comprehensive lifestyle modification plan. The use of cigarettes is reported to determine a 4-mmHg increase in systolic blood pressure and a 3-mmHg increase in diastolic blood pressure [18], probably by increasing the resting heart rate [19]. Furthermore, hypertensive patients who smoke are at an additional increased risk for cardiovascular events (ischemic stroke and hemorrhagic stroke) compared with those who do not smoke, and this risk correlates directly with the number of cigarettes smoked [20, 21].

15.3.2 Diet

A diet effective in the treatment of hypertension must include vegetables, fruits, and low-fat dairy products and should be low in saturated fat and refined grains/carbohydrates, not high in sodium, but rich in potassium, magnesium, calcium, and fiber.

Two very well-studied diets for hypertension prevention and control are the Mediterranean [14] and DASH (Dietary Approach to Stop Hypertension) [5] diets.

15.3.2.1 Mediterranean Diet

The Mediterranean diet's antihypertensive effect was evaluated in the SUN study, a prospective cohort study conducted from 1999 to 2005 in 9,408 men and women [22]. The study documented a mean systolic BP reduction of 3.1 mmHg (95% confidence interval [CI] 5.4 to −0.8) and mean diastolic BP decrease of 1.9 mmHg (95% CI 3.6 to −0.1) [22].

The benefits of the Mediterranean diet are beyond the anti-hypertensive effect taken in isolation. Foods that we introduce into the diet are not only a source of calories, but are important modulators of the nervous, endocrine, and immune systems [14]. Thus, beyond hypertension, it has been demonstrated that the Mediterranean diet has favorable effects on lipoprotein levels, endothelium vasodilation, insulin resistance, metabolic syndrome, anti-oxidant capacity, myocardial and cardiovascular mortality, and cancer incidence in obese patients and in those with previous myocardial infarction [23, 24].

Additionally, adherence to the Mediterranean diet was demonstrated to be associated with approximately a 20% reduction in all-cause mortality in both men and women [25]. This percentage doubles in the elderly population [26].

One of the main components of the Mediterranean diet is olive oil, rich in healthy polyphenols and monounsaturated fatty acids (oleic acid) with an anti-hypertensive effect [27, 28]. In addition, phenolic compounds in olive oil prevent lipoperoxidation, improve the lipid profile and endothelial function (inducing nitric oxide-mediated endothelium-dependent relaxation [29, 30]), and have antithrombotic properties [31].

The Food and Drug Administration (FDA) confirms that consuming approximately two tablespoons (23 g) of olive oil per day may reduce the risk of heart disease [5].

Another very famous part of the Mediterranean diet is linked to the consumption of red wine. Although alcohol consumption can cause multiple organ damage and raise BP, red wine consumption is inversely associated with mortality from cardiovascular diseases [32], risk reduction being greatest in the case of low to moderate intake [33, 34]. Studies performed with de-alcoholized red, but not white wine confirm short-term cardiovascular benefits [35]. This is because grape skins, seeds, and stems from which the red wine is produced [36] contain many bioactive polyphenols, including flavonoids (quercetin, catechin, and epicatechin), pro-anthocyanidins, and anthocyanins, phenolic acids (gallic, caftaric, and caffeic acid), and the trihydroxystilbene termed *resveratrol*.

More than a purely anti-hypertensive effect [37, 38], the red wine polyphenols improve endothelial function, leading to decreased arterial damage, decreased angiotensin-II activity, increased nitric oxide, decreased platelet aggregation, decreased LDL oxidation, and the stimulation of the anti-senescence factor sirtuin [35].

The Mediterranean diet is rich in fibers that are extremely effective in reducing both systolic and diastolic BP in hypertensive patients [39].

15.3.2.2 DASH Diet

The Dietary Approaches to Stop Hypertension (DASH) diet (Table 15.3) is an analog of the Mediterranean diet coded in the context of the US alimentation system, with the specific aim of lowering blood pressure.

Table 15.3 The Dietary Approaches to Stop Hypertension (DASH) diet

Food group	Daily servings	Serving sizes	Examples and notes	Significance of each food group to the DASH eating plan
Grains and grain products	7–8	1 slice bread 1 oz dry cereal[a] ½ C cooked rice, pasta, or cereal	Whole wheat bread, English muffin, pita bread, bagel, cereals, grits, oatmeal, crackers, unsalted pretzels, and popcorn	Major sources of energy and fiber
Vegetables	4–5	1 C raw leafy vegetable ½ C cooked vegetable 6 oz vegetable juice	Tomatoes, potatoes, carrots, green peas, squash, broccoli, turnip greens, collards, kale, spinach, artichokes, green beans, lima beans, sweet potatoes	Rich sources of potassium, magnesium, and fiber
Fruits	4–5	6 oz fruit juice 1 medium fruit ¼ C dried fruit ½ C fresh, frozen, or canned fruit	Apricots, bananas, dates, grapes, oranges, orange juice, grapefruit, grapefruit juice, mangoes, melons, peaches, pineapples, prunes, raisins, strawberries, tangerines	Important sources of potassium, magnesium, and fiber
Low-fat or fat-free dairy foods	2–3	8 oz milk 1 C yogurt 1.5 oz cheese	Fat-free (skim) or low-fat (1%) milk, fat-free or low-fat buttermilk, fat-free or low-fat regular or frozen yogurt, low-fat and fat-free cheese	Major sources of calcium and protein
Meats, poultry, and fish	2 or less	3 oz cooked meats, poultry, or fish	Select only lean; trim away visible fat; broil, roast, or boil instead of frying; remove skin from poultry	Rich sources of protein and magnesium
Nuts, seeds, and dry beans	4–5 per week	1.5 oz or ⅓C nuts ½ oz or 2 Tbsp seeds ½ C cooked dry beans and peas	Almonds, filberts, mixed nuts, peanuts, walnuts, sunflower seeds, kidney beans, lentils	Rich sources of energy, magnesium, potassium, protein, and fiber
Fats and oils[b]	2–3	1 tsp soft margarine 1 Tbsp low-fat mayonnaise 2 Tbsp light salad dressing 1 tsp vegetable oil	Soft margarine, low-fat mayonnaise, light salad dressing, vegetable oil (such as olive, corn, canola, or safflower)	In DASH 27% of the calories are fat, including that in or added to foods
Sweets	5 per week	1 Tbsp sugar I Tbsp jelly or jam ½ oz jelly beans 8 oz lemonade	Maple syrup, sugar, jelly, jam, fruit-flavored gelatin, jelly beans, hard candy, fruit punch, sorbet, ices	Sweets should be low in fat

From the DASH study, as published by the Joint National Committee on Prevention, Detection, Evaluation, and Treatment of High Blood Pressure and the National High Blood Pressure Education Program Coordination Committee The sixth report of the Joint National Committee on prevention, detection, evaluation and treatment of high blood pressure. (Modified from Rakel [5])

[a]Equals ½ to 1-¼ C, depending on cereal type. Check the product nutrition label

[b]Fat content changes serving counts for fat and oils. For example, 1 Tbsp of regular salad dressing equals 1 serving; 1 Tbsp of low-fat dressing equals ½ a serving; 1 Tbsp of a fat-free dressing equals 0 servings

As described by Plotnikoff and Dusek (cited in Rakel [5]): "the DASH diet trial enrolled 459 participants and provided each with all his or her food for 11 weeks. For the first 3 weeks, the participants were provided with a control diet that was low in fruits, vegetables, and dairy products, with a fat content typical of the average diet in the USA. Participants were then randomly assigned to receive the control diet, a diet rich in fruits and vegetables, or a "combination" diet rich in fruits, vegetables, and low-fat dairy products and with reduced saturated and total fat for 8 weeks. Sodium intake and body weight were maintained at constant levels. For the 326 participants with prehypertension, the DASH diet resulted in reduced SBP and DBP of 3.5 mmHg ($P < 0.001$) and 2.1 mmHg ($P = 0.003$), respectively. Among the 133 subjects with stage 1 hypertension, the DASH diet reduced SBP and DBP by 11.4 and 5.5 mmHg respectively, more than the control diet ($P < 0.001$ for each)" [40].

15.3.2.3 Anti-ACE Peptides

Observational and epidemiological studies demonstrate a consistent association between high protein intake and a reduction in BP [41]. The source of protein is important, being animal protein (milk, chicken, and fish, such as sardine [42] or bonito fish, a member of the tuna family [43]) less effective than non-animal protein [44] (such as soy, which contains isoflavones, saponins, phytic acid, amino acids, trypsin inhibitors, fiber, and globulins with an anti-hypertensive effect [45]).

15.3.2.4 Omega-3 Fatty Acids

A diet rich in omega-3 polyunsaturated fatty acids (contained in cold water fatty fish or grass-fed animals) may prevent the development of hypertension [46] and is an effective remedy in the early stages of the disease [47]. Omega-3 fatty acid deficiency contributed to the development of hypertension in animal models [48].

Furthermore, as the omega-3 fatty acids are effective at improving insulin sensitivity and dyslipidemia, they may be particularly useful in patients with the metabolic syndrome [1].

15.3.2.5 Cocoa (*Theobroma cacao*)

Regular intake of cocoa-containing foods is linked to lower cardiovascular and all-cause mortality and is inversely associated with BP [49, 50]. Regular cocoa (dark chocolate) intake demonstrated significant reductions in the values of both systolic and diastolic BP, in healthy subjects and in cases of prehypertension or grade 1 hypertension [5, 51].

In the studies cited, regular consumption of cocoa has not resulted in an increase in body weight, plasma levels of lipids, glucose, and 8-isoprostane (a measure of oxidative stress). The BP decrease was also accompanied by a sustained increase in the vasodilatory nitric oxide donor, *S*-nitrosoglutathione. In comparison, the polyphenol-free white chocolate intake caused no changes in BP or plasma biomarkers [51].

The benefit of flavanol-containing cocoa appears to extend to persons with diabetes as well [52]. For all these reasons, it is possible to consider recommending one-fourth of a standard-sized dark chocolate bar consisting of 70% cocoa daily [5].

15.3.3 Supplements

The quality of the studies related to the possible beneficial effect of selective supplementation of certain elements is poor. This is because it is very difficult to determine whether the baseline value of an alleged deficient state is to trace in the blood, at an intracellular or simply at a functional level. Given the interindividual and intra-individual variability (for example, linked to the activation of the stress axis as a function of psycho-emotional states [3, 14, 15]), these forms of insufficiency can also be additive. Then, the question is that we often dose elements blindly: in some people, poor blood levels of a certain element can be traced back without this causing specific problems (the intracellular stores could be in order and functionally normal), whereas other people possess normal blood levels of the same element at the expense of the intracellular store or have functional deficits.

Table 15.4 Nutritional supplements in hypertension. Modified from Devries and Dalen [44]

Supplements	Daily intake
Coenzyme Q10	120–150 mg 2× a day
Fish oil	3–4 g a day
Nattokinase (NSK-SD)	50–100 mg if dietary natto is not consumed
Magnesium	400–800 mg a day
Organic garlic	1,000 mg if not taken in diet
Hawthorn	1,000 to 1,500 mg per day
Quercetin	500–1,000 mg per day 2× a day
Vitamin D3	2000 units per day
Vitamin B6	100 mg 1–2× a day
Vitamin C	250–500 mg 2× a day

Therefore, it is difficult to establish a critical value of a nutrient that can be good for all people, below which supplementation is necessary. There is also individual variability in bioavailability, uptake, and metabolism that are often not considered in the available literature. The result is that much of the interventional nutrition research does not answer the very important clinical question, "Does replenishment of a deficiency to a given serum level result in an improved clinical outcome?" A summary of nutritional supplements in hypertension is presented in Table 15.4.

15.3.3.1 Potassium and Sodium

Diet low in potassium and high in sodium is linked to hypertension, cardiovascular diseases, and cancer [43]. Natural diets rich in fruit and vegetables provide the correct intake of potassium and sodium, although potassium supplementation with a good anti-hypertensive effect may be required [53–56]. Potassium should be used with caution in patients with kidney disease or those taking digitalis, potassium-sparing diuretics, and angiotensin-converting enzyme inhibitor anti-hypertensive drugs.

15.3.3.2 Magnesium

Magnesium homeostasis is so closely linked to that of potassium that some forms of hypokalemia result from a magnesium-deficient intake. Magnesium is a well-understood and frequently used intervention for the hypertension of pre-eclampsia. With a proper diet, such as the Mediterranean or DASH (natural sources of magnesium including pumpkin seeds, nuts, quinoa, spinach, bran cereal, buckwheat, and beans), the intake of magnesium should be sufficient not to require supplementation, as suggested by the JNC 7 guidelines [2].

However, several reports have demonstrated a link between higher intake of magnesium and lower blood pressure [57, 58]. On the other hand, low dietary intake of magnesium correlates strongly with high BP [59].

An important source of magnesium is water: water with many minerals such as magnesium is called "hard water" and there is an inverse correlation between water hardness and high blood pressure. Magnesium supplementation can be very beneficial in hypertensive subjects who take diuretics or who have high levels of renin. Magnesium may be administered in different formulations, but it seems to be better absorbed and more effective when linked to the intermediates of the Krebs cycle (aspartate, malate, succinate, fumarate, or citrate). It should keep in mind that serum magnesium levels do not reflect intracellular magnesium and the many forms of magnesium may have different bioavailability and physiological activity [60]. To quote Rakel: "The result is a 'one-size-fits-all' approach to magnesium studies of varying dosing and varying type of magnesium that prevents any meta-analysis of existing randomized trials. Despite these limitations, magnesium appears to be beneficial and nontoxic" [5].

15.3.4 Dosage

Starting at a low dose of the non-oxide forms of magnesium (120–200 mg/day) and slowly increase the dose to 400–1,200 mg/day) as tolerated, monitoring serum levels [54].

15.3.5 Precautions

Magnesium is well tolerated in general, but can sometimes cause looser stool; supplements must be used with great care in patients with kidney disease or severe heart disease (atrio-ventricular block) [1].

15.3.5.1 Calcium

Hypertension is linked to a low intake of calcium, but this evidence is not as strong as from magnesium or potassium [54, 61]. There are conflicting opinions [62] about the antihypertensive effect of calcium supplementation: it seems to be more effective in blacks, in salt-sensitive patients, and in elderly hypertensive patients [63, 64]. Calcium citrate is more effective than calcium carbonate.

15.3.5.2 Vitamins C, B6, and D

Vitamins C and B6 have a lowering BP effect in people with mild hypertension [43]. Vitamin C (with its antioxidant effect) promotes lead excretion, which is linked to hypertension and cardiovascular mortality [65–67]. Vitamin B6 supplementation (oral dosage 5 mg/kg) is linked to decreased serum norepinephrine [68, 69].

Calcitriol, also known as 1,25-dihydroxy vitamin D, is the activated form of vitamin D, controlling hundreds of genes, and an almost ubiquitous effect in the cardiovascular [70, 71] and renal system [72].

Although vitamin D deficiency is associated with an increased risk for hypertension [73, 74], its supplementation did not appear sufficient to be able to recommend its extensive use for the treatment of hypertension [75–77]. For this hormone, the considerations made at the beginning of the paragraph are of paramount importance. BP is finely regulated in a complex integrated system made of cytokines, hormones, and neurotransmitters [3, 14, 15]. It is difficult to establish a cutoff value to apply to all individuals (regardless of their psychological, emotional, and environmental characteristics), on which to base an effective supplementary intervention. As suggested by Plotnikoff and Dusek (cited in Rakel [5]): "the most important question at this time is whether a threshold serum level is needed to reduce the risk of incident hypertension or to reduce already elevated BPs" [5]. Additionally, the length of time of vitamin D sufficiency required for prevention or reduction must be defined.

15.3.5.3 Coenzyme Q10

Coenzyme Q10 (CoQ10, ubiquinone, or ubiquinol) is synthesized within the body, and is a crucial cofactor for the production of adenosine triphosphate (ATP), exerting a potent anti-oxidant effect. The highest tissue concentration is found in the heart, and the highest cellular concentration is on the inner membrane of the mitochondrion. Thirty-nine percent of hypertensive patients show a deficiency in this element [43, 78], as it occurs during aging or in the case of hyperthyroidism, cardiovascular disease, total parenteral nutrition, aerobic training, and ultraviolet exposure [79].

The supplementation of CoQ10 has the potential to significantly reduce both systolic and diastolic hypertension after 4–12 weeks of therapy [80], with concomitant improvements in cardiovascular functional status (New York Heart Association (NYHA) functional class) and medication requirements [81]. After an average of 4.4 months, 37% of patients were able to discontinue one antihypertensive drug, 11% discontinued two drugs, and 4% discontinued three drugs. Only 3% required the addition of one antihypertensive drug, and none required the addition of more than one antihypertensive drug. Twenty-five percent of all patients were able to control their BP with only CoQ10 supplementation [81] and had significant side effects [82]. In many studies, patients were able to discontinue medications [82].

Some medications commonly prescribed for the treatment of cardiovascular diseases undermine the reserves of CoQ10: statins and some beta blockers, such as propranolol, can reduce endogenous production of CoQ10 by as much as 40% [83].

The effect of CoQ10 on hypertension is still unknown: it does not affect the levels of renin, sodium, or aldosterone but can reduce two significant drivers of hypertension, oxidative stress and hyperinsulinemia [84], improving cholesterol values and peripheral vascular resistance [43].

15.3.5.4 Dosage

The dose to achieve a serum level greater than 2.0 μg/mL is 75–350 mg a day taken with meals that contain some fat [5].

15.3.5.5 Precautions

Side effects are not infrequent, but include abdominal discomfort, nausea, vomiting, diarrhea, anorexia, rash, and headache. CoQ10 has an antiplatelet effect; thus, theoretically it can increase the risk of bleeding with antiplatelet or anticoagulant agents. Excretion is through the bile, and accumulation can occur in patients with hepatic impairment or biliary obstruction [5, 43].

15.3.6 Weight Loss and Exercise

Dietary interventions to reduce body weight result in better BP reduction compared with prescription drugs, such as orlistat or sibutramine. Weight loss of 4 kg (10 lb) by diet seems to reduce systolic BP by approximately 6 mmHg [85].

All the main cardiovascular guidelines recommend aerobic endurance exercise for the primary prevention, treatment, and control of hypertension and cardiovascular diseases [1, 86]. The effect of BP reduction varies from 5 to 10 mmHg after an exercise session and can last up to 22 h following endurance exercise. The higher the initial BP, the greater is the response [86].

Hypertensive patients should perform a moderate (40% to less than 60% oxygen consumption reserve [VO_2R]) aerobic exercise (endurance physical activity supplemented by resistance exercise) on most, preferably all, days of the week, for at least 30 min of continuous or accumulated physical activity per day [86].

15.3.7 Phytotherapy

Many patients, despite being in chronic therapy with hypotensive drugs, fail to maintain adequate blood pressure values. On the other hand, there are patients who refuse standard drug therapy and begin to take herbs without telling their doctor, without any prescription or guarantees of effectiveness. Scientific research in the field of herbal medicine has produced valuable evidence: e.g., *licorice* can cause pseudo-aldosteronism from glycyrrhizin, with high blood pressure [87]; we know that there are ACE inhibitors, such as some vegetable tannins [88] and oleacin [89]. Some plants are commonly used for the treatment of hypertension, sometimes without sufficient scientific evidence, such as mistletoe.

Mistletoe (*Viscum album*) is widely used in traditional medicine in Germany [90]. This plant contains flavonoids, polyphenols, alkaloids, and polysaccharides, and cytotoxic and immunostimulant proteins (viscotoxin and lecithin) [91–95]. The mechanism of action is still unclear: it may act centrally and has diuretic properties. It is used in powder or dyes. Mistletoe is poorly absorbed orally.

Hibiscus tea and extracts prepared from the dried flowers (calyces) of *Hibiscus sabdariffa* have demonstrated anti-hypertensive properties in clinical trials [96–99], similar to those observed with captopril (9.6 mg of total anthocyanins compared with 50 mg of captopril) [100] or lisinopril (250 mg of total anthocyanins/day compared with 10 mg of lisinopril) [101].

Garlic (*Allium sativum*). Despite the tradition and its extensive use as a hypotensive, scientific data have only recently emerged. The indication for its use concerns elderly hypertensive and dyslipidemic patients, in the form of dry extract standardized to allicin, and is capable of lowering the blood pressure by about 10 mmHg at both systolic and diastolic levels.

Hawthorn (*Crataegus monogyna* or *Crataegus oxyacantha*) is another plant traditionally used as a mild hypotensive and is known and appreciated as a mild sedative. The drug is present in the flowers and contains polyphenols (vitexin, hyperoside, pro-anthocyanidins, epicatechin, amines, and triterpenes). The hypotensive effectiveness of hawthorn (at a diastolic level) was demonstrated in a study by Walker et al. [102] conducted in diabetic patients using 1,200 mg of dry extract. The pharmacological effects of the hawthorn require at least 2–4 weeks and determine a reduction in coronary spasm with an increase in blood flow in that area, a positive inotropic action, a reduction in peripheral resistance, and modest central sedative action [103–105]. The latter helps to reduce blood pressure: its pro-anthocyanidins inhibit the synthesis of cyclic AMP phosphodiesterase [88]. Some flavonoids (also contained in passionflower) interact with benzodiazepine receptors and are also capable of acting as antagonists of oxygen radicals. The formulation most suitable for a clinical purpose is the dry extract standardized and titrated at 2% in flavonoids. Side effects are rare, and hawthorn should be used with caution in patients with bradycardia. There are also possible interactions with digitalis and anti-arrhythmic agents [1].

In Mediterranean folk medicine, infusion of olive leaves (*Olea europaea*) was used as a hypotensive agent. The glycerin macerate of the olive leaf has shown a hypotensive action with a calcium channel blocker mechanism [106]. High doses of olive derivatives have a negative chronotropic and inotropic action [88]. Best results are produced with the use of all the extracts of the plant, where flavonoids, such as rutin and hesperidin are present [88]. Oleacin compound, a substance with ACE-inhibitory action, was also isolated [89].

Many plants possess calcium-antagonist activity: *Ligusticum wallichii, Jatropha podagrica, Stephania tetrahedron, Panax notoginseng, Salvia miltiorrhiza, Uncaria rhynchophylla, Artemisia capillaris, Peucedanum praeruptorin,* members of the *Gentianaceae* family, and *Paeonia suffruticosa* [107].

In the case of hypertension, the plants with diuretic activity are *Equisetum arvense* [108, 109], hawkweed (*Hieracium pilosella*) [110], couch grass (*Triticum repens*), and *Ribes nigrum* [88], *Taraxacum officinale* [111], birch (*Betula alba*) [112], and orthosiphon [113, 114], usable as a fluid extract or better, in dry extracts. In particular, the extract from *Ribes nigrum* leaves in vitro activates endothelial nitric oxide synthase (eNOS) [115].

Herbs to avoid and that require close monitoring in the treatment of patients with hypertension include licorice, ephedra, and *Panax ginseng* [88]. These have the capacity to raise blood pressure significantly.

15.3.7.1 Dosage and Precautions for Garlic

The dosage for raw garlic cloves is one half to two per day. Supplements can help prevent garlic breath. Consider a standardized dose of 350 mg twice a day (4,000 μg of allicin) [5], or 4,000 mg of fresh garlic q.d [43]. Adverse effects include the following: diaphoresis dizziness; mouth, esophagus, and stomach irritation; nausea; and vomiting. Allergic reactions are rare. Doses greater than for culinary use may increase the risk of bleeding if they are taken with anticoagulants or antiplatelet agents.

15.3.7.2 Dosage and Precautions for Hawthorn

The German Commission E Monographs cites the use of standardized extracts containing 30–169 mg of pro-anthocyanidins (18.75%) calculated as epicatechin or 3.5–19.8 mg of flavonoids (2.2%) calculated as hyperoside taken in two to three individual doses for a total of 750–1,500 mg of hawthorn per day [5].

Transient side effects including dizziness, gastrointestinal complaints, headaches, and heart palpitations have been reported [105]. *Crataegus* extract WS 1442 may determine an initial progression of heart failure, but the risk decreases over time [116].

15.3.7.3 Tricks of the Trade

Hawthorn, garlic, olive tree, and mistletoe are those most frequently used in practice. Based on our experience we can say that the hawthorn is most effective when hypertension is linked to stress and the pressure is not stable, but goes up and down depending on the nervous tension. Garlic is more effective in elderly subjects with arteriosclerosis and a tendency toward high cholesterol. The olive tree seems to be more effective in people with a tendency towards excessive weight, high cholesterol, high triglycerides, and high blood sugar: in practice the "blood" subjects of the Hippocratic tradition. Mistletoe works better when taken in the form of a decoction prepared with fresh leaves.

15.3.8 Mind–Body Therapy

It is a fact that the mind–body disciplines are associated with lowering blood pressure. The scientific path that led to this evidence [117–122] was complex and very often hampered by a lack of understanding that the researchers have of statistical confidence intervals and thresholds (for a further discussion of this issue, see our recent review and related bibliography [15]). Even those who have questioned the effectiveness of the methods [123] have surprisingly concluded that mind–body practices produced only modest benefits in reducing SBP, even though the investigators reported a roughly 5.5-mmHg reduction in SBP and a 3.5-mmHg reduction in DBP [122]. It should be taken into consideration that systolic BP reductions between 2 and 5 mmHg result in decreased mortality from stroke (14%), coronary heart disease (9%), and total mortality (7%) [6].

As we recently described [14]: "Verifying the effects of a medium such as meditation, mind–body therapies or music is particularly hard." Numerous subjective biases are lurking and difficult to measure or inevitable. Moreover, different meta-analyses of high-quality studies can arrive at different conclusions based on authors' end-point and selection of studies [124]. Randomized clinical trials (RCTs) can only be carried out, by definition, with patients and individuals who are willing to be randomized. Therefore, such trials are excluding the potentially most beneficial therapeutic agents: conscious choice and active engagement. Thus, by default, RCTs can only test and describe the minimum effect on people who use a certain intervention, as if it were delivered to them as a passive recipient, like a medication. However, listening to or playing music is not a medication. It requires active involvement and the decision to regularly dedicate a specific amount of time, over a longer period to change one's habits, attitudes, and physiological responses. This can only be assessed in long-term comparative cohort studies that in other conditions and occasions have shown reliable results comparable with RCTs [125]. To explore correctly many faces of the so-called alternative medicines, the scientific input should conform to the basic ancient principles and philosophies of the remedies under consideration, investigating them "as they are". Such research requires the already discussed "whole system biology and physics approaches," global participation with protocols evolved through intense interface with modern science, and regulatory reforms to eliminate cultural and economic barriers [126].

Nowadays, well-designed randomized controlled trials have demonstrated the efficacy of mind–body interventions, including elicitation of relaxation response [127], biofeedback [128], transcendental meditation (TM) [129, 130], yoga [131], qi gong [132, 133], and tai chi [134], on the reduction of SBP or DBP. Aggregating these studies, average reductions of roughly 10 mmHg and 7 mmHg are found for SBP and DBP respectively.

Moreover, an American Heart Association scientific statement provided a recommendation of class IIB, level of evidence B for TM implementation in clinical practice for hypertension treatment, based on the available level of evidence from the published literature [135].

15.4 Therapies to Consider: Ayurveda and Traditional Chinese and East Asian Medicine

Ayurveda and traditional Asian medicine and Chinese medicine are complete health systems with an ancient tradition, which modern Western medicine can use to draw valuable information on treatment and prevention. According to the Eastern medical traditions mentioned, the treatment of hypertension is based on a holistic approach and aims to "rebalance" the sick person.

In the case of Ayurveda, hypertension seems to derive from an imbalance of the doshas vata and pitta and requires a diet that "pacifies" such elements, breathing exercises (pranayama) [136–140], aromatherapy [141, 142], massage [143–145], yoga [146], and meditation. In addition to the herbs already mentioned, Ayurvedic medicine has used *Rauvolfia serpentina* (its active ingredient is reserpine) for over 1,500 years as one of the most active plants for hypertension. Given the risk of toxicity, its use was banned in the food and herbal industry in many countries, including Italy, and further research is needed to validate it as a medical treatment, either the plant alone, or in combination with other herbs.

Similar observations can be made in the case of traditional Chinese medicine (TCM). For TCM, a hypertensive patient may have a yin deficiency of the liver and kidney, ascendant liver yang, phlegm stagnation, or blood stagnation. The treatment is based on the use of herbs [5] (in the case of hypertension treatment: Gouteng [*Uncaria* species], Niu Xi [*Cyathae* species], Tianma [*Gastrodia* species], Chuanxiong [*Ligustrum sinense*], Fuling [*Poria cocos* Wolf], Zexie [*Alismatis* species], Juha [chrysanthemum], and Danshen [*Salvia miltiorrhiza*]), massage [147], acupuncture [148], and moxibustion [149].

References

1. Camm AJ, Luscher TF, Serruys PW (2009) ESC textbook of cardiovascular medicine (2nd edn). Oxford Med, 1–1398
2. Chobanian AV et al (2003) Seventh report of the Joint National Committee on Prevention, Detection, Evaluation, and Treatment of High Blood Pressure. Hypertension 42:1206–1252
3. Dal Lin C et al (2015) Coronary microvascular and endothelial function regulation: crossroads of psychoneuroendocrine immunitary signals and quantum physics [Part A]. J Integr Cardiol 1:132–163
4. Vasan RS et al (2002) Residual lifetime risk for developing hypertension in middle-aged women and men: The Framingham Heart Study. JAMA 287:1003–1010
5. Rakel D (2012) Integrative medicine (3rd edn). Elsevier, pp 1–1039
6. Whelton PK et al (2002) Primary prevention of hypertension: clinical and public health advisory from The National High Blood Pressure Education Program. JAMA 288:1882–1888
7. Tuffs A (2002) Three out of four Germans have used complementary or natural remedies. BMJ 325:990
8. Kitiyakara C, Wilcox CS (1998) Antioxidants for hypertension. Curr Opin Nephrol Hypertens 7:531–538
9. Nayak DU, Karmen C, Frishman WH, Vakili BA (2001) Antioxidant vitamins and enzymatic and synthetic oxygen-derived free radical scavengers in the prevention and treatment of cardiovascular disease. Heart Dis 3:28–45
10. Vaziri ND, Liang K, Ding Y (1999) Increased nitric oxide inactivation by reactive oxygen species in lead-induced hypertension. Kidney Int 56:1492–1498
11. Lacy F, O'Connor DT, Schmid-Schönbein GW (1998) Plasma hydrogen peroxide production in hypertensives and normotensive subjects at genetic risk of hypertension. J Hypertens 16:291–303
12. Kumar KV, Das UN (1993) Are free radicals involved in the pathobiology of human essential hypertension? Free Radic Res Commun 19:59–66
13. McIntyre M, Bohr DF, Dominiczak AF (1999) Endothelial function in hypertension: the role of superoxide anion. Hypertension 34:539–545
14. Dal Lin C et al (2015) Coronary microvascular and endothelial function regulation: crossroads of psychoneuroendocrine immunitary signals and quantum physics [Part C]. J Integr Cardiol 1:189–209
15. Dal Lin C et al (2015) Coronary microvascular and endothelial function regulation: crossroads of psychoneuroendocrine immunitary signals and quantum physics [Part B]. J Integr Cardiol 1:164–188
16. Pipe AL, Papadakis S, Reid RD (2010) The role of smoking cessation in the prevention of coronary artery disease. Curr Atheroscler Rep 12:145–150
17. Siasos G et al (2014) Smoking and atherosclerosis: mechanisms of disease and new therapeutic approaches. Curr Med Chem 21:3936–3948
18. Benowitz NL, Hansson A, Jacob P (2002) Cardiovascular effects of nasal and transdermal nicotine and cigarette smoking. Hypertension 39:1107–1112
19. Linneberg A et al (2015) Effect of smoking on blood pressure and resting heart rate: a Mendelian randomization meta-analysis in the CARTA Consortium. Circ Cardiovasc Genet 8:832–841
20. Yamagishi K et al (2003) Smoking raises the risk of total and ischemic strokes in hypertensive men. Hypertens Res 26:209–217
21. Kurth T et al (2003) Smoking and the risk of hemorrhagic stroke in men. Stroke 34:1151–1155
22. Núñez-Córdoba JM, Valencia-Serrano F, Toledo E, Alonso A, Martínez-González MA (2009) The Mediterranean diet and incidence of hypertension: the

Seguimiento Universidad de Navarra (SUN) Study. Am J Epidemiol 169:339–346
23. Estruch R et al (2013) Primary prevention of cardiovascular disease with a Mediterranean diet. N Engl J Med 368:1279–1290
24. Serra-Majem L, Roman B, Estruch R (2006) Scientific evidence of interventions using the Mediterranean diet: a systematic review. Nutr Rev 64:S27–47
25. Mitrou PN et al (2007) Mediterranean dietary pattern and prediction of all-cause mortality in a US population: results from the NIH-AARP Diet and Health Study. Arch Intern Med 167:2461–2468
26. Knoops KTB et al (2004) Mediterranean diet, lifestyle factors, and 10-year mortality in elderly European men and women: the HALE project. JAMA 292:1433–1439
27. Terés S et al (2008) Oleic acid content is responsible for the reduction in blood pressure induced by olive oil. Proc Natl Acad Sci U S A 105:13811–13816
28. Estruch R et al (2006) Effects of a Mediterranean-style diet on cardiovascular risk factors: a randomized trial. Ann Intern Med 145:1–11
29. Schini-Kerth VB, Auger C, Etienne-Selloum N, Chataigneau T (2010) Polyphenol-induced endothelium-dependent relaxations role of NO and EDHF. Adv Pharmacol 60:133–175
30. Galleano M, Pechanova O, Fraga CG (2010) Hypertension, nitric oxide, oxidants, and dietary plant polyphenols. Curr Pharm Biotechnol 11:837–848
31. López-Miranda J et al (2010) Olive oil and health: summary of the II international conference on olive oil and health consensus report, Jaén and Córdoba (Spain) 2008. Nutr Metab Cardiovasc Dis 20:284–294
32. Brown L et al (2009) The biological responses to resveratrol and other polyphenols from alcoholic beverages. Alcohol Clin Exp Res 33:1513–1523
33. Rotondo S, Di Castelnuovo A, de Gaetano G (2001) The relationship between wine consumption and cardiovascular risk: from epidemiological evidence to biological plausibility. Ital Heart J 2:1–8
34. Grønbaek M (2002) Alcohol, type of alcohol, and all-cause and coronary heart disease mortality. Ann N Y Acad Sci 957:16–20
35. Opie LH, Lecour S (2007) The red wine hypothesis: from concepts to protective signalling molecules. Eur Heart J 28:1683–1693
36. Soleas GJ, Diamandis EP, Goldberg DM (1997) Wine as a biological fluid: history, production, and role in disease prevention. J Clin Lab Anal 11:287–313
37. Mizutani K, Ikeda K, Kawai Y, Yamori Y (2001) Protective effect of resveratrol on oxidative damage in male and female stroke-prone spontaneously hypertensive rats. Clin Exp Pharmacol Physiol 28:55–59
38. Baur JA, Sinclair DA (2006) Therapeutic potential of resveratrol: the in vivo evidence. Nat Rev Drug Discov 5:493–506
39. Whelton SP et al (2005) Effect of dietary fiber intake on blood pressure: a meta-analysis of randomized, controlled clinical trials. J Hypertens 23:475–481
40. Appel LJ et al (1997) A clinical trial of the effects of dietary patterns on blood pressure. N Engl J Med 336:1117–1124
41. Obarzanek E, Velletri PA, Cutler JA (1996) Dietary protein and blood pressure. JAMA 275:1598–1603
42. Kawasaki T et al (2000) Antihypertensive effect of valyl-tyrosine, a short chain peptide derived from sardine muscle hydrolyzate, on mild hypertensive subjects. J Hum Hypertens 14:519–523
43. Pizzorno JE, Murray MT (2013) Textbook of natural medicine, 4th edn. Elsevier, Seattle
44. Devries S, Dalen J (2011) Integrative cardiology. Oxford University Press, Oxford
45. Hasler CM, Kundrat S, Wool D (2000) Functional foods and cardiovascular disease. Curr Atheroscler Rep 2:467–475
46. Xun P et al (2011) Fish oil, selenium and mercury in relation to incidence of hypertension: a 20-year follow-up study. J Intern Med 270:175–186
47. Mori TA et al (2009) The effects of omega-3 fatty acids and coenzyme Q10 on blood pressure and heart rate in chronic kidney disease: a randomized controlled trial. J Hypertens 27:1863–1872
48. Begg DP et al (2010) Hypertension induced by omega-3 polyunsaturated fatty acid deficiency is alleviated by alpha-linolenic acid regardless of dietary source. Hypertens Res 33:808–813
49. Buijsse B, Feskens EJM, Kok FJ, Kromhout D (2006) Cocoa intake, blood pressure, and cardiovascular mortality: the Zutphen Elderly Study. Arch Intern Med 166:411–417
50. Taubert D, Roesen R, Schömig E (2007) Effect of cocoa and tea intake on blood pressure: a meta-analysis. Arch Intern Med 167:626–634
51. Taubert D, Roesen R, Lehmann C, Jung N, Schömig E (2007) Effects of low habitual cocoa intake on blood pressure and bioactive nitric oxide: a randomized controlled trial. JAMA 298:49–60
52. Balzer J et al (2008) Sustained benefits in vascular function through flavanol-containing cocoa in medicated diabetic patients a double-masked, randomized, controlled trial. J Am Coll Cardiol 51:2141–2149
53. Whelton PK, He J (1999) Potassium in preventing and treating high blood pressure. Semin Nephrol 19:494–499
54. Patki PS et al (1990) Efficacy of potassium and magnesium in essential hypertension: a double-blind, placebo controlled, crossover study. BMJ 301:521–523
55. Fotherby MD, Potter JF (1997) Long-term potassium supplementation lowers blood pressure in elderly hypertensive subjects. Int J Clin Pract 51:219–222
56. Fotherby MD, Potter JF (1992) Potassium supplementation reduces clinic and ambulatory blood

pressure in elderly hypertensive patients. J Hypertens 10:1403–1408

57. Hatzistavri LS et al (2009) Oral magnesium supplementation reduces ambulatory blood pressure in patients with mild hypertension. Am J Hypertens 22:1070–1075
58. Guerrero-Romero F, Rodríguez-Morán M (2009) The effect of lowering blood pressure by magnesium supplementation in diabetic hypertensive adults with low serum magnesium levels: a randomized, double-blind, placebo-controlled clinical trial. J Hum Hypertens 23:245–251
59. Song Y et al (2006) Dietary magnesium intake and risk of incident hypertension among middle-aged and older US women in a 10-year follow-up study. Am J Cardiol 98:1616–1621
60. Baker WL et al (2009) Effect of magnesium L-lactate on blood pressure in patients with an implantable cardioverter defibrillator. Ann Pharmacother 43:569–576
61. Cappuccio FP et al (1995) Epidemiologic association between dietary calcium intake and blood pressure: a meta-analysis of published data. Am J Epidemiol 142:935–945
62. Meese RB et al (1987) The inconsistent effects of calcium supplements upon blood pressure in primary hypertension. Am J Med Sci 294:219–224
63. Sowers JR, Zemel MB, Standley PR, Zemel PC (1989) Calcium and hypertension. J Lab Clin Med 114:338–348
64. Takagi Y, Fukase M, Takata S, Fujimi T, Fujita T (1991) Calcium treatment of essential hypertension in elderly patients evaluated by 24 H monitoring. Am J Hypertens 4:836–839
65. Hajjar IM, George V, Sasse EA, Kochar MS (2002) A randomized, double-blind, controlled trial of vitamin C in the management of hypertension and lipids. Am J Ther 9:289–293
66. Fotherby MD, Williams JC, Forster LA, Craner P, Ferns GA (2000) Effect of vitamin C on ambulatory blood pressure and plasma lipids in older persons. J Hypertens 18:411–415
67. Galley HF, Thornton J, Howdle PD, Walker BE, Webster NR (1997) Combination oral antioxidant supplementation reduces blood pressure. Clin Sci (Lond) 92:361–365
68. van Dijk RA, Rauwerda JA, Steyn M, Twisk JW, Stehouwer CD (2001) Long-term homocysteine-lowering treatment with folic acid plus pyridoxine is associated with decreased blood pressure but not with improved brachial artery endothelium-dependent vasodilation or carotid artery stiffness: a 2-year, randomized, placebo-contr. Arterioscler Thromb Vasc Biol 21:2072–2079
69. Aybak M, Sermet A, Ayyildiz MO, Karakilçik AZ (1995) Effect of oral pyridoxine hydrochloride supplementation on arterial blood pressure in patients with essential hypertension. Arzneimittelforschung 45:1271–1273
70. Kawashima H (1987) Receptor for 1,25-dihydroxyvitamin D in a vascular smooth muscle cell line derived from rat aorta. Biochem Biophys Res Commun 146:1–6
71. Dal Lin C, Tona F, Osto E (2015) Coronary microvascular function and beyond: the crosstalk between hormones, cytokines, and neurotransmitters. Int J Endocrinol 17:312848
72. Li YC et al (2002) 1,25-Dihydroxyvitamin D(3) is a negative endocrine regulator of the renin-angiotensin system. J Clin Invest 110:229–238
73. Forman JP et al (2007) Plasma 25-hydroxyvitamin D levels and risk of incident hypertension. Hypertension 49:1063–1069
74. Anderson JL et al (2010) Relation of vitamin D deficiency to cardiovascular risk factors, disease status, and incident events in a general healthcare population. Am J Cardiol 106:963–968
75. Pfeifer M, Begerow B, Minne HW, Nachtigall D, Hansen C (2001) Effects of a short-term vitamin D (3) and calcium supplementation on blood pressure and parathyroid hormone levels in elderly women. J Clin Endocrinol Metab 86:1633–1637
76. Beveridge LA et al (2015) Effect of vitamin D supplementation on blood pressure: a systematic review and meta-analysis incorporating individual patient data. JAMA Intern Med 175:745–754
77. Jorde R, Sneve M, Torjesen P, Figenschau Y (2010) No improvement in cardiovascular risk factors in overweight and obese subjects after supplementation with vitamin D3 for 1 year. J Intern Med 267:462–472
78. Yamagami T, Shibata N, Folkers K (1975) Bioenergetics in clinical medicine. Studies on coenzyme Q10 and essential hypertension. Res Commun Chem Pathol Pharmacol 11:273–288
79. Digiesi V et al (1994) Coenzyme Q10 in essential hypertension. Mol Aspects Med 15(Suppl):s257–263
80. Ho MJ, Bellusci A, Wright JM (2009) Blood pressure lowering efficacy of coenzyme Q10 for primary hypertension. Cochrane Database Syst Rev, CD007435
81. Langsjoen P, Willis R, Folkers K (1994) Treatment of essential hypertension with coenzyme Q10. Mol Aspects Med 15(Suppl):S265–272
82. Rosenfeldt FL et al (2007) Coenzyme Q10 in the treatment of hypertension: a meta-analysis of the clinical trials. J Hum Hypertens 21:297–306
83. Ghirlanda G et al (1993) Evidence of plasma CoQ10-lowering effect by HMG-CoA reductase inhibitors: a double-blind, placebo-controlled study. J Clin Pharmacol 33:226–229
84. Singh RB, Niaz MA, Rastogi SS, Shukla PK, Thakur AS (1999) Effect of hydrosoluble coenzyme Q10 on blood pressures and insulin resistance in hypertensive patients with coronary artery disease. J Hum Hypertens 13:203–208
85. Horvath K et al (2008) Long-term effects of weight-reducing interventions in hypertensive patients:

systematic review and meta-analysis. Arch Intern Med 168:571–580
86. Pescatello LS et al (2004) American College of Sports Medicine position stand. Exercise and hypertension. Med Sci Sports Exerc 36:533–553
87. Kario K, Suzuki T, Nakagawa Y, Mitsuhashi T, Shimada K (1997) White-coat hypertension triggered by iatrogenic hypertension. Lancet 349:1330
88. Firenzuoli, F. (2009) Fitoterapia. Guida all'uso clinico delle piante medicinali. Elsevier
89. Hansen K et al (1996) Isolation of an angiotensin converting enzyme (ACE) inhibitor from Olea europaea and Olea lancea. Phytomedicine 2:319–325
90. Orhan DD, Küpeli E, Yesilada E, Ergun F (2006) Anti-inflammatory and antinociceptive activity of flavonoids isolated from Viscum album ssp album. Zeitschrift fur Naturforsch – Sect C J Biosci 61:26–30
91. Önay-Uçar E, Karagöz A, Arda N (2006) Antioxidant activity of Viscum album ssp. album. Fitoterapia 77:556–560
92. Gupta G et al (2012) Sedative, antiepileptic and antipsychotic effects of Viscum album L. (Loranthaceae) in mice and rats. J Ethnopharmacol 141:810–816
93. Gardin NE (2009) Immunological response to mistletoe (Viscum album L.) in cancer patients: a four-case series. Phyther Res 23:407–411
94. Tenorio FA, Del Valle L, González A, Pastelín G (2005) Vasodilator activity of the aqueous extract of Viscum album. Fitoterapia 76:204–209
95. Deliorman D et al (2000) Studies on the vascular effects of the fractions and phenolic compounds isolated from Viscum album ssp album. J Ethnopharmacol 72:323–329
96. McKay DL, Chen C-Y O, Saltzman E, Blumberg JB (2010) Hibiscus sabdariffa L. tea (tisane) lowers blood pressure in prehypertensive and mildly hypertensive adults. J Nutr 140:298–303
97. Mozaffari-Khosravi H, Jalali-Khanabadi B-A, Afkhami-Ardekani M, Fatehi F, Noori-Shadkam M (2009) The effects of sour tea (Hibiscus sabdariffa) on hypertension in patients with type II diabetes. J Hum Hypertens 23:48–54
98. Mozaffari-Khosravi H, Ahadi Z, Barzegar K (2013) The effect of green tea and sour tea on blood pressure of patients with type 2 diabetes: a randomized clinical trial. J Diet Suppl 10:105–115
99. Haji Faraji M, Haji Tarkhani A (1999) The effect of sour tea (Hibiscus sabdariffa) on essential hypertension. J Ethnopharmacol 65:231–236
100. Herrera-Arellano A, Flores-Romero S, Chávez-Soto MA, Tortoriello J (2004) Effectiveness and tolerability of a standardized extract from Hibiscus sabdariffa in patients with mild to moderate hypertension: a controlled and randomized clinical trial. Phytomedicine 11:375–382
101. Herrera-Arellano A et al (2007) Clinical effects produced by a standardized herbal medicinal product of Hibiscus sabdariffa on patients with hypertension. A randomized, double-blind, lisinopril-controlled clinical trial. Planta Med 73:6–12
102. Walker AF et al (2006) Hypotensive effects of hawthorn for patients with diabetes taking prescription drugs: a randomised controlled trial. Br J Gen Pract 56:437–443
103. Müller A, Linke W, Zhao Y, Klaus W (1996) Crataegus extract prolongs action potential duration in guinea-pig papillary muscle. Phytomedicine 3:257–261
104. Schüssler M, Hölzl J, Fricke U (1995) Myocardial effects of flavonoids from Crataegus species. Arzneimittelforschung 45:842–845
105. Daniele C, Mazzanti G, Pittler MH, Ernst E (2006) Adverse-event profile of Crataegus spp.: a systematic review. Drug Saf 29:523–535
106. Zarzuelo A, Duarte J, Jiménez J, González M, Utrilla MP (1991) Vasodilator effect of olive leaf. Planta Med 57:417–419
107. Castaldo S (1996) Plant derived calcium antagonists and their possible clinical application. Phyther Res 10, sup//1; Soc. Ital. di Farmacogn. Congr. Naz. 8, Soc. Ital. di Farmacogn. S199–S201.
108. Carneiro DM et al. (2014) Randomized, double-blind clinical trial to assess the acute diuretic effect of equisetum arvense (field horsetail) in healthy volunteers. Evidence-based Complement Altern Med 2014:760683
109. Mimica-Dukic N et al (2008) Phenolic compounds in field horsetail (Equisetum arvense L.) as natural antioxidants. Molecules 13:1455–1464
110. Beaux D, Fleurentin J, Mortier F (1999) Effect of extracts of Orthosiphon stamineus Benth, Hieracium pilosella L., Sambucus nigra L. and Arctostaphylos uva-ursi (L.) Spreng. in rats. Phyther Res 13:222–225
111. Clare BA, Conroy RS, Spelman K (2009) The diuretic effect in human subjects of an extract of Taraxacum officinale folium over a single day. J Altern Complement Med 15:929–934
112. Krasutsky PA (2006) Birch bark research and development. Nat Prod Rep 23:919–942
113. Luo C et al (2013) Protection of H9c2 rat cardiomyoblasts against oxidative insults by total paeony glucosides from Radix Paeoniae Rubrae. Phytomedicine 21:20–24
114. De Bruyne B et al (2003) Intracoronary and intravenous adenosine 5′-triphosphate, adenosine, papaverine, and contrast medium to assess fractional flow reserve in humans. Circulation 107:1877–1883
115. Luzak B et al (2014) Extract from Ribes nigrum leaves in vitro activates nitric oxide synthase (eNOS) and increases CD39 expression in human endothelial cells. J Physiol Biochem 70:1007–1019
116. Zick SM, Gillespie B, Aaronson KD (2008) The effect of Crataegus oxycantha Special Extract WS 1442 on clinical progression in patients with mild to moderate symptoms of heart failure. Eur J Heart Fail 10:587–593

117. Frankel BL, Patel DJ, Horwitz D, Friedewald WT, Gaarder KR (1978) Treatment of hypertension with biofeedback and relaxation techniques. Psychosom Med 40:276–293
118. Hafner RJ (1982) Psychological treatment of essential hypertension: a controlled comparison of meditation and meditation plus biofeedback. Biofeedback Self Regul 7:305–316
119. Linden W, Lenz JW, Con AH (2001) Individualized stress management for primary hypertension: a randomized trial. Arch Intern Med 161:1071–1080
120. McGrady AV, Yonker R, Tan SY, Fine TH, Woerner M (1981) The effect of biofeedback-assisted relaxation training on blood pressure and selected biochemical parameters in patients with essential hypertension. Biofeedback Self Regul 6:343–353
121. Patel C, North WR (1975) Randomised controlled trial of yoga and bio-feedback in management of hypertension. Lancet 2:93–95
122. Seer P, Raeburn JM (1980) Meditation training and essential hypertension: a methodological study. J Behav Med 3:59–71
123. Dickinson H et al (2008) Relaxation therapies for the management of primary hypertension in adults: a Cochrane review. J Hum Hypertens 22:809–820
124. Cramer H, Lauche R, Haller H, Dobos G, Michalsen A (2015) A systematic review of yoga for heart disease. Eur J Prev Cardiol 22:284–295
125. Rutledge T, Mills P, Schneider R (2014) Meditation intervention reviews. JAMA Intern Med 174:1193
126. Singh RH (2010) Exploring issues in the development of Ayurvedic research methodology. J Ayurveda Integr Med 1:91–95
127. Dusek JA et al (2008) Stress management versus lifestyle modification on systolic hypertension and medication elimination: a randomized trial. J Altern Complement Med 14:129–138
128. Blanchard EB et al (1996) Controlled evaluation of thermal biofeedback in treatment of elevated blood pressure in unmedicated mild hypertension. Biofeedback Self Regul 21:167–190
129. Schneider RH et al (2005) A randomized controlled trial of stress reduction in African Americans treated for hypertension for over one year. Am J Hypertens 18:88–98
130. Schneider RH et al (1995) A randomised controlled trial of stress reduction for hypertension in older African Americans. Hypertension 26:820–7
131. Murugesan R, Govindarajulu N, Bera TK (2000) Effect of selected yogic practices on the management of hypertension. Indian J Physiol Pharmacol 44:207–210
132. Lee MS, Lee MS, Kim H-J, Choi E-S (2004) Effects of qigong on blood pressure, high-density lipoprotein cholesterol and other lipid levels in essential hypertension patients. Int J Neurosci 114:777–786
133. Lee M-S, Lee MS, Kim H-J, Moon S-R (2003) Qigong reduced blood pressure and catecholamine levels of patients with essential hypertension. Int J Neurosci 113:1691–1701
134. Lee MS, Pittler MH, Guo R, Ernst E (2007) Qigong for hypertension: a systematic review of randomized clinical trials. J Hypertens 25:1525–1532
135. Brook RD et al (2013) Beyond medications and diet: alternative approaches to lowering blood pressure: a scientific statement from the American Heart Association. Hypertension 61:1360–183
136. Anderson DE, McNeely JD, Windham BG (2010) Regular slow-breathing exercise effects on blood pressure and breathing patterns at rest. J Hum Hypertens 24:807–813
137. Bhavanani AB, Sanjay Z, Madanmohan (2011) Immediate effect of sukha pranayama on cardiovascular variables in patients of hypertension. Int J Yoga Therap 2011(21):73–76
138. Kaushik RM, Kaushik R, Mahajan SK, Rajesh V (2006) Effects of mental relaxation and slow breathing in essential hypertension. Complement Ther Med 14:120–126
139. Lee JS et al (2003) Effects of diaphragmatic breathing on ambulatory blood pressure and heart rate. Biomed Pharmacother 57(Suppl 1):87s–91s
140. Bhavanani AB, Madanmohan, Sanjay Z (2012) Immediate effect of chandra nadi pranayama (left unilateral forced nostril breathing) on cardiovascular parameters in hypertensive patients. Int J Yoga 5:108–11
141. Price S, Price L (2012) Aromatherapy for health professionals, 4edn. Elsevier, 1–355
142. Stein RA, Mehmet CO (2004) Complementary and alternative cardiovascular medicine. Springer, Berlin
143. Walaszek R (2015) Impact of classic massage on blood pressure in patients with clinically diagnosed hypertension. J Tradit Chin Med 35:396–401
144. Basler AJ (2011) Pilot study investigating the effects of Ayurvedic Abhyanga massage on subjective stress experience. J Altern Complement Med 17:435–440
145. Dhuri KD, Bodhe PV, Vaidya AB (2013) Shirodhara: a psycho-physiological profile in healthy volunteers. J Ayurveda Integr Med 4:40–44
146. Cohen DL et al (2011) Iyengar yoga versus enhanced usual care on blood pressure in patients with prehypertension to stage I hypertension: a randomized controlled trial. Evid Based Complement Alternat Med 2011(546428)
147. Xiong XJ, Li SJ, Zhang YQ (2015) Massage therapy for essential hypertension: a systematic review. J Hum Hypertens 29:143–151
148. Flachskampf FA et al (2007) Randomized trial of acupuncture to lower blood pressure. Circulation 115:3121–3129
149. Kim J-I, Choi J-Y, Lee H, Lee MS, Ernst E (2010) Moxibustion for hypertension: a systematic review. BMC Cardiovasc Disord 10:33

16 Integrated Approach to Coronary Artery Disease

Carlo Dal Lin, Marco Silvestro, Raffaele Migliorini, Francesco Tona, and Massimo Fioranelli

16.1 Introduction

About 20 million persons in the USA have coronary heart disease (CHD):10.2 million with angina pectoris and 8.5 million with myocardial infarction [1]. The lifetime risk for developing coronary artery disease for people in middle age is 50% for men and 30% for women [2]. According to a 2013–2014 World Health Organization study, over 4 million deaths annually are due to cardiovascular disease, for which ischemic heart disease is the main factor [3]. Mortality from CHD is expected to increase in developing countries from an estimated 9 million in 1990 to a projected 19 million by 2020 [4].

The American Heart Association estimates that 1.1 million myocardial infarctions occur in the USA alone and that 40% of these patients will die [5]. Indeed, CHD is responsible for more than 2,000 deaths every day in Western society [6] and one of three US residents is destined to die of a cardiovascular cause [6]. Approximately half of the deaths occur before the patient receives medical attention [5]. The incidence of myocardial infarction is within the range of 1 per 250 to 1 per 500 of the population per year [5].

Clearly, we still have a lot of work to do. The main causes of CHD and its risk factors are related to lifestyle and environment, as demonstrated by the Interheart Study [7, 8] (Table 16.1).

Nutritional imbalance, sedentary lifestyle, stress and depression, smoking, and air pollution play a key role in the pathogenesis of risk factors for CHD and the onset and progression of atherosclerotic disease [9, 10]. Also, what is commonly called "genetic predisposition" seems to be increasingly linked to genome activation patterns in response to environmental influences, as demonstrated by the acquisition of the local, most high-profile, cardiovascular risk of migrants from areas with a low incidence of coronary heart disease [11, 12]. The concept of an epigenetic modulation of coronary artery disease, with traces that can be transmitted transgenerationally, is taking hold [9]. These traces are stable but reversible, and this indicates the importance of prevention with an integrated approach to the care of CHD [9, 11–13].

Currently, it is thought that one of three children born in the year 2000 will go on to develop diabetes during his or her lifetime [14]. Consequently, for the first time in history, it is possible for children to have a shorter life expectancy than their parents [12, 15].

As stated by Stephen Devries [8, 16]: "an integrative approach acknowledges the great

C. Dal Lin, M.D. (✉) • M. Silvestro, N.D. • R. Migliorini, M.D. • F. Tona, M.D., Ph.D.
Department of Cardiological, Thoracic and Vascular Sciences, Padua University Medical School, Padova, Italy
e-mail: carlodallin@libero.it

M. Fioranelli, M.D.
Department of Nuclear Physics, Sub-Nuclear and Radiation, Guglielmo Marconi University, Rome, Italy

M. Fioranelli (ed.), *Integrative Cardiology*, DOI 10.1007/978-3-319-40010-5_16

Table 16.1 Results of the Interheart Study. Modified from [8]

Cardiovascular risk factor	Relative risk
Smoking	2.87
Hypertension	1.91
Elevated Apo B/ Apo A1	3.25
Diabetes	2.37
Abdominal obesity	1.12
Psychosocial factors	2.67
Daily consumption of fruits and vegetables	0.7
Regular physical activity	0.86

value and potentially lifesaving benefits of modern pharmacology and procedures, while at the same time recognizing the limitations of these approaches when they are used in isolation." Most drug and interventional therapy patterns are studied in the context of acute illness and do not fit or even fall into the context of chronic disease [9, 11, 12, 17].

Devries [16] states, "an integrative approach is ideally suited for prevention and treatment of coronary disease because it addresses many of the root causes, especially those influenced by lifestyle." Thus, cardiologists should become familiar with a broader spectrum of therapies beyond those that typically constitute conventional cardiovascular care (Fig. 16.1).

The Coronary Artery Surgery Study (CASS) demonstrated that patients with healthy hearts, but with one, two, or three stenotic major heart vessels, did surprisingly well without surgery, regardless of the number or severity of blockages [18]. This result correlates with what has emerged from the COURAGE study, where the benefits of coronary revascularization compared with optimal medical therapy were lacking, in the case of stable coronary artery disease, although angiographically critical [19–22]. Moreover, there is evidence that prolonged dual antiplatelet therapy following placement of a drug-eluting stent increases major bleeding but is not associated with a decrease in composite rates of death or myocardial infarction [23, 24]. From these observations coronary artery stenosis does not estimate correctly the possible presence of a reduction of flow in the artery. Furthermore, acute coronary events often arise from "mild" coronary lesions that are far less than 50% obstructive [25]. These seemingly harmless plaques are more "vulnerable," having a large lipid core and thin fibrous cap, which make them likely to rupture and evolve into a complete thrombotic occlusion and a potentially lethal cardiac event [26]. This is the explanation for the anecdotal familiar to most clinicians and patients about the individual who sailed through a stress test with "normal" results, only to suffer a cardiac catastrophe a short time later.

But what determines the catastrophe precisely at some point in the patient's history?

A possible answer to this question comes from the study of coronary microcirculation to understand the dense network of factors that, adjusting endothelial function, can maintain the balance between health and cardiovascular disease. For an extended discussion of the issue, please see our recent reviews [9, 11–13]. Briefly, we focus on the *functional* restriction to blood flow, which may lead to ischemia even in the absence of atherosclerotic plaques or angiographically critical plaques. The mechanism that drives myocardial ischemia concerns the regulation of coronary microcirculation in which several factors converge: neurotransmitters, cytokines, and hormones. In turn, these mediators are involved in the activation and operation of the integrated chronic stress axis, on which the psychological and emotional profiles and lifestyle of the subjects play a key role [9, 11, 12].

We agree with Stephen Devries when he says [16]: "The finding that a coronary event can rapidly develop from what angiographically appears to be a 'mild' coronary lesion emphasizes the need to prevent coronary lesions from developing, rather than to focus on reducing the severity of severe stenoses with interventional procedures." We would add that more resources should be invested in the field of preventive medical research and basic research into understanding the origin of these phenomena.

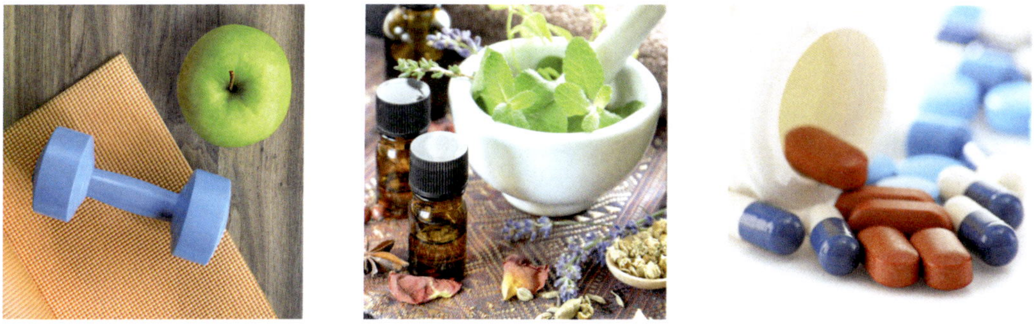

Minimize obstacles to healing →

- Lifestyle indications: eliminate smoking, alcohol and caffeine.

- Stress: stress management through relaxation, meditation, yoga, biofeedback.

- Diet: minimize saturated fats, fried foods, simple carbohydrates, food allergens.

- Sedentary lifestyle: carefully graded progressive exercise.

Tailor natural interventions to patient needs →

- Dietary imbalances: increase fiber, garlic, onions, vegetables, fish, high potency vitamin-mineral.

- Low antioxidant status: antioxidants.

- Coronary vasospasm; hypertension: Magnesium, Potassium, CoQ10, Crataegus.

- Hyperlipidemia: panthetine.

- Poor exercise tollerance: CoQ10, L-carnitine, panthetine, Crataegus, Ammi visnaga.

Determine need for conventional therapy

- Unstable angina or severe vascular occlusion: refer for hospidalization.

- Patient chooses angiogram, angioplasty, bypass: avoid garlic, additional vitamins and supplements.

Fig. 16.1 In summary: staged integrative approach to coronary heart disease. Don't smoke, promote risk factors reduction (diabetes, hypertension, hyperlipidemia), regular exercise, provide a comprehensive nutritional plan (adding fiber and omega-3 fatty acids, vegetables, whole grain bread, and cereals), evaluate for depression, anxiety or anger proneness, and manage stress

16.2 Nutrition

From Hippocrates, we know that "food is medicine." Nutrition represents the best tool available for prevention and treatment of CHD as demonstrated by the striking results of the Lyon Diet Heart study [27]. This study, conducted in individuals who survived myocardial infarction, shows that a Mediterranean-style diet leads to a 73% reduction in cardiovascular events, including myocardial infarction and cardiac death, after 27 months in comparison with controls. After 5 years of follow-up the benefit of the Mediterranean-style diet was maintained with a 72% reduction in cardiovascular events [28].

The cornerstone of the Mediterranean diet consists in eating a lot of vegetables (especially dark green leafy vegetables [29]) and fruit, nuts, and fish, in using olive oil and in a low to moderate intake of red meat and refined carbohydrates. Thus, it is possible to recommend a daily consumption of five servings of vegetables and two servings of fruit [16].

A single high-fat meal transiently impairs endothelial function and blood flow [30].

In the Mediterranean diet, chicken or fish substitute red meat, reducing the risk of CHD of 30% [31, 32] to 40% [33].

The Mediterranean diet emphasizes the consumption of whole grains to reduce CHD risk [34]. Indeed, refined grains favor atherosclerosis, releasing more glucose into the circulation and triggering higher insulin levels. This process is accompanied by reduced levels of high-density lipoprotein (HDL) and increased levels of atherogenic small dense low-density lipoprotein (LDL) [35]. Examples of whole grains include barley, buckwheat, quinoa, polenta, and brown rice.

As suggested by Hallfrisch et al. [36]: "the manner in which grains are prepared also has important health implications. Consuming pulverized grains, even whole grains, results in a higher blood glucose level than when the intact grain is eaten. Therefore, boiled whole grains are typically a healthier choice than bread made from the flour of whole grains."

Moreover, increasing consumption of nuts, another key element of the Mediterranean diet, to two handfuls per day reduces LDL [37] and the risk of CHD [38]. The nutmeg oil contains substances with platelet anti-aggregating action [39]: eugenol, isoeugenol, safrole, elemicin, myristicin, and limonene. The mechanism of action is the inhibition of cyclooxygenase [40, 41].

Finally, curcumin, soy beans extracts protect heart function against myocardial ischemia–reperfusion injury by activation of the JAK2/STAT3 signaling pathway [42–44].

16.3 Exercise

Along with nutrition, exercise is the other natural cornerstone to be added for cardiovascular health maintenance and for the treatment of CHD and its consequences. It must be emphasized that the intensity of exercise is less important than the frequency and consistency [45]. The two best forms of exercise to reduce cardiovascular risk are aerobic exercise (30 min of brisk walking every day) and resistance training (two to three sessions per week of light resistance training interspersed with stretching [45] or yoga [46, 47]).

In patients with ischemic heart disease or cardiovascular risk factors, it is good practice to run a stress test or a cardiopulmonary test for proper exercise prescription [5].

As we recently described [9, 11, 12], exercise alone is not enough: we have to take care of the mental aspects of our patients. Bergh et al. [48] have shown exercise to be an effective advantage in terms of prevention and treatment of cardiovascular diseases, must be accompanied by good psychological resistance to stress. In fact, low-stress resilience in adolescence is associated with increased risk of CVD in middle age. The association remains after adjustment for physical fitness: higher physical fitness is inversely associated with CVD risk; however, this is significantly attenuated by low-stress resilience [48].

16.4 Supplements

Change in lifestyle is the basis of a program of primary and secondary prevention of cardiovascular disease. The optimization of lifestyle is vital, to treat dyslipidemia before it is necessary to use statins. We want to recall that 33% of heart attacks occur in individuals with a total cholesterol above 200 mg/dL [49]. For the integrated care of dyslipidemia see Chap. 14.

We would like to focus attention on the availability of some lipid-lowering supplements only (Table 16.2) that can be employed in patients philosophically opposed to the use of statins or who are not able to tolerate them for the onset of side effects (myalgia). They are: *fiber* (psyllium 10 g per day) [50, 51]; *plants*

Table 16.2 Alternative therapies for reduction of low-density lipoprotein cholesterol. Modified from Rakel [16]

Product	Percentage of reduction
Psyllium (10 g/day)	7 %
Sterol and stanol (1.8 g/day)	14 %
Niacin (up to 2 g/day)	15–20 %
Red yeast rice (2,400 mg/day)	20–30 %

containing phytosterols and stanols (1.8 g per day as a single dose, added to certain margarines or in pill form) [52]; *niacin*, a vitamin B (500 mg per day, titrated upward by 500-mg increments every 6–8 weeks as needed, to a maximum of 2,000 mg per day, checking liver function and flushing. To avoid niacin flush, niacin must be taken with dinner or after dinner with apple sauce or with aspirin. Flush-free niacin compounds are ineffective) [53, 54], *red yeast rice* (600 mg twice daily, then 1,200 mg b.i.d) [55–59], and *fish oil* (not the total fish oil, but its eicosapentaenoic (EPA) and docosahexaenoic (DHA) acids lower triglyceride values with a dosage of 1,000 mg per day for prevention and 1,000 mg to 4,000 mg for the treatment of hypertriglyceridemia) [60].

Coenzyme Q10 (CoQ10) is an essential component of mitochondrial energy production and is commonly deficient in elderly people, in subjects taking statins and beta-blockers, and in patients with heart diseases in general [61]. Its supplementation could be useful for improving myalgia in patients with a history of statin-related muscle symptoms [62–65]. Moreover, CoQ10 (100 mg to 200 mg per day) seems to improve systolic function in the case of heart failure [66], to halve the frequency of angina attacks in stable patients, and to increase treadmill exercise tolerance [67].

The action of *vitamin D* receptors regulates blood pressure and vascular arterial function [68] and a deficiency in vitamin D correlates with higher cardiovascular risk, especially in hypertensive subjects [69]. However, even if data about the efficacy of its supplementation are inconclusive, values higher than 30 ng/mL are desirable [16]. It can be helpful in reducing the risk of muscle pain associated with statins [70].

Selective *folic acid* supplementation has not proven to be useful for the prevention of cardiovascular events, but foods rich in folate (dark green leafy vegetables) are associated with significant benefit [71–73].

Vitamin E exists in eight isomers: four tocopherols and four tocotrienols. Studies have focused only on the alpha-tocopherol fraction of vitamin E, with no cardiovascular benefit [74–77]. Probably, in the future, gamma and delta tocopherols may be more beneficial [78, 79].

Heart ischemia reduces the levels of *carnitine* (see Chap. 17 on heart failure) increasing the risk for angina [61]. Its supplementation (900 mg q.d.) improves angina and CHD [80–84], allowing the heart muscle to utilize limited oxygen more efficiently, improves exercise tolerance, exerts a cardioprotective and slightly anti-extrasystolic beats function, and represents a good alternative to drugs in patients with stable angina pectoris [18].

Pantethine is a component of coenzyme A that decreases during ischemia: its supplementation 900 mg q.d. determines a lipid-lowering effect [18]. It could be useful in treating angina [85].

Magnesium deficiency may produce coronary vasospasms and non-occlusive myocardial infarction [86–89]. Magnesium supplementation in the first hour after an acute infarction reduces immediate and long-term complications and death rates, dilating coronary arteries, inhibiting platelet aggregation, reducing infarct size, and helping to manage arrhythmias and angina [90–92].

Arginine supplementation (3–6 g/day) could be effective in cases of angina pectoris because of its ability to increase nitric oxide levels, thereby improving blood flow, reducing thrombosis and improving rheology [93–96]. Higher doses could be unsafe [97].

16.5 Phytomedicine

In cardiovascular medicine, there are many compounds of herbal medicine that can be used for therapy [98] and many drugs used in hospitals in western standard clinical practice are derived from plants, such as digitalis, hypericum, valerian, or senna [99]. On the other hand, we are discovering in plants new principles and extracts potentially active on the cardiovascular system that can be used as herbal medicines or become the basis for new drug products [100], such as *astragaloside IV* [101–104] and *naringenin* [105], compounds with anti- inflammatory activity, that inhibit the NF-kB factor.

The epidemiological evidence reported above on the use of herbs and these introductory examples serve to demonstrate how the cardiologist or internist should familiarize themselves with the use of herbs because: many herbal remedies interfere with most of the antiplatelet agents, anticoagulants, anti-arrhythmics and diuretics [106, 107]; many sub-clinical diseases find in herbal medicine an helpful and economic help, that can be integrated into standard clinical practice [99]; many substances of plant origin, anti-oxidants, or food (Mediterranean diet [108, 109] or plant-based diets [110, 111]), are useful in the prevention of endothelial damage from atherosclerosis or other risk factors (smoking, free reactive oxygen radicals, hypercholesterolemia) [112, 113].

16.5.1 Dark Chocolate

Regular consumption of dark chocolate is associated with low serum concentrations of C-reactive protein [114, 115], blood pressure-lowering [116], platelet anti-aggregation effects [117], endothelial protection [118, 119], coronary vasomotion improvement [120], and insulin sensitivity increase [121, 122].

16.5.2 Green Tea, Black Tea, and Coffee

As revealed by Kuriyama et al. [123–125], green tea consumption reduces mortality from cardiovascular disease of all causes, acting on the control of inflammation and vascular atherosclerosis. Moreover, epidemiological studies have shown a reduction in the risk of stroke derived from the intake of coffee or tea, independently of known cardiovascular risk factors [126, 127]. The anti-oxidant properties of coffee, cocoa, and tea [128] are well known for their benefits for the cardiovascular system, the coronary area in particular, owing to the action of the polyphenols contained in these foods [129]. Coffee contains over a thousand chemicals, many formed during the roasting process. From a physiological point of view, the potential bioactives are caffeine, the diterpenes cafestol and kahweol, found in the oil, and the polyphenols, most notably chlorogenic acid [130, 131]. Black tea consumption, with its anti-oxidant flavonoids, reverses endothelial dysfunction in patients with coronary artery disease [132–134].

Experimental data show that the polyphenols in green and black tea protect the endothelium in an equivalent manner [135, 136] and that the consumption of tea causes rapid improvements in the hemorheological parameters and in the function of endothelial progenitor cells, and may represent an important factor for cardiovascular protection, especially in smokers [137, 138]. The age of an individual correlates with the state of his arteries: during life, risk factors (smoking, hypertension, diabetes, hyperlipidemia, stress) cause damage to the endothelium of the vascular system in several places, constituting the first event of a series of processes that lead to the formation of atheroma and thrombus. The elements located under the endothelium, mainly collagen fibers, mediate the response and activation of platelets in a process in which platelet activating factor (PAF) plays and important role, being involved in the pathogenesis of thrombosis, vascular permeability, and endothelial damage.

16.5.3 *Vitis vinifera* and *Polygonum cuspidatum*

Another plant that recently entered the handbook of cardiovascular herbal medicine is *Vitis vinifera*: from its seeds resveratrol and of procyanidins are extracted [139, 140]. Procyanidins are indicated in the prevention of post-ischemic myocardial injury [141, 142], disorders of peripheral venous insufficiency, and in protecting endothelial cells, performing an anti-oxidant action that may also be useful in the treatment and prevention of many degenerative and chronic inflammatory conditions [143, 144]. Resveratrol is a phytoalexin, also present in other plants (such as in *Polygonum cuspidatum*), which has an anti-inflammatory activity (COX-2 inhibitor) [145] and a weak phyto-estrogenic action [146], prevents certain stages of carcinogenesis and also increases the activity of some anti-HIV drugs, such as zidovudine and didanosine [99]. Moreover, the anti-oxidant properties of red wine were demonstrated, also capable of inhibiting the formation of NF-kB, implicated in the pathogenesis of atherosclerosis [147]. Resveratrol has an antiplatelet activity and inhibits the oxidation of lipoproteins [146]. In summary, the grape contains a number of substances very useful in the prevention of cardiovascular disease [148, 149]. The resveratrol is present in the husk of the grains of grapes in a dose of 50–100 mg/g, while in wine it is present in an amount equal to 0.1–0.15 mg/L [99].

16.5.4 *Salvia miltiorrhiza*

There are some interesting therapeutic perspectives regarding the use of *Salvia miltiorrhiza* (*Bunge*), a typical plant of traditional Chinese medicine (Danshen) from which extracts of roots are used [150]. The plant contains a number of fat-soluble substances (tanshinones I, IIA, and IIB) and soluble (salvianolic acids A and B), which have the following properties: antiplatelet activity [151]; they release nitric oxide by endothelial cells [152]; they protect the myocardium from ischemic damage and reduce the area of myocardial necrosis by activation of the JAK2/STAT3 signaling pathway [42–44, 153]; and they stimulate coronary vasodilation and protect the central nervous system from ischemic damage [100]. According to current scientific evidence, despite the interesting results, there is not sufficient security to be able to definitively recommend the use of *Salvia miltiorrhiza* because of the poor methodological quality of the studies available. However, it is a very promising medicinal plant for preventing cardiovascular and cerebrovascular ischemic diseases. There may be interactions with antiplatelet drugs and oral anticoagulants.

16.5.5 *Ginkgo biloba*

In recent decades, the *Ginkgo biloba* leaves have been studied and used as a source of active metabolites able to treat atherosclerosis: in fact, they contain a mixture of flavonoid glycosides and terpene derivatives, which have vascular properties [154]. In particular, the terpene derivatives called ginkgolides and bilobalides, named according to their chemical structure with the letters of the alphabet (A, B, C, M, J) are potent antagonists of PAF [155]; they also antagonize coronary PAF-induced vasoconstriction, PAF-induced thrombus formation, and appear to significantly reduce the consequences of stroke [99]. Flavonoids of ginkgo biloba, in addition to reducing arteriolar spasm and inducing anti-inflammatory activity, increase the release of insulin from Langerhans cells [156].

Ginkgo (*Ginkgo biloba*) is an ornamental plant of eastern origin that has been growing since the Mesozoic. Traditional Chinese medicine also uses its fruits, whereas Western herbalism only uses the leaves, which contain the aforementioned terpenic derivatives with anti-PAF function and flavonoids with specific action on the microcirculation [157]. The latter, in fact, protect cell membranes by the action of oxygen free radicals and reduce endothelial progenitor cell senescence through augmentation of telomerase activity [158]; reduce arteriolar spasm; play an anti-inflammatory action [156]; reduce capillary permeability; increase the resistance of the capillaries; optimize the use of oxygen and glucose by the tissues; and regulate nitric oxide synthesis [159, 160]. Although there are conflicting data in the literature [161–163], and it is therefore necessary to gather additional evidence to establish the correct indications and timing of use in various cardiovascular diseases, the extracts of the plant could be employed for the treatment of atherosclerosis and its clinical manifestations (ischemic heart disease [164], peripheral vasculopathy [165, 166], cerebrovascular disease [167]), diabetes mellitus [168], vasculitis [169], angiosclerosis of the elderly brain [170], in Raynaud's disease and dizzy syndromes [171]. Ginkgo is also indicated in the prevention of vascular damage from high blood pressure and smoking, and in the prevention of deep vein thrombosis. Caution should be exercised when treating patients with liver disease [172], those with coagulation disorders or who are pregnant. There may be interactions with antiplatelet drugs and anticoagulants [173]. Clinical use involves the administration of the dry extract standardized to 24 % flavonoids and 6 % ginkgolides (substances that are more concentrated in the fruit can cause allergic or toxic reactions). The average dosage of standardized dry extract is 80 mg, 2–3 times a day [99].

16.5.6 *Vaccinium myrtillus*

Other plants studied with regard to modern cardiovascular herbalism are the blueberry (*Vaccinium myrtillus*) and the cranberry [174, 175]. The extracts of the berries were once considered only for their actions in reinforcing the capillaries. Today, the whole plant is used as a medicine that contains anthocyanins (cyanidin, delphinidin, pelargonidin, malvidin, peonidin, petunidin, and hirsutidin) and glycosides, including anthocyanidins, which give the purple color to the berries (and to numerous flowers of other plants) [99, 176]. Furthermore, the plant contains flavonoids and tannins [177]. The plant protects the endothelial cells because of its inhibitory action on the elastases and collagenases, making the connective tissue more stable and elastic [178]. Anthocyanosides inhibit platelet aggregation mediated by adenosine diphosphate, collagen, arachidonic acid, and PAF through the inhibition of thromboxane A2 and the degradation of AMP-c (a mechanism that appears similar to that of garlic) [99]. An antagonistic action on angiotensin II and the stimulation of the prostacyclin synthesis by the vascular wall [176, 179] have also been demonstrated. The anti-oxidant properties [180] of blueberry flavonoids are indicated in the prevention of ischemic heart disease and stroke [181–183]. Procyanidins inhibit xanthine oxidase in a non competitive way [184]. Blueberry extract also protects the arteriovenous microcirculation from damage related to the process of ischemia-–reperfusion [185]. The clinical efficacy of blueberry extract was primarily detected in the retinal area [186], where the plant's ability to sharpen night vision and to regenerate rhodopsin by increasing the activity of retinal LDH has been shown. Its active ingredients, finally, contrast capillary fragility, reducing vascular permeability, even at the peripheral level [178]. The blueberry can be employed in the treatment of patients with hypertensive retinopathy and/or diabetic and smoking patients with initial signs of micro- and macrovascular arteriosclerotic damage.

16.5.7 *Allium sativum*

Garlic (*Allium sativum*) has been used in medicine for thousands of years and has interesting cardiovascular properties [187]. These include the ability to inhibit platelet aggregation and the fibrinolytic, hypofibrinogenic, lipid-lowering, hypoglycemic, and hypotensive activities [188–190]. The German Ministry of Health has officially recognized the specific role of garlic in the treatment and prevention of atherosclerosis [99, 191, 192]. In addition, the plant is the most frequently used in the presence of heart disease [193] and for cardiovascular risk reduction [194, 195]. The main constituent of fresh garlic is alliin, which is transformed in turn into allicin as soon as the bulb is bruised by the action of an enzyme called allinase [196]. Allicin, being very unstable, is partly transformed quickly into another compound called ajoene [196]. Other important constituents are vinylditin, thiosulfinates, essential oil, deoxy-fructopyranosyl-allyl-cysteine sulfoxide) and allixin [196]. Platelet aggregation is inhibited by membrane receptor blocking and has been documented in vitro and in vivo with a dose-dependent mechanism [99].

The reduced platelet aggregation, the increased fibrinolysis, and the lipid-lowering action reduce the thrombotic risk [197–200]. Furthermore, the molecules of ajoene determine in vitro the inhibition of the cyclo- and lipo-oxygenase equal to indomethacin [99]. Garlic enhances the inhibitory action of prostacyclin 2 and of forskolin on platelet aggregation [201]. Furthermore, adenosine deaminase is inhibited, with a consequent increase in the adenosine available on the vascular endothelium, with vasodilatory and antiplatelet activity [202, 203]. The antiplatelet activity is very effective in vitro [204], but may not be the same in vivo, because the active substances are rapidly metabolized by tissues and are themselves quite unstable [205]. Some extracts also have reduced activity in vivo: the oils distilled in a current of steam have an activity of 35 % and macerated oil 12 % [99]. The fluid extracts would be inactive after only 6 months. In animals, the extracts of garlic have been shown to prevent damage from ischemia–reperfusion injury, owing to a calcium channel blocker activity and thanks to the anti-radical properties of allylcysteine, allylmercapto-cysteine, and alliin [206, 207]. The intake of the dry extract, carefully titrated, seem to have positive effects on the elasticity of the aorta of elderly patients [99, 208, 209]. The calcium channel blocker action may explain the hypotensive effect of garlic [210]. Garlic has many other pharmacological properties: cholesterol-lowering [211, 212], hypoglycemic, prevention of carcinogenesis (stomach, colon, and bladder), prevention of inflammatory and infectious diseases of the respiratory and digestive systems; immunostimulant; antimicrobial action (bacteria and viruses); reduction in the animal secretion of thyroid hormones and increased thyroid-stimulating hormone [99, 188, 195, 213]. Garlic is therefore indicated in the prevention and treatment of atherosclerosis [214], dyslipidemia [215], and hypertension [216]. Numerous preparations are available on the market; only the fresh-crushed bulbs of garlic, and some preparations of garlic powder contain sufficient allicin to be active and effective [217]. Macerated oils or essential oils are inactive [99]. For therapeutic purposes, the use of 4 g per day of fresh bulbs of garlic is recommended, which contains about 40 mg of alliin, which shed 20 mg of allicin. Dried garlic extract obtained from fresh bulbs exists, titrated and standardized in alliin and allicin to 10 %. They are preferred because they allow enough of a supply to exert adequate pharmacological action. High doses of garlic may lead to gastritis, nausea, vomiting, and diarrhea, and its use is contraindicated in cases of peptic ulcer, gastritis, cross-allergies (onion), and hypothyroidism [218]. Allergic reactions are possible in the form of contact dermatitis or asthma from garlic powder inhalation [218]. It is not recommended for use during pregnancy and lactation, and when patients are undergoing surgery because it can increase the risk of postoperative bleeding [99]. In the treatment of atherosclerosis use of the onion can be indicated (*Allium cepa*), which shares some of the properties of garlic [198].

16.5.8 Hawthorn and *Ammi visnaga* (Khella)

Extracts from hawthorn berries and flowering tops reduce angina attacks, lower blood pressure and serum cholesterol levels [219–223]; enhance cardiac contractility; and improve heart energetic–metabolic processes and blood and oxygen supply, causing coronary vasodilation [99]. Dosages (t.i. d.): berries or flowers (dried): 3–5 g or as a tea; tincture (1:5): 4–6 mL (1–1.5 tsp); fluid extract (1:1): 1:2 mL (0.25–0.5 tsp), solid extract (10 % procyanidins or 1.8 % vitexin-4'-rhamoside): 100–250 mg [18].

Ammi visnaga (khella) is an ancient Mediterranean medicinal plant used historically to treat angina [224]. The mechanism of action of its constituent "*khellin*," is similar to calcium channel blocking drugs and is extremely effective in relieving angina symptoms and improving exercise tolerance [225, 226]. It works synergistically with hawthorn. Dosages (t.i.d): dried powdered extract (12 % khellin content): 100 mg [18].

16.5.9 *Paeonia lactiflora* and *Pueraria lobata*

Total glucosides of paeony (TPGs), compounds extracted from the roots of *Paeonia lactiflora Pall*, have been used as an anti-inflammatory drug for the treatment of rheumatoid arthritis (RA) in China and is finding application in the treatment of atherosclerotic vascular disease [227]. In an animal model, it has been found that TPGs significantly ameliorate myocardial ischemia and their action may occur by reducing oxidative stress in ischemic myocardium [228, 229].

Puerarin is one of the most important effective components of *Pueraria lobata*, which exhibited classic estrogen-like biological activities and had remarkable cardiovascular protective effects in in vivo and in vitro experiments [230]. The beneficial effects of puerarin for CHD treatment purposes may be due to its wide spectrum of pharmacological properties, such as vasodilation and vascular protection [231], cardioprotection [232], anti-atherosclerotic (anti-inflammation, attenuating insulin resistance, and anti-oxidant) [233] neuroprotection, alleviating pain, and inhibiting alcohol intake [234].

16.5.10 Arnica comp.-Heel® Tablets

Recently [235], the effectiveness of treatment with a tablet a day of a low-dose composite drug (Arnica comp.-Heel® tablets) has been demonstrated to reduce the risk of cardiovascular events in patients with clinically stable coronary disease. This drug contains many compounds with anti-inflammatory properties (*Achillea millefolium*, *Aconitum napellus*, *Arnica montana*, *Atropa belladonna*, *Bellis perennis*, *Calendula officinalis*, *Chamomilla*, *Echinacea angustifolia*, *Echinacea purpurea*, *Hamamelis virginiana*, *Hepar sulfuris*, *Hypericum perforatum*, *Mercurius solubilis Hahnemanni*, and *Symphytum*) able to prevent plaque instability, improving the outcome of patients with stable coronary artery disease in addition to standard therapy [235].

16.5.11 Tricks of the Trade

Hawthorn, Chinese sage, and ginkgo work well, as described in the scientific literature. Good results can be achieved in the "senile" heart with a combination of hawthorn and ginseng, when there are symptoms such as palpitations and shortness of breath with minimal exertion, sweating at the slightest effort, dizziness, very marked weakness, and weak pulse.

Pueraria is an excellent plant for preventing or treating cardiovascular problems, especially when they are linked to smoking and alcohol consumption. In our experience, it is very effective in helping the body to detoxify from alcohol and nicotine and reducing its dependence on these substances (http://www.ordfarmacistips.it/prof.asp?id=94).

There is a need for more scientific research to clarify the effectiveness of the bud extracts traditionally used in the treatment of cardiovascular disorders. In any case, Pol Henry points out the possible use of *Cornus sanguinea* + *Syringa vulgaris* + *Crataegus oxyacantha* to prevent myocardial infarction; *Cornus sanguinea* + *Zea mais* the first week after infarction; *Alnus glutinosa* + *Zea mais* maize after the first week (http://www.ibs.it/code/9788871723167/piteragrave/compendio-gemmoterapia-clinica.html).

16.5.12 Future Perspective for Research

The Ayurvedic system of medicine uses several other plants of Indian origin for the prevention and treatment of CHD. For example: *Acorus calamus* (*vaca*), *Aegle marmelos* (*bilva*), *Emblica officinalis* (*amalaki*), *Glycyrrhiza glabra* (*yastimadhu*), *Centella asiatica* (*mandukaparni*), *Nardostachys jatamansi* (*jatamansi*), *Ocimum sanctum* (*tulasi*), *Saussurea lappa* (*kustha or puskaramula*), *Terminalia arjuna* (*arjuna*), *Withania somnifera* (*asvagandha*), and rudraksa. Their description and methods of use are beyond the scope of this chapter, but it is possible to gain a clear overview in the book by Dr Vaidya Bhagwan Dash [236].

Finally, Chen et al. [237] recently described more than 50 natural products for antithrombosis according to their anticoagulation, antiplatelet aggregation, and fibrinolysis activity.

16.6 Mind–Body Therapies and Psychological Risk

The important contributions of psycho-neuro-endocrine immunology and integrative medicine approaches to the field of cardiology is the description of the intimate mind–body connection in heart health. It is a common experience in the daily clinical practice of every cardiologist to find people who are aware of how a particular mood or difficult experiences of life "have made them sick." But most conventional medical encounters do not include assessment of the patient's emotional state, let alone offer therapies directed at mind–body interventions.

As we recently described [9, 11, 12]: "our inner dialogue modulates cardiovascular function. At the same event, people experience different emotional reactions and a same person during his/her life and maturation could react differently in similar, specific situations. Between event and emotion there is no automatic link."

> According to Rozanski et al. [238], specific personalities and their characteristic psychological traits (depression, anxiety, character traits, social isolation, and chronic life stress) contribute significantly to the pathogenesis and expression of coronary artery disease (CAD) because of adverse health behaviors (such as poor diet and smoking) and direct biological mechanisms, such as immune, neuroendocrine, and platelet activation. Thus, the concept of "personality" (namely "the individual differences in characteristic patterns of thinking, feeling and behaving" [239]) represents a key factor in regulating the health of the cardiovascular system.
>
> Emotions do not automatically take away from what happens in people's lives, but are derived from the type of internal dialogue that is done facing what happens. Different personalities are more or less vulnerable to stress, with relationships existing between different personalities and the function of the hypothalamic–pituitary–adrenal (HPA) axis [240–244] and immune [245, 246] and nervous systems [247]. Different patterns of thinking, feeling, and behaving essentially modulate the cross-talk between the nervous, endocrine, and immune systems. It is just as true that the nervous, endocrine, immune, and metabolic systems and their functions could influence mental attitude [248]. In particular, "type D" personality or the "type A coronary-prone behavior," according to Rozanski and Mittleman, are related to a higher incidence of CVD [238, 249].
>
> Although with many nuances, it can be said that every human being can only try two great emotions in their lifetime: love (serenity, tranquility) or fear, but never both at the same time [250]. This oscillates constantly between the two poles. An inner dialogue oriented to the past or the future that is full of anxiety, distrust, jealousy, envy, ambition, regret, etc., produces fear, in its various emotional colors. An inner dialogue turned to the present, concrete, confident, proactive, compassionate, conscious, etc., produces feelings of "love," serenity, and tranquility [250].

Thus, the emotional states most commonly linked to heart disease are stress, anxiety, and depression [251, 252]. Psychological stress alone is comparable with strenuous exercise in reducing coronary blood flow [252] or is able to mimic a heart attack (Takotsubo cardiomyopathy) [253]. The drug therapies do not appear to protect against ischemia-induced mental stress; ergometric tests are not able to detect this form of ischemia either [9, 11, 12].

Moreover, stress is a contributor to chronic dyslipidemia and increases total cholesterol by 7 mg/dL and LDL-C by 5 mg/dL within an hour of acute psychological stress [254].

The other side of the coin reveals how the methods of stress prevention and management play a vital role in the care of patients with CHD. Meditation practiced by individuals with coronary disease over 5 years was demonstrated to reduce the combined risk of a cardiovascular event and death by 43% [255, 256]. The practice of meditation reduces the cardiac workload and the levels of circulating molecular mediators of stress, blunting the expected increase in heart rate associated with infusion of isoproterenol [252].

There are many arrows in the quiver of a cardiologist. Many mind–body techniques can be recommended to patients with CHD to manage their stress and anxiety more effectively: conventional psychoactive medication or cognitive behavioral therapy, many forms of meditation, yoga, biofeedback, healing touch, Reiki, massage, and acupuncture.

As suggested by Stephen Devries [16]: "no one resource is generically superior to another. Instead, referral should be made based on an individualized assessment including the patient's prior knowledge or history with a particular approach, the patient's philosophical inclination, local expertise, and cost. This 'matching' process is truly one of the arts of integrative medicine."

16.7 Can Lifestyle Changes Reverse CHD? The Lifestyle Heart Trial

As stated by Winston Churchill: "however beautiful the strategy, you should occasionally look at the results."

Focus on lifestyle and especially on diet and stress management leads to very interesting results. Ornish et al. showed regression of atherosclerosis after only a year of change in lifestyle, without the use of lipid-lowering drugs [257, 258]. After 5 years, the myocardial perfusion is improved more than in the controls who were underwent conventional treatment [259].

16.8 Conventional Therapies

In addition to the change of lifestyle based on nutrition, exercise, and stress management, patients with symptomatic CHD should receive treatments according to European Society of Cardiology (ESC) or American Heart Association/American College of Cardiology (AHA/ACC) guidelines.

Milestones for the drug treatment of CHD are: aspirin, nitrates, beta blockers, and calcium channel blockers, angiotensin-converting enzyme inhibitors, and statins.

Interventional and invasive procedures, such as angioplasty and stenting or coronary bypass heart surgery, could be life-saving.

A detailed discussion of these therapies is beyond the scope of this chapter, but can be found in the ESC/AHA/ACC guideline statements [5].

References

1. Lloyd-Jones D et al (2010) Executive summary: heart disease and stroke statistics-2010 update: a report from the American Heart Association. Circulation 121:948–954
2. Lerner DJ, Kannel WB (1986) Patterns of coronary heart disease morbidity and mortality in the sexes: a 26-year follow-up of the Framingham population. Am Heart J 111:383–390
3. Nichols M, Townsend N, Scarborough P, Rayner M (2013) Cardiovascular disease in Europe: epidemiological update. Eur Heart J 34:3028–3034
4. Okrainec K, Banerjee DK, Eisenberg MJ (2004) Coronary artery disease in the developing world. Am Heart J 148:7–15
5. John Camm A, Luscher TF, Serruys PW (2009) ESC textbook of cardiovascular medicine, 2nd edn. Oxford University Press, Oxford
6. Go AS et al (2013) Heart disease and stroke statistics—2013 update: a report from the American Heart Association. Circulation 127:e6–e245
7. Ogden CL et al (2006) Prevalence of overweight and obesity in the United States, 1999–2004. JAMA 295:1549–1555
8. Devries S, Dalen J (2011) Integrative cardiology. Oxford University Press, Oxford, pp 1–324
9. Dal Lin C et al (2015) Coronary microvascular and endothelial function regulation: crossroads of psychoneuroendocrine immunitary signals and quantum physics [Part A]. J Integr Cardiol 1:132–163
10. Goldstein BI et al (2015) Major depressive disorder and bipolar disorder predispose youth to accelerated atherosclerosis and early cardiovascular disease. Circulation 132:965–986
11. Dal Lin C et al (2015) Coronary microvascular and endothelial function regulation: crossroads of psychoneuroendocrine immunitary signals and quantum physics [Part B]. J Integr Cardiol 1:164–188
12. Dal Lin C et al (2015) Coronary microvascular and endothelial function regulation: crossroads of psychoneuroendocrine immunitary signals and quantum physics [Part C]. J Integr Cardiol 1:189–209
13. Dal Lin C, Tona F, Osto E (2015) Coronary microvascular function and beyond: the crosstalk between hormones, cytokines, and neurotransmitters. Int J Endocrinol 2015:1–17
14. Narayan KMV, Boyle JP, Thompson TJ, Sorensen SW, Williamson DF (2003) Lifetime risk for diabetes mellitus in the United States. JAMA 290:1884–1890
15. Olshansky SJ et al (2005) A potential decline in life expectancy in the United States in the 21st century. N Engl J Med 352:1138–1145
16. Rakel D (2012) Integrative medicine, 3rd edn. Elsevier, Amsterdam
17. Fani Marvasti F, Stafford RS (2012) From sick care to health care – reengineering prevention into the US System. N Engl J Med 367:889–891
18. Pizzorno JE, Murray MT, Herb JB (2008) The clinician's handbook of natural medicine, 2nd edn. Churchill Livingstone, Edinburgh
19. Riaz IB et al (2014) Meta-analysis of revascularization versus medical therapy for atherosclerotic renal artery stenosis. Am J Cardiol 114:1116–1123
20. Bangalore S, Pursnani S, Kumar S, Bagos PG (2013) Percutaneous coronary intervention versus optimal medical therapy for prevention of spontaneous myocardial infarction in subjects with stable ischemic heart disease. Circulation 127:769–781
21. Thomas S, Gokhale R, Boden WE, Devereaux PJ (2013) A meta-analysis of randomized controlled

trials comparing percutaneous coronary intervention with medical therapy in stable angina pectoris. Can J Cardiol 29:472–482
22. Boden WE et al (2009) Impact of optimal medical therapy with or without percutaneous coronary intervention on long-term cardiovascular end points in patients with stable coronary artery disease (from the COURAGE Trial). Am J Cardiol 104:1–4
23. El-Hayek G et al (2014) Meta-analysis of randomized clinical trials comparing short-term versus long-term dual antiplatelet therapy following drug-eluting stents. Am J Cardiol 114:236–242
24. Brieger DB, Redfern J (2013) Contemporary themes in acute coronary syndrome management: from acute illness to secondary prevention. Med J Aust 199:174–178
25. Mann JM, Davies MJ (1996) Vulnerable plaque. Relation of characteristics to degree of stenosis in human coronary arteries. Circulation 94:928–931
26. Falk E, Shah PK, Fuster V (1995) Coronary plaque disruption. Circulation 92:657–671
27. De Lorgeril M et al (1994) Mediterranean alpha-linolenic acid-rich diet in secondary prevention of coronary heart disease. Lancet 343:1454–1459
28. De Lorgeril M et al (1999) Mediterranean diet, traditional risk factors, and the rate of cardiovascular complications after myocardial infarction: final report of the Lyon Diet Heart Study. Circulation 99:779–7785
29. Joshipura KJ et al (2001) The effect of fruit and vegetable intake on risk for coronary heart disease. Ann Intern Med 134:1106–1114
30. Vogel RA, Corretti MC, Plotnick GD (1997) Effect of a single high-fat meal on endothelial function in healthy subjects. Am J Cardiol 79:350–354
31. Hu FB et al (1999) Dietary saturated fats and their food sources in relation to the risk of coronary heart disease in women. Am J Clin Nutr 70:1001–1008
32. Daviglus ML et al (1997) Fish consumption and the 30-year risk of fatal myocardial infarction. N Engl J Med 336:1046–1053
33. Burr ML, et al (1989) Effects of changes in fat, fish, and fibre intakes on death and myocardial reinfarction: diet and reinfarction trial (DART). Lancet (London, England) 2:757–761
34. Mellen PB, Walsh TF, Herrington DM (2008) Whole grain intake and cardiovascular disease: a meta-analysis. Nutr Metab Cardiovasc Dis 18:283–290
35. Welsh JA et al (2010) Caloric sweetener consumption and dyslipidemia among US adults. JAMA 303:1490–1497
36. Hallfrisch J, Behall KM (2000) Mechanisms of the effects of grains on insulin and glucose responses. J Am Coll Nutr 19:320S–325S
37. Sabaté J, Ang Y (2009) Nuts and health outcomes: new epidemiologic evidence. Am J Clin Nutr 89:1643S–1648S
38. Ros E, Tapsell LC, Sabaté J (2010) Nuts and berries for heart health. Curr Atheroscler Rep 12:397–406
39. Janssens J et al (1990) Nutmeg oil: identification and quantitation of its most active constituents as inhibitors of platelet aggregation. J Ethnopharmacol 29:179–188
40. Su L et al (2007) Total phenolic contents, chelating capacities, and radical-scavenging properties of black peppercorn, nutmeg, rosehip, cinnamon and oregano leaf. Food Chem 100:990–997
41. Calliste CA et al (2010) A new antioxidant from wild nutmeg. Food Chem 118:489–496
42. Duan W et al (2012) The effects of curcumin post-treatment against myocardial ischemia and reperfusion by activation of the JAK2/STAT3 signaling pathway. Basic Res Cardiol 107:263
43. Zhang M, Cai S, Ma J (2015) Evaluation of cardioprotective effect of soybean oligosaccharides. Gene 555:329–334
44. Ge G et al (2014) Protective effect of Salvia miltiorrhiza aqueous extract on myocardium oxidative injury in ischemic-reperfusion rats. Gene 546:97–103
45. Tanasescu M et al (2002) Exercise type and intensity in relation to coronary heart disease in men. JAMA 288:1994–2000
46. Madanmohan UK, Bhavanani AB, Shatapathy CC, Sahai A (2004) Modulation of cardiovascular response to exercise by yoga training. Indian J Physiol Pharmacol 48:461–465
47. Yeung A et al (2014) Randomised controlled trial of a 12 week yoga intervention on negative affective states, cardiovascular and cognitive function in post-cardiac rehabilitation patients. BMC Complement Altern Med 14:411
48. Bergh C, Udumyan R, Fall K, Almroth H, Montgomery S (2015) Stress resilience and physical fitness in adolescence and risk of coronary heart disease in middle age. Heart 101:623–629
49. Castelli WP (1996) Lipids, risk factors and ischaemic heart disease. Atherosclerosis 124 (Suppl):S1–9
50. Brown L, Rosner B, Willett WW, Sacks FM (1999) Cholesterol-lowering effects of dietary fiber: a meta-analysis. Am J Clin Nutr 69:30–42
51. Anderson JW et al (2000) Long-term cholesterol-lowering effects of psyllium as an adjunct to diet therapy in the treatment of hypercholesterolemia. Am J Clin Nutr 71:1433–1438
52. Miettinen TA, Puska P, Gylling H, Vanhanen H, Vartiainen E (1995) Reduction of serum cholesterol with sitostanol-ester margarine in a mildly hypercholesterolemic population. N Engl J Med 333:1308–1312
53. Norris RB (2006) Flush-free niacin': dietary supplement may be 'benefit-free'. Prev Cardiol 9:64–65
54. Papaliodis D, Boucher W, Kempuraj D, Theoharides TC (2008) The flavonoid luteolin inhibits niacin-induced flush. Br J Pharmacol 153:1382–1387
55. Heber D et al (1999) Cholesterol-lowering effects of a proprietary Chinese red-yeast-rice dietary supplement. Am J Clin Nutr 69:231–236
56. Becker DJ et al (2008) Simvastatin vs therapeutic lifestyle changes and supplements: randomized primary prevention trial. Mayo Clin Proc 83:758–764
57. Gordon RY, Cooperman T, Obermeyer W, Becker DJ (2010) Marked variability of monacolin levels in

commercial red yeast rice products: buyer beware! Arch Intern Med 170:1722–1727
58. Becker DJ et al (2009) Red yeast rice for dyslipidemia in statin-intolerant patients: a randomized trial. Ann Intern Med 150(830–839): W147–149
59. Lu Z et al (2008) Effect of Xuezhikang, an extract from red yeast Chinese rice, on coronary events in a Chinese population with previous myocardial infarction. Am J Cardiol 101:1689–1693
60. Hokanson JE, Austin MA (1996) Plasma triglyceride level is a risk factor for cardiovascular disease independent of high-density lipoprotein cholesterol level: a meta-analysis of population-based prospective studies. J Cardiovasc Risk 3:213–219
61. Pizzorno JE, Murray MT (2013) Textbook of natural medicine, 4th edn. Elsevier, Amsterdam
62. Young JM et al (2007) Effect of coenzyme Q (10) supplementation on simvastatin-induced myalgia. Am J Cardiol 100:1400–1403
63. Caso G, Kelly P, McNurlan MA, Lawson WE (2007) Effect of coenzyme q10 on myopathic symptoms in patients treated with statins. Am J Cardiol 99:1409–1412
64. Marcoff L, Thompson PD (2007) The role of coenzyme Q10 in statin-associated myopathy: a systematic review. J Am Coll Cardiol 49:2231–2237
65. Hathcock JN, Shao A (2006) Risk assessment for coenzyme Q10 (Ubiquinone). Regul Toxicol Pharmacol 45:282–288
66. Sander S, Coleman CI, Patel AA, Kluger J, White CM (2006) The impact of coenzyme Q10 on systolic function in patients with chronic heart failure. J Card Fail 12:464–472
67. Kamikawa T, Kobayashi A, Yamashita T, Hayashi H, Yamazaki N (1985) Effects of coenzyme Q10 on exercise tolerance in chronic stable angina pectoris. Am J Cardiol 56:247–251
68. Holick MF (2007) Vitamin D deficiency. N Engl J Med 357:266–281
69. Wang TJ et al (2008) Vitamin D deficiency and risk of cardiovascular disease. Circulation 117:503–511
70. Ahmed W et al (2009) Low serum 25 (OH) vitamin D levels (<32 ng/mL) are associated with reversible myositis-myalgia in statin-treated patients. Transl Res 153:11–16
71. Homocysteine Studies Collaboration (2002) Homocysteine and risk of ischemic heart disease and stroke: a meta-analysis. JAMA 288:2015–2022
72. Bønaa KH et al (2006) Homocysteine lowering and cardiovascular events after acute myocardial infarction. N Engl J Med 354:1578–1588
73. Lonn E et al (2006) Homocysteine lowering with folic acid and B vitamins in vascular disease. N Engl J Med 354:1567–1577
74. Stephens NG et al. (1996) Randomised controlled trial of vitamin E in patients with coronary disease: Cambridge Heart Antioxidant Study (CHAOS). Lancet (London, England) 347: 781–786
75. Yusuf S, Dagenais G, Pogue J, Bosch J, Sleight P (2000) Vitamin E supplementation and cardiovascular events in high-risk patients. The Heart Outcomes Prevention Evaluation Study Investigators. N Engl J Med 342:154–160
76. Gruppo Italiano per lo Studio della Sopravvivenza nell'Infarto miocardico (1999) Dietary supplementation with n-3 polyunsaturated fatty acids and vitamin E after myocardial infarction: results of the GISSI-Prevenzione trial. Lancet (London, England) 354: 447–455
77. Sesso HD et al (2008) Vitamins E and C in the prevention of cardiovascular disease in men: the Physicians' Health Study II randomized controlled trial. JAMA 300:2123–2133
78. Huang H-Y, Appel LJ (2003) Supplementation of diets with alpha-tocopherol reduces serum concentrations of gamma- and delta-tocopherol in humans. J Nutr 133:3137–3140
79. Dietrich M et al (2006) Does gamma-tocopherol play a role in the primary prevention of heart disease and cancer? A review. J Am Coll Nutr 25:292–299
80. Lagioia R et al (1992) Propionyl-L-carnitine: a new compound in the metabolic approach to the treatment of effort angina. Int J Cardiol 34:167–172
81. Bartels GL, Remme WJ, Pillay M, Schönfeld DH, Kruijssen DA (1994) Effects of L-propionylcarnitine on ischemia-induced myocardial dysfunction in men with angina pectoris. Am J Cardiol 74:125–310
82. Cacciatore L et al (1991) The therapeutic effect of L-carnitine in patients with exercise-induced stable angina: a controlled study. Drugs Exp Clin Res 17:225–235
83. Davini P, Bigalli A, Lamanna F, Boem A (1992) Controlled study on L-carnitine therapeutic efficacy in post-infarction. Drugs Exp Clin Res 18:355–365
84. Kamikawa T et al (1984) Effects of L-carnitine on exercise tolerance in patients with stable angina pectoris. Jpn Heart J 25:587–597
85. Hayashi H et al (1985) Effects of pantethine on action potential of canine papillary muscle during hypoxic perfusion. Jpn Heart J 26:289–296
86. Turlapaty PD, Altura BM (1980) Magnesium deficiency produces spasms of coronary arteries: relationship to etiology of sudden death ischemic heart disease. Science 208:198–200
87. Altura BM (1988) Ischemic heart disease and magnesium. Magnesium 7:57–67
88. McLean RM (1994) Magnesium and its therapeutic uses: a review. Am J Med 96:63–76
89. Purvis JR, Movahed A (1992) Magnesium disorders and cardiovascular diseases. Clin Cardiol 15:556–568
90. Hampton EM, Whang DD, Whang R (1994) Intravenous magnesium therapy in acute myocardial infarction. Ann Pharmacother 28:212–219
91. Teo KK, Yusuf S (1993) Role of magnesium in reducing mortality in acute myocardial infarction. A review of the evidence. Drugs 46:347–359

92. Shechter M, Kaplinsky E, Rabinowitz B (1992) The rationale of magnesium supplementation in acute myocardial infarction. A review of the literature. Arch Intern Med 152:2189–2196
93. Bednarz B et al (2000) Effects of oral L-arginine supplementation on exercise-induced QT dispersion and exercise tolerance in stable angina pectoris. Int J Cardiol 75:205–210
94. Kobayashi N, Nakamura M, Hiramori K (1999) Effects of infusion of L-arginine on exercise-induced myocardial ischemic ST-segment changes and capacity to exercise of patients with stable angina pectoris. Coron Artery Dis 10:321–326
95. Ceremuzyński L, Chamiec T, Herbaczyńska-Cedro K (1997) Effect of supplemental oral L-arginine on exercise capacity in patients with stable angina pectoris. Am J Cardiol 80:331–333
96. Tripathi P, Chandra M, Misra MK (2009) Oral administration of L-arginine in patients with angina or following myocardial infarction may be protective by increasing plasma superoxide dismutase and total thiols with reduction in serum cholesterol and xanthine oxidase. Oxid Med Cell Longev 2:231–237
97. Schulman SP et al (2006) L-arginine therapy in acute myocardial infarction: the Vascular Interaction With Age in Myocardial Infarction (VINTAGE MI) randomized clinical trial. JAMA 295:58–64
98. Rangel-Huerta O, Pastor-Villaescusa B, Aguilera C, Gil A (2015) A systematic review of the efficacy of bioactive compounds in cardiovascular disease: phenolic compounds. Nutrients 7:5177
99. Fabio Firenzuoli (2009) Fitoterapia. Guida all'uso clinico delle piante medicinali. Elsevier, Milan
100. Gao Z, Xu H, Shi D, Wen C, Liu B (2012) Analysis on outcome of 5284 patients with coronary artery disease: the role of integrative medicine. J Ethnopharmacol 141:578–583
101. Ren S, Zhang H, Mu Y, Sun M, Liu P (2013) Pharmacological effects of Astragaloside IV: a literature review. J Tradit Chin Med 33:413–416
102. Zhang WD et al (2006) Astragaloside IV from Astragalus membranaceus shows cardioprotection during myocardial ischemia in vivo and in vitro. Planta Med 72:4–8
103. Chen P et al (2011) Astragaloside IV attenuates myocardial fibrosis by inhibiting TGF-β1 signaling in coxsackievirus B3-induced cardiomyopathy. Eur J Pharmacol 658:168–174
104. Qu YZ et al (2009) Astragaloside IV attenuates cerebral ischemia-reperfusion-induced increase in permeability of the blood-brain barrier in rats. Eur J Pharmacol 606:137–141
105. Chtourou Y et al (2015) Naringenin reduces cholesterol-induced hepatic inflammation in rats by modulating matrix metalloproteinases-2, 9 via inhibition of nuclear factor kB pathway. Eur J Pharmacol 746:96–105
106. Izzo AA, Di Carlo G, Borrelli F, Ernst E (2005) Cardiovascular pharmacotherapy and herbal medicines: the risk of drug interaction. Int J Cardiol 98:1–14
107. Valli G, Giardina EGV (2002) Benefits, adverse effects and drug interactions of herbal therapies with cardiovascular effects. J Am Coll Cardiol 39:1083–1095
108. Sofi F, Cesari F, Abbate R, Gensini GF, Casini A (2008) Adherence to Mediterranean diet and health status: meta-analysis. BMJ 337:a1344
109. Kushi LH, Meyer KA, Jacobs DR (1999) Cereals, legumes, and chronic disease risk reduction: evidence from epidemiologic studies. Am J Clin Nutr 70:451S–458S
110. Kottler BM, Ferdowsian HR, Barnard ND (2009) Effects of plant-based diets on plasma lipids. Am J Cardiol 104:947–956
111. Sabaté J (1999) Nut consumption, vegetarian diets, ischemic heart disease risk, and all- cause mortality: evidence from epidemiologic studies. in. Am J Clin Nutr 70:500S–503S
112. Nasri H, Baradaran A, Shirzad H, Rafieian-Kopaei M (2014) New concepts in nutraceuticals as alternative for pharmaceuticals. Int J Prev Med 5:1487–1499
113. Shukla SK, Gupta S, Ojha SK, Sharma SB (2010) Cardiovascular friendly natural products: a promising approach in the management of CVD. Nat Prod Res 24:873–898
114. Di Giuseppe R et al (2008) Regular consumption of dark chocolate is associated with low serum concentrations of C-reactive protein in a healthy Italian population. J Nutr 138:1939–1945
115. Corti R, Flammer AJ, Hollenberg NK, Luscher TF (2009) Cocoa and cardiovascular health. Circulation 119:1433–1441
116. Desch S et al (2010) Low vs higher-dose dark chocolate and blood pressure in cardiovascular high-risk patients. Am J Hypertens 23:694–700
117. Innes AJ, Kennedy G, McLaren M, Bancroft AJ, Belch JJF (2003) Dark chocolate inhibits platelet aggregation in healthy volunteers. Platelets 14:325
118. Vinson JA, Proch J, Zubik L (1999) Phenol antioxidant quantity and quality in foods: Cocoa, dark chocolate, and milk chocolate. J Agric Food Chem 47:4821–4824
119. Grassi D et al (2012) Protective effects of flavanol-rich dark chocolate on endothelial function and wave reflection during acute hyperglycemia. Hypertension 60:827–832
120. Flammer AJ et al (2007) Dark chocolate improves coronary vasomotion and reduces platelet reactivity. Circulation 116:2376–2382
121. Grassi D, Lippi C, Necozione S, Desideri G, Ferri C (2005) Short-term administration of dark chocolate is followed by a significant increase in insulin sensitivity and a decrease in blood pressure in healthy persons. Am J Clin Nutr 81:611–614
122. Sirtori CR, Galli C, Anderson JW, Sirtori E, Arnoldi A (2009) Functional foods for dyslipidaemia and cardiovascular risk prevention. Nutr Res Rev 22:244–261

123. Kuriyama S (2008) The relation between green tea consumption and cardiovascular disease as evidenced by epidemiological studies. J Nutr 138:1548S–1553S
124. Sone T et al (2011) Randomized controlled trial for an effect of catechin-enriched green tea consumption on adiponectin and cardiovascular disease risk factors. Food Nutr Res 55:8326
125. Kuriyama S et al (2006) Green tea consumption and mortality due to cardiovascular disease, cancer, and all causes in Japan: the Ohsaki study. JAMA 296:1255–1265
126. Larsson SC (2014) Coffee, tea, and cocoa and risk of stroke. Stroke 45:309–314
127. Larsson SC et al (2008) Coffee and tea consumption and risk of stroke subtypes in male smokers. Stroke 39:1681–1687
128. Grassi D et al (2013) Tea, flavonoids, and cardiovascular health: endothelial protection. Am J Clin Nutr 98:1660S
129. Bonita JS, Mandarano M, Shuta D, Vinson J (2007) Coffee and cardiovascular disease: in vitro, cellular, animal, and human studies. Pharmacol Res 55:187–198
130. Gensini GF, Lippi D, Conti AA (2007) Past, present and future of green tea: from pleasant beverage to drug in pills? Recenti Prog Med 98:347–351
131. Sofi F et al (2007) Coffee consumption and risk of coronary heart disease: a meta-analysis. Nutr Metab Cardiovasc Dis 17:209–223
132. Duffy SJ et al (2001) Short- and long-term black tea consumption reverses endothelial dysfunction in patients with coronary artery disease. Circulation 104:151
133. Geleijnse JM, Launer LJ, Hofman A, Pols HA, Witteman JC (1999) Tea flavonoids may protect against atherosclerosis: the Rotterdam Study. Arch Intern Med 159:2170–2174
134. Geleijnse JM, Launer LJ, Van Der Kuip DAM, Hofman A, Witteman JCM (2002) Inverse association of tea and flavonoid intakes with incident myocardial infarction: The Rotterdam Study. Am J Clin Nutr 75:880–886
135. Alexopoulos N et al (2008) The acute effect of green tea consumption on endothelial function in healthy individuals. Eur J Cardiovasc Prev Rehabil 15:300–305
136. Jochmann N et al (2008) The efficacy of black tea in ameliorating endothelial function is equivalent to that of green tea. Br J Nutr 99:863–868
137. Kim W et al (2006) Effect of green tea consumption on endothelial function and circulating endothelial progenitor cells in chronic smokers. Circ J 70:1052–1057
138. Arab L, Khan F, Lam H (2013) Tea consumption and cardiovascular disease risk. Am J Clin Nutr 98:1651S–1659S
139. Bombardelli E, Morazzoni P (1995) Vitis vinifera L. Fitoterapia 66:291–317
140. De Bruyne T et al (1999) Biological evaluation of proanthocyanidin dimers and related polyphenols. J Nat Prod 62:954–958
141. Maffei Facinó R et al (1996) Procyanidines from Vitis vinifera seeds protect rabbit heart from ischemia/reperfusion injury: antioxidant intervention and/or iron and copper sequestering ability. Planta Med 62:495–502
142. Sato M, Maulik G, Ray PS, Bagchi D, Das DK (1999) Cardioprotective effects of grape seed proanthocyanidin against ischemic reperfusion injury. J Mol Cell Cardiol 31:1289–1297
143. Serafini M, Ghiselli A, Ferro-Luzzi A (1994) Red wine, tea, and antioxidants. Lancet 344:626
144. Bagchi D et al (2000) Free radicals and grape seed proanthocyanidin extract: importance in human health and disease prevention. Toxicology 148:187–197
145. Opie LH, Lecour S (2007) The red wine hypothesis: from concepts to protective signalling molecules. Eur Heart J 28:1683–1693
146. Bhat KPL, Kosmeder JW, Pezzuto JM (2001) Biological effects of resveratrol. Antioxid Redox Signal 3:1041–1064
147. Blanco-Colio LM et al (2000) Red wine intake prevents nuclear factor-kappaB activation in peripheral blood mononuclear cells of healthy volunteers during postprandial lipemia. Circulation 102:120–126
148. Baur JA, Sinclair DA (2006) Therapeutic potential of resveratrol: the in vivo evidence. Nat Rev Drug Discov 5:493–506
149. Das M, Das DK (2010) Resveratrol and cardiovascular health. Mol Aspects Med 31:503–512
150. Cheng B, Hung CT, Chiu W (2002) Herbal medicine and anaesthesia in Hong Kong. Med J 8:123–130
151. Fasinu PS, Bouic PJ, Rosenkranz B (2012) An overview of the evidence and mechanisms of herb-drug interactions. Front Pharmacol 3:69
152. Zhang J et al (2008) Compound Salvia droplet pill, a traditional Chinese medicine, for the treatment of unstable angina pectoris: a systematic review. Med Sci Monit 14:RA1–7
153. Wu T, Ni J, Wu J (2008) Danshen (Chinese medicinal herb) preparations for acute myocardial infarction. Cochrane database Syst Rev CD004465
154. Zatalia SR, Sanusi H (2013) The role of antioxidants in the pathophysiology, complications, and management of diabetes mellitus. Acta Med Indones 45:141–7
155. Smith PF, Maclennan K, Darlington CL (1996) The neuroprotective properties of the Ginkgo biloba leaf: a review of the possible relationship to platelet-activating factor (PAF). J Ethnopharmacol 50:131–139
156. Silvio S, Loggia RD, Tubaro A, Bombardelli E (1993) Anti-inflammatory activity of Ginkgo biloba flavonoids. Planta Med 59:588
157. Singh B, Kaur P, Gopichand Singh RD, Ahuja PS (2008) Biology and chemistry of Ginkgo biloba. Fitoterapia 79:401–418

158. Dong XX et al (2007) Ginkgo biloba extract reduces endothelial progenitor-cell senescence through augmentation of telomerase activity. J Cardiovasc Pharmacol 49:111–115
159. Diamond BJ et al (2000) Ginkgo biloba extract: mechanisms and clinical indications. Arch Phys Med Rehabil 81:668–678
160. Calapai G et al (2000) Neuroprotective effects of Ginkgo biloba extract in brain ischemia are mediated by inhibition of nitric oxide synthesis. Life Sci 67:2673–2683
161. Vellas B et al (2012) Long-term use of standardised ginkgo biloba extract for the prevention of Alzheimer's disease (GuidAge): a randomised placebo-controlled trial. Lancet Neurol 11:851–859
162. Kuller LH et al (2010) Does ginkgo biloba reduce the risk of cardiovascular events? Circ Cardiovasc Qual Outcomes 3:41–47
163. Weinmann S, Roll S, Schwarzbach C, Vauth C, Willich SN (2010) Effects of Ginkgo biloba in dementia: systematic review and meta-analysis. BMC Geriatr 10:14
164. Mahady GB (2002) Ginkgo biloba for the prevention and treatment of cardiovascular disease: a review of the literature. J Cardiovasc Nurs 16:21–32
165. Wang J, Zhou S, Bronks R, Graham J, Myers S (2007) Supervised exercise training combined with ginkgo biloba treatment for patients with peripheral arterial disease. Clin Rehabil 21:579–586
166. Pittler MH, Ernst E (2005) Complementary therapies for peripheral arterial disease: systematic review. Atherosclerosis 181:1–7
167. Schweizer J, Hautmann C (1999) Comparison of two dosages of ginkgo biloba extract EGb 761 in patients with peripheral arterial occlusive disease Fontaine's stage IIb. A randomised, double-blind, multicentric clinical trial. Arzneimittelforschung 49:900–904
168. Lim S et al (2011) Egb761, a ginkgo biloba extract, is effective against atherosclerosis in vitro, and in a rat model of type 2 diabetes. PLoS One 6:E20301
169. Köse K, Doğan P, Aşçioğlu M, Aşçioğlu O (1997) In vitro antioxidant effect of Ginkgo biloba extract (EGb 761) on lipoperoxidation induced by hydrogen peroxide in erythrocytes of Behçet's patients. Jpn J Pharmacol 75:253–258
170. Le Bars PL et al (1997) A placebo-controlled, double-blind, randomized trial of an extract of Ginkgo biloba for dementia. North American EGb Study Group. JAMA 278:1327–1332
171. Hopfenmüller W (1994) Evidence for a therapeutic effect of Ginkgo biloba special extract. Meta-analysis of 11 clinical studies in patients with cerebrovascular insufficiency in old age. Arzneimittelforschung 44:1005–1013
172. Guo L, Mei N, Liao W, Chan P-C, Fu PP (2010) Ginkgo biloba extract induces gene expression changes in xenobiotics metabolism and the Myc-centered network. OMICS 14:75–90
173. Gardner CD, Zehnder JL, Rigby AJ, Nicholus JR, Farquhar JW (2007) Effect of Ginkgo biloba (EGb 761) and aspirin on platelet aggregation and platelet function analysis among older adults at risk of cardiovascular disease: a randomized clinical trial. Blood Coagul Fibrinolysis 18:787–793
174. McKay DL, Blumberg JB (2007) Cranberries (Vaccinium macrocarpon) and cardiovascular disease risk factors. Nutr Rev 65:490–502
175. Blumberg JB et al (2013) Cranberries and their bioactive constituents in human health. Adv Nutr 4:618–632
176. Morazzoni P, Livio S, Scilingo A, Malandrino S (1991) Vaccinium myrtillus anthocyanosides pharmacokinetics in rats. Arzneimittelforschung 41:128–131
177. Rimando AM, Kalt W, Magee JB, Dewey J, Ballington JR (2004) Resveratrol, pterostilbene, and piceatannol in Vaccinium berries. J Agric Food Chem 52:4713–4719
178. Chu W, Cheung SCM, Lau R et al. (2008) Bilberry (Vaccinium myrtillus L.). In: Benzie IFF and Wachtel-Galor S (eds) Herbal medicine: biomolecular and clinical aspects, 2nd edn. CRC Press/Taylor and Francis, Boca Raton, FL
179. Persson IA-L, Persson K, Andersson RGG (2009) Effect of Vaccinium myrtillus and its polyphenols on angiotensin-converting enzyme activity in human endothelial cells. J Agric Food Chem 57:4626–4629
180. Wilson T, Porcari JP, Harbin D (1998) Cranberry extract inhibits low density lipoprotein oxidation. Life Sci 62:PL381–386
181. Hertog MG, Feskens EJ, Hollman PC, Katan MB, Kromhout D (1993) Dietary antioxidant flavonoids and risk of coronary heart disease: the Zutphen Elderly Study. Lancet 342:1007–1011
182. Hertog MG et al (1995) Flavonoid intake and long-term risk of coronary heart disease and cancer in the seven countries study. Arch Intern Med 155:381–386
183. Keli SO, Hertog MG, Feskens EJ, Kromhout D (1996) Dietary flavonoids, antioxidant vitamins, and incidence of stroke: the Zutphen study. Arch Intern Med 156:637–642
184. Costantino L, Albasini A, Rastelli G, Benvenuti S (1992) Activity of polyphenolic crude extracts as scavengers of superoxide radicals and inhibitors of xanthine oxidase. Planta Med 58:342–344
185. Bertuglia S, Malandrino S, Colantuoni A (1995) Effect of vaccinium myrtillus anthocyanosides on ischaemia reperfusion injury in hamster cheek pouch microcirculation. Pharmacol Res 31:183–187
186. Matsunaga N, Chikaraishi Y, Shimazawa M, Yokota S, Hara H (2010) Vaccinium myrtillus (bilberry) extracts reduce angiogenesis in vitro and in vivo. Evid Based Complement Altern Med 7:47–56
187. Rivlin RS (2001) Historical perspective on the use of garlic. J Nutr 131:951S–954
188. Rana SV, Pal R, Vaiphei K, Sharma SK, Ola RP (2011) Garlic in health and disease. Nutr Res Rev 24:60–71

189. Shouk R, Abdou A, Shetty K, Sarkar D, Eid AH (2014) Mechanisms underlying the antihypertensive effects of garlic bioactives. Nutr Res 34:106–115
190. Capraz M, Dilek M, Akpolat T (2007) Garlic, hypertension and patient education. Int J Cardiol 121:130–131
191. Tattelman E (2005) Health effects of garlic. Am Fam Physician 72:103–106
192. Orekhov AN, ünwald J (1997) Effects of garlic on atherosclerosis. Nutrition 13:656–663
193. Gardiner P, Graham RE, Legedza ATR, Eisenberg DM, Phillips RS (2006) Factors associated with dietary supplement use among prescription medication users. Arch Intern Med 166:1968–1974
194. Gorinstein S et al (2007) The atherosclerotic heart disease and protecting properties of garlic: contemporary data. Mol Nutr Food Res 51:1365–1381
195. Tsai CW, Chen HW, Sheen LY, Lii CK (2012) Garlic: health benefits and actions. Biomed 2:17–29
196. Agarwal KC (1996) Therapeutic actions of garlic constituents. Med Res Rev 16:111–124
197. Jung F, Jung E, Pindur G, Kiesewetter H (2007) Effect of different garlic preparations on the fluidity of blood, fibrinolytic activity, and peripheral microcirculation in comparison with placebo. Planta Med 56:668–668
198. Banerjee SK, Maulik SK (2002) Effect of garlic on cardiovascular disorders: a review. Nutr J 1:4
199. Beretz A, Cazenave JP (1991) Old and new natural products as the source of modern antithrombotic drugs. Planta Med 57:S68–S72
200. Legnani C et al (1993) Effects of a dried garlic preparation on fibrinolysis and platelet aggregation in healthy subjects. Arzneimittelforschung 43:119–122
201. Bordia A, Verma SK, Srivastava KC (1998) Effect of garlic (Allium sativum) on blood lipids, blood sugar, fibrinogen and fibrinolytic activity in patients with coronary artery disease. Prostaglandins, Leukot Essent Fat Acids 58:257–263
202. Rahman K (2007) Effects of garlic on platelet biochemistry and physiology. Mol Nutr Food Res 51:1335–1344
203. Srivastava KC (1986) Evidence for the mechanism by which garlic inhibits platelet aggregation. Prostaglandins Leukot Med 22:313–321
204. Bordia A (1978) Effect of garlic on human platelet aggregation in vitro. Atherosclerosis 30:355–360
205. Bordia A, Verma SK, Srivastava KC (1996) Effect of garlic on platelet aggregation in humans: a study in healthy subjects and patients with coronary artery disease. Prostaglandins Leukot Essent Fat Acids 55:201–205
206. Pittler MH, Ernst E (2007) Clinical effectiveness of garlic (Allium sativum). Mol Nutr Food Res 51:1382–1385
207. Pedraza-Chaverrí J, Medina-Campos ON, Ávila-Lombardo R, Berenice Zúñiga-Bustos A, Orozco-Ibarra M (2006) Reactive oxygen species scavenging capacity of different cooked garlic preparations. Life Sci 78:761–770
208. Mahdavi-Roshan M et al (2015) Effect of garlic powder tablet on carotid intima-media thickness in patients with coronary artery disease: a preliminary randomized controlled trial. Nutr Health 22:143–155
209. Breithaupt-Grügler K, Ling M, Boudoulas H, Belz GG (1997) Protective effect of chronic garlic intake on elastic properties of aorta in the elderly. Circulation 96:2649–2655
210. Ried K, Frank OR, Stocks NP, Fakler P, Sullivan T (2008) Effect of garlic on blood pressure: a systematic review and meta-analysis. BMC Cardiovasc Disord 8:13
211. Stevinson C, Pittler MH, Ernst E (2000) Garlic for treating hypercholesterolemia. A meta-analysis of randomized clinical trials. Ann Intern Med 133:420–429
212. Warshafsky S, Kamer RS, Sivak SL (1993) Effect of garlic on total serum cholesterol. A meta-analysis. Ann Intern Med 119:599–605
213. Rahman K (2010) in Bioact Foods Promot Heal 235–244. doi:10.1016/B978-0-12-374628-3.00016-5
214. Budoff M (2006) Aged garlic extract retards progression of coronary artery calcification. J Nutr 136:741S–744S
215. Ried K, Toben C, Fakler P (2013) Effect of garlic on serum lipids: an updated meta-analysis. Nutr Rev 71:282–299
216. Silagy CA, Neil HA (1994) A meta-analysis of the effect of garlic on blood pressure. J Hypertens 12:463–468
217. Scharbert G, Kalb ML, Duris M, Marschalek C, Kozek-Langenecker SA (2007) Garlic at dietary doses does not impair platelet function. Anesth Analg 105:1214–1218
218. Owens C, Baergen R, Puckett D (2014) Online sources of herbal product information. Am J Med 127:109–115
219. Ammon HP, Händel M (1981) Crataegus, toxicology and pharmacology. I. Toxicity. Planta Med 43:105–120
220. Ammon HP, Händel M (1981) Crataegus, toxicology and pharmacology. II. Pharmacodynamics. Planta Med 43:209–239
221. Ammon HP, Händel M (1981) Crataegus, toxicology and pharmacology. III. Pharmacodynamics and pharmacokinetics. Planta Med 43:313–322
222. Blesken R (1992) Crataegus in cardiology. Fortschr Med 110:290–292
223. Nasa Y, Hashizume H, Hoque AN, Abiko Y (1993) Protective effect of crataegus extract on the cardiac mechanical dysfunction in isolated perfused working rat heart. Arzneimittelforschung 43:945–949
224. Osher HL, Katz KH, Wagner DJ (1951) Khellin in the treatment of angina pectoris. N Engl J Med 244:315–321
225. Anrep GV, Kenawy MR, Barsoum GS (1949) The coronary vasodilator action of khellin. Am Heart J 37:531–542

226. Conn JJ, Kissane RW, Koon RA, Clark TE (1953) The treatment of angina pectoris with khellin. Ann Intern Med 38:23–27
227. Li J, Chen CX, Shen YH (2011) Effects of total glucosides from paeony (Paeonia lactiflora Pall) roots on experimental atherosclerosis in rats. J Ethnopharmacol 135:469–475
228. Long J et al (2012) Cardioprotective effect of total paeony glycosides against isoprenaline-induced myocardial ischemia in rats. Phytomedicine 19:672–676
229. Luo C et al (2013) Protection of H9c2 rat cardiomyoblasts against oxidative insults by total paeony glucosides from Radix Paeoniae Rubrae. Phytomedicine 21:20–24
230. Wei S (2015) Progress on cardiovascular protections and mechanism research of puerarin. Zhongguo Zhong Yao Za Zhi 40:2278–2284
231. Lu Q et al (2014) Puerarin attenuates calcification of vascular smooth muscle cells. Am J Chin Med 42:337–347
232. Yu W et al (2014) Flos Puerariae extract prevents myocardial apoptosis via attenuation oxidative stress in streptozotocin-induced diabetic mice. PLoS One 9, e98044
233. Bao L et al (2015) The anti-atherosclerotic effects of puerarin on induced-atherosclerosis in rabbits. Biomed Pap Med Fac Univ Palacký, Olomouc, Czechoslov 159:53–59
234. Zhou Y-X, Zhang H, Peng C (2014) Puerarin: a review of pharmacological effects. Phytother Res 28:961–975
235. Fioranelli M et al. (2016) Efficacia di Arnica Comp.-Heel® nel ridurre il rischio di eventi cardiovascolari in pazienti con coronaropatia stabile. Minerva Cardioangiol 64:1–8
236. Dash B (2006) Herbal treatment for heart disease. Health Armony B. Jain Publisher Ltd, New Delhi
237. Chen C et al (2015) Natural products for anti-thrombosis. Evidence-Based Complement Altern Med 2015, 876426
238. Rozanski A, Blumenthal JA, Kaplan J (1999) Impact of psychological factors on the pathogenesis of cardiovascular disease and implications for therapy. Circulation 99:2192–2217
239. Balestri M, Calati R, Serretti A, De Ronchi D (2014) Genetic modulation of personality traits: a systematic review of the literature. Int Clin Psychopharmacol 29:1–15
240. Rademaker AR, Kleber RJ, Geuze E, Vermetten E (2009) Personality dimensions harm avoidance and self-directedness predict the cortisol awakening response in military men. Biol Psychol 81:177–183
241. Dimopoulou C et al (2013) Increased prevalence of anxiety-associated personality traits in patients with Cushing's disease: a cross-sectional study. Neuroendocrinology 97:139–145
242. Yoda N et al (2008) Classification of adult patients with type 2 diabetes using the Temperament and Character Inventory. Psychiatry Clin Neurosci 62:279–285
243. Joyce PR, Mulder RT, Cloninger CR (1994) Temperament and hypercortisolemia in depression. Am J Psychiatry 151:195–198
244. Wang S et al (1997) Relationships between hormonal profile and novelty seeking in combat-related posttraumatic stress disorder. Biol Psychiatry 41:145–151
245. Simic I et al (2013) A preliminary evaluation of leukocyte phospho-glucocorticoid receptor as a potential biomarker of depressogenic vulnerability in healthy adults. Psychiatry Res 209:658–664
246. Capitanio JP et al (2008) Personality and serotonin transporter genotype interact with social context to affect immunity and viral set-point in simian immunodeficiency virus disease. Brain Behav Immun 22:676–689
247. Carnevali L, Sgoifo A (2014) Vagal modulation of resting heart rate in rats: the role of stress, psychosocial factors, and physical exercise. Front Physiol 5: 118
248. Ader R (2011) Psychoneuroimmunology, Two-Volume Set. Elsevier
249. Mittleman MA et al (1995) Triggering of acute myocardial infarction onset by episodes of anger. Determinants of Myocardial Infarction Onset Study Investigators. Circulation 92:1720–5
250. Stegano L (2009) Psicofisiologia. Dalla genetica comportamentale alle attività cognitive. Zanichelli
251. Janszky I, Ahnve S, Lundberg I, Hemmingsson T (2010) Early-onset depression, anxiety, and risk of subsequent coronary heart disease: 37-year follow-up of 49,321 young Swedish men. J Am Coll Cardiol 56:31–37
252. Dimsdale JE (2008) Psychological stress and cardiovascular disease. J Am Coll Cardiol 51: 1237–1246
253. Wittstein IS et al (2005) Neurohumoral features of myocardial stunning due to sudden emotional stress. N Engl J Med 352:539–548
254. Steptoe A, Brydon L (2005) Associations between acute lipid stress responses and fasting lipid levels 3 years later. Health Psychol 24:601–607
255. Schneider RH et al (2012) Stress reduction in the secondary prevention of cardiovascular disease: randomized, controlled trial of transcendental meditation and health education in blacks. Circ Cardiovasc Qual Outcomes 5:750–758
256. Giltay EJ, Kamphuis MH, Kalmijn S, Zitman FG, Kromhout D (2006) Dispositional optimism and the risk of cardiovascular death: the Zutphen Elderly Study. Arch Intern Med 166:431–436
257. Ornish D et al (1990) Can lifestyle changes reverse coronary heart disease? The Lifestyle Heart Trial. Lancet 336:129
258. Ornish D et al (1998) Intensive lifestyle changes for reversal of coronary heart disease. JAMA 280:2001–2007
259. Gould KL et al (1995) Changes in myocardial perfusion abnormalities by positron emission tomography after long-term, intense risk factor modification. JAMA 274:894–901

Integrated Approach to Heart Failure 17

Carlo Dal Lin, Marco Silvestro, Raffaele Migliorini, Francesco Tona, and Massimo Fioranelli

17.1 Introduction

Congestive heart failure (CHF) is the inability of the heart to pump blood effectively throughout the body. Such dysfunction may concern myocardial contractility, the ventricular preload, the end-diastolic volume, an obstacle to cardiac ejection, or excessive afterload and heart rate. The main causes of heart failure are long-term hypertension, previous myocardial infarction, disorders of the heart valves, cardiomyopathies, and chronic lung disease. A condition of compensation can be precipitated by some aggravating factors such as increased metabolic demand, as in the case of thyrotoxicosis, anemia, arteriovenous shunt, fever, fluid overload, increased sodium intake, environmental temperature that is too high or too low, renal or hepatic failure, respiratory insufficiency, emotional stress, pregnancy, obesity, arrhythmias, pulmonary embolism, alcohol ingestion, nutrient deficiency, uncontrolled hypertensive states, and beta-blockers, anti-arrhythmic drugs, and sodium-retaining drugs such as steroids and nonsteroidal anti-inflammatory drugs (NSAIDs) [1].

The state of failure is determined by a reduction in cardiac output leading to renal compensation (retention of sodium and fluids) and activation of the angiotensin–aldosterone system that increases peripheral resistance and afterload to maintain an adequate perfusion pressure. In parallel, the heart rate tends to increase under the sympathetic drive and the heart begins to dilate via the Frank–Starling mechanism. This establishes a vicious cycle leading to a gradual deterioration of the general cardiovascular state and systemic perfusion [2–6]. The symptomatology reported by patients varies according to the heart section affected: if the left ventricle is failing, symptoms prevail related to pulmonary congestion and systemic low output (exertional dyspnea, cough, fatigue, orthopnea, rales, gallop rhythm); if it is the right ventricle, systemic venous congestion is observed, with elevated venous pressure, peripheral edema, and hepatomegaly/ascites. In both cases, the clinical picture is dominated by fatigue, asthenia, and dyspnea.

Framing the symptoms is very important for a functional classification of the patient, enshrining the prognosis and the course of therapy (Table 17.1).

The diagnosis is confirmed by echocardiography and cardiac catheterization.

Despite pharmacological and technological progress, morbidity, mortality, and the escalating financial burden to society associated with heart

C. Dal Lin, M.D. (✉) • M. Silvestro, N.D. • R. Migliorini, M.D. • F. Tona, M.D., Ph.D.
Department of Cardiological, Thoracic and Vascular Sciences, Padua University Medical School, Padova, Italy
e-mail: carlodallin@libero.it

M. Fioranelli, M.D.
Department of Nuclear Physics, Sub-Nuclear and Radiation, Guglielmo Marconi University, Rome, Italy

M. Fioranelli (ed.), *Integrative Cardiology*, DOI 10.1007/978-3-319-40010-5_17

Table 17.1 New York Heart Association (NYHA) functional classification system [1]

NYHA class	Description
I	Physical activity not limited by symptoms such as shortness of breath, fatigue, or palpitations
II	Physical exertion mildly limited, with symptoms of shortness of breath, fatigue, or palpitations developing with typical daily activities
III	Physical activity severely curtailed; symptoms of shortness of breath, fatigue, or palpitations developing with any kind of activity
IV	Symptoms and physical discomfort present even at rest

Table 17.2 Stages of heart failure (HF)

ACC/AHA stage	Description
A	At risk for HF, but without structural heart disease or HF symptoms
B	Structural heart disease, but without signs or symptoms of HF
C	Structural heart disease with prior or current symptoms of HF
D	Refractory heart failure requiring specialized intervention

Modified from Hunt SA, et al. ACC/AHA 2005 guideline update for the diagnosis and management of chronic heart failure in the adult – summary article: a report of the American College of Cardiology/American Heart Association Task Force on Practice Guidelines (Writing Committee to Update the 2001 Guidelines for the Evaluation and Management of Heart Failure). J Am Coll Cardiol. 2005;46:1116–1143

failure remain unacceptably high. At 40 years of age, the lifetime risk of developing heart failure for both men and women is 20%. A conservative estimate of the direct and indirect costs of heart failure in the USA for 2010 is $39.2 billion [7]. The 1-year mortality rate for heart failure is 20% [8, 9]. The incidence of heart failure is expected to increase with the increase in the average age of the population and survival following heart attacks [1].

With regard to the integrative medicine approach, the single best way to treat heart failure is to prevent its development and its inexorable vicious cycle, leading toward progressive greater infirmity and death within a few years. As stated by Russell and Greenfield (cited in Rakel [7]): "*Prevention, prevention, prevention must be our mantra with respect to heart failure management. Do everything to prevent the disease from ever developing in the first place. Integrative means to help prevent or at least aggressively treat disorders that contribute to development of heart failure (including hypertension, coronary artery disease, diabetes, and dyslipidemia).*"

It is essential to strengthen the educational interventions aimed at cardiovascular health early in life and carefully oversee and control the main cardiovascular risks, such as hypertension, diabetes, obesity, coronary artery disease, and stress [10–12].

As we will see, the integrated approach has great advantages in New York Heart Association (NYHA) classes I and II and in the early stages of heart failure (stages A to C in Table 17.2). For people who have already developed symptomatic heart failure, and in NYHA stages III and IV, the emphasis rests squarely on conventional medical therapy. Complementary medical therapies with the promise of efficacy and evidence for safety can be used as adjuncts, to the benefit of most patients.

Although the main objective of integrative cardiology is the prevention of heart failure, in patients with established heart failure progressive cardiovascular deterioration has to be prevented, symptoms minimized, quality of life enhanced, and survival rates increased.

In Fig. 17.1a and b the treatment algorithm for heart failure by stage of the disease is shown.

17.2 Lifestyle and Nutrition

In addition to all the programs for prevention and care, especially in the context of CHF, close attention must be paid to tobacco and alcohol cessation and weight management, educating patients and their family regarding the adverse effects of smoking, excessive alcohol intake, and obesity. The heart is a muscle and needs to be trained: the condition of heart failure is not a contraindication to exercise. There is great deal of evidence [13–16] regarding the safety [17] and benefits of cardiological rehabilitation with

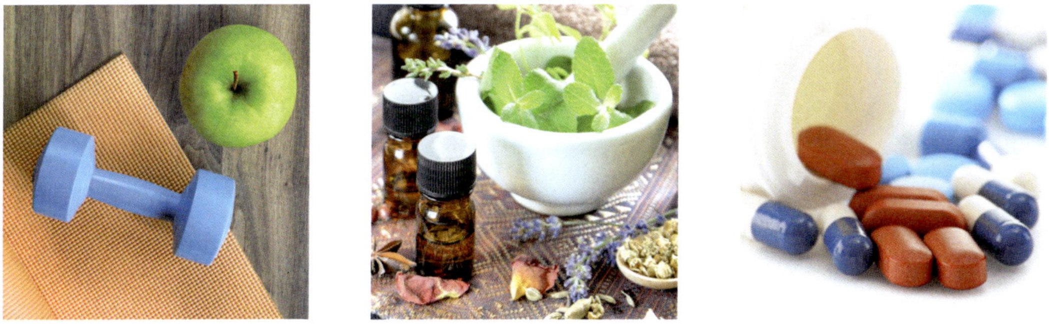

Minimize obstacles to healing ⟶ **Tailor natural interventions to patient needs** ⟶ **Determine need for conventional therapy**

Minimize obstacles to healing

Control precipitating factors (such as hypertension and other risk factors, nonsteroideal antiinflammatory medications and first generation calcium channel blockers): see the chapter on hypertension.

Obesity: weight management program to achieve ideal body weight.

Diet: attention on fluids ammount, eliminate refined processed foods, reduce saturated animal fats, emphasize whole plant foods, restrict sodium<1,8 g q.d.

Stress and depression management

Spirituality

Bioenergetics (Acupuncture)

Graded exercise: enroll patients in a certified rehabilitation program.

Tailor natural interventions to patient needs

Indications of magnesium deficiency or use conventional drugs: magnesium.

Increase myocardial energy production: Thiamin, Carnitine, CoQ10.

Improve cardiac output: Crataegus, Terminalia.

Enhance peripheral vascular flow: arginine.

Determine need for conventional therapy

Severe CHF (NYHA stage III or IV): refer for conventional adjunctive medication.

See Fig.1-B

Fig. 17.1 (**a**) In summary: staged integrative approach to heart failure. Don't smoke, follow an anti-inflammatory or Mediterranean diet, control weight, perform regular physical fitness activities, manage stress, treat depression, take care of spirituality, work to manage medical conditions that may lead to heart failure (high blood pressure, coronary artery disease, dyslipidemia, and diabetes), avoid overuse of nonsteroidal anti-inflammatory medications. (**b**) Clinical pathway: management of congestive heart failure (*CHF*). *CAD* coronary artery disease, *CRT* cardiac resynchronization therapy, *DM* diabetes mellitus, *EF* ejection fraction, *HF* heart failure, *ICD* implantable cardioverter defibrillator, *NYHA* New York Heart Association. Modified from Rakel [7]

graded exercise programming in patients with cardiac dysfunction in terms of functional improvement [18] and quality of life [19, 20]. The combination of exercise and proper diet helps to maintain a proper body weight by reducing the workload of a dysfunctional heart. Rest is important and patients should be advised to sleep at least 7–8 h per night [7, 21].

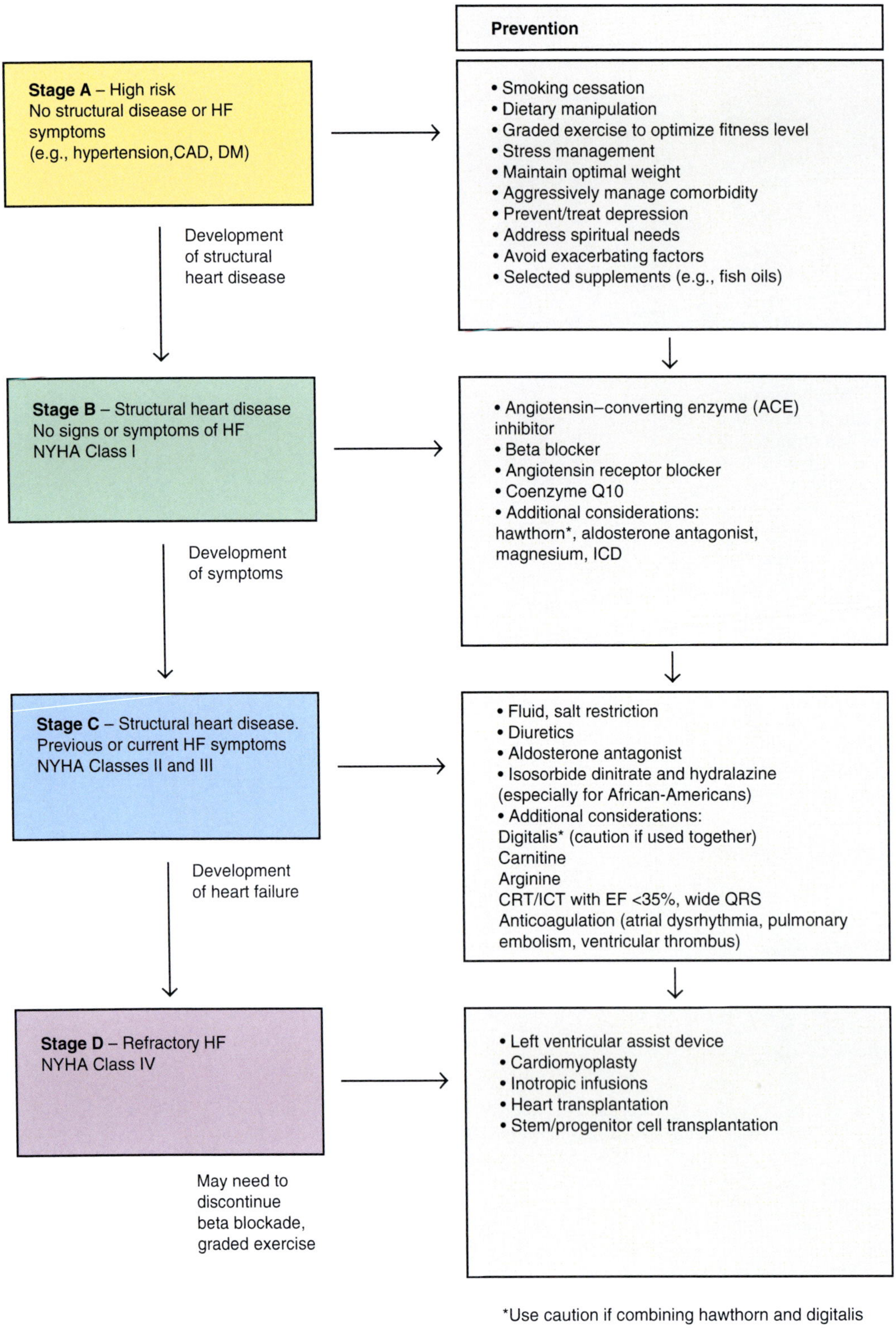

Fig. 17.1 (continued)

The doctors and professionals who care for patients with CHF should also pay attention to their spiritual side [22–25]. Indeed, many patients with CHF struggle with their spirituality, "*a struggle that adds to an already stressful situation and perhaps leads to morbidity*" [7, 26, 27]. The spiritual challenges associated with heart failure have been equated with those experienced by people with cancer [28]. As suggested by Russel and Greenfield (cited in Rakel [7]): "*attention to spiritual needs can help people adjust to their new circumstances, address specific regrets with regard to prior lifestyle choices, and search for present meaning and future hope*" [29, 30].

Dietary recommendations for hypertension are appropriate for most CHF patients. In particular, a Mediterranean or Dietary Approaches to Stop Hypertension (DASH) diet, low in sodium and high in potassium, paying attention to the ingestion of fluids, may help prevent development of heart failure and slow progression of established disease. Patients with CHF may need to limit sodium intake to 2 g/day and daily ingestion of water to 1.5–2 L.

17.3 Supplements

Nutritional supplements improve myocardial energy production and this is a very important effect in a pathological scenario always characterized by energy depletion, often due to nutrient or coenzyme deficiency [21].

17.3.1 Magnesium

Magnesium is a key element for adenosine triphosphate (ATP) production. In the case of CHF, magnesium levels correlate directly with survival rates [31] and deficiency is linked to arrhythmias, reduced cardiovascular prognosis, worsened ischemia, and increased mortality in acute myocardial infarction [1]. The deficiency of this mineral is probably caused by inadequate intake, increased wasting owing to the overactivation of renin–angiotensin–aldosterone system typical of CHF [32], and by conventional drug therapy such as digitalis, diuretics, beta-blockers, and calcium-channel blockers [33–36]. Magnesium supplementation produces positive effects in patients with CHF on conventional drugs, even if serum magnesium is normal [32]. The recommended dosage is: 200–400 mg t.i.d. (magnesium citrate).

17.3.2 Thiamine

Thiamine, or vitamin B1 deficiency, has remarkable cardiovascular effects, leading to the so-called wet beri-beri disease, a condition related to sodium retention, peripheral vasodilation, and heart failure [1]. A common important drug used in CHF treatment, such as furosemide, causes B1 deficiency [37], although it is uncommon to have a significant lack of thiamine, except in alcoholics [38].

Many people, especially elderly and hospitalized patients, however, do not reach the recommended daily dose of 1.5 mg [38]. A daily dose of 80–240 mg of vitamin B1 improves the clinical condition of CHF, as it improves patients' ejection fraction by as much as 13–22% [39, 40]. Its use at doses of 200–250 mg qd, in the context of CHF, is recommendable, given the lack of risk and the low cost [21].

17.3.3 L-Carnitine

Carnitine is an important factor for the production of ATP, being a carrier of fatty acids into the myocardial mitochondria [21]. The myocardium stores considerable stocks of carnitine and coenzyme Q10, in excess of the metabolic standard needs, but this quantity is dramatically depleted in the course of ischemia and CHF [41–48]. Carnitine supplementation improves myocardial performance [47, 49–54] and outcome [55] in the case of CHF [56–59] in proportion to the duration of its use [60]: the longer it is used, the greater the improvement. When administered 500 mg t.i.d. for 6 months, the maximum exercise time improves by 16–25% and the ejection fraction by 12–13% [60]. When carnitine is given in an acute setting, it lowers pulmonary artery and capillary wedge pressures [59].

17.3.4 Coenzyme Q10

Coenzyme Q10 (CoQ10) is present in small amounts in most diets and is also synthesized within the body from tyrosine, partially through a common pathway shared with cholesterol synthesis. It is found in its highest concentrations within the mitochondrial membranes of organs that have significant energy requirements, especially the heart, where is involved with energy production [7, 61, 62]. CoQ10 exerts anti-oxidant and membrane-stabilizing effects as well [7, 63].

The amount of CoQ10 is reduced in patients with CHF and the deficit is greater, the worse the NYHA class [7, 64].

For CoQ10 the considerations made in the case of hypertension are also valid. In particular, it appears to be a key factor to be added to conventional CHF drugs [21, 65], because it improves the clinical picture and quality of life of patients with CHF [66–69]. In particular, the clinical signs of CHF (cyanosis, peripheral and pulmonary edema, hepatomegaly, venous congestion, palpitations, sweating, insomnia, dizziness, nocturia) improved by 50–80% with few and mild side effects [70]. Two recent studies failed to show clinical efficacy [71, 72].

The optimal dosage of CoQ10 in the setting of heart failure is as yet undetermined. Studies have used doses ranging from 30 to 600 mg/day, but most practitioners initially prescribe 100–200 mg daily. Softgel capsules of CoQ10 appear to provide superior bioavailability [73] and rare side effects (gastrointestinal upset) [74]. CoQ10 is reduced in those who take statins [75–79]. Care should be taken in the case of concomitant warfarin consumption [7, 80, 81], possibly necessitating dose adjustment.

17.3.5 L-Arginine

Arginine is a valuable amino acid in the treatment of CHF, improving hemodynamics and endothelial function [82–86], exercise tolerance [82, 87, 88], kidney function [89], and quality of life [90]. In fact, from arginine the body synthesizes nitric oxide with a vasodilatory effect. The administration of 5.6–12.6 g of arginine per day (mean dosage recommended 2–6 g [7]) leads to an increase in peripheral blood flow of 30% and an 8% increase in the distance traveled during the 6-min walking test [82].

17.3.6 Vitamin E

Questions persist about the safety of high-dose vitamin E in patients with established cardiovascular disease [91].

17.4 Phytotherapy

Herbs and supplements require in 4–6 weeks to obtain an evident clinical benefit and are useful in the early stages of heart failure (ACC/AHA stages A to C and NYHA classes I to III). Thus, the use of these agents is not appropriate for acutely worsening heart failure.

17.4.1 Hawthorn (*Crataegus oxyacantha, laevigata,* and *monogyna*)

The herbal medicinal plants and their derivatives are used as a complementary therapy for heart failure [92]; among these, in addition to those with diuretic and hypotensive activity, hawthorn plays an important role. The tops (flowers and leaves) of this plant are used and are obtained from the species *Crataegus oxyacantha, laevigata, and monogyna*.

Hawthorn (*Crataegus oxyacantha*) was considered a "cardio-sedative" folk medicine, but evidence proves that it has the opposite effect enough to be recommended in the complementary therapy of heart failure NYHA classes I and II (Table 17.3).

Several pharmacological studies on hawthorn extract reveal a protective function on ischemic heart and myocardial damage related to hypertension. In particular, its flavonoids have an ACE inhibitory action with hypotensive effects [94, 96, 97] and protect the cardiomyocytes

Table 17.3 Effects of hawthorn [93–95]

Increased coronary artery blood flow
Enhanced pumping efficiency of the heart (improved contractility)
Anti-oxidant activity
Phosphodiesterase inhibition
Angiotensin-converting enzyme inhibition
Anti-dysrhythmic effects (lengthens the effective refractory period, unlike many cardiac drugs)
Mild reduction in systemic vascular resistance (lowered blood pressure)

following ischemia-reperfusion [98]. Luteolin, hyperoside, vitexin, and rutin increase the coronary flow significantly, have a mildly positive inotropic effect, and optimize the speed of relaxation of heart myocells [99]. Anthocyanosides determine the liberation of PGI2, a prostaglandin with endothelial vasodilatory activity [100]. We recommend a dosage of 5–20 mg/day of flavonoids present in 250–1,000 mg/day of dry extract 2%.

In addition to its positive inotropic and lusitropic effects, the polyphenols, amines, and triterpenic acid content in hawthorn have a negative chronotropic action (reducing the heart rate), a positive dromotropic effect (reducing the conduction time), and a negative bathmotropic action (lengthening the refractory period) [101]. In arterial and coronary areas a decrease in peripheral and coronary resistance was observed, with a modest hypotensive action, an anti-oxidant, anti-inflammatory, and endothelial protective effect, and antiplatelet activity [100].

Different clinical trials featuring the hawthorn have followed over time [102, 103], confirming the effectiveness of the extracts of this plant in increasing the force of contraction of the heart, reducing the symptoms and dyspnea, and improving exercise tolerance, particularly in patients in NYHA classes I–II [28, 104–111]. In the various studies mentioned, two types of hawthorn extracts were employed, standardized in flavonoids to 2.2% or procyanidins 18.8%, with variable dosage from 160 mg to 1,800 mg/day. Most practitioners believe that therapeutic efficacy is greater with higher doses (600–1,800 mg/day) [7]. Again, no noticeable improvement may occur for 6–12 weeks.

Most of the studies with positive results, however, did not include treatment with drugs now accepted as standard medical therapy, such as ACE inhibitors and beta-blockers. Later studies employing hawthorn in the setting of CHF in combination with current standard medical therapy reported less successful outcomes [103, 112, 113]. Even in these studies a modest improvement in the left ventricular ejection fraction was identified along with a trend toward reduced cardiac mortality, most notably for those with significantly impaired left ventricular function [103, 112, 113].

Hawthorn is well tolerated and has few side effects (3% incidence) such as headache, fatigue, dizziness, palpitations, rash, drowsiness, agitation, and gastrointestinal disorders. It may interact with drugs such as digitalis, beta-blockers, diuretics, ACE inhibitors, and platelet anti-aggregants [114]. Nevertheless, the results of a retrospective safety analysis should be reported, where hawthorn use not only failed to impede the progression of the disease, but also appeared in some patients to increase the risk of early heart failure progression. In light of a previously good safety record, these findings are puzzling and concerning. Probably, the use of hawthorn in a holistic program that includes nutritional care and adequate stress management could avoid these outcomes [10–12].

In future, as suggested by Russel and Greenfield (cited in Rakel [7]): "*because the purported beneficial actions of hawthorn overlap some of those inherent to medications such as ACE inhibitors and beta blockers, combination therapy possibly would permit the use of lower doses with no diminution of therapeutic effectiveness.*"

Nowadays, the digital and pharmaceutical formulations based on hawthorn find elective indications in patients with impaired myocardial contractile force only in the case of atrial fibrillation; otherwise, the mortality of patients with heart failure increases [1]. Most conventional medical practitioners reflexively state that hawthorn should not be given to people taking digitalis for heart failure [115]. In the past, sparteine, an extract of the broom (*Sarothamnus scoparius*), was also used, but then abandoned for toxicity reasons [100].

17.4.2 *Terminalia arjuna*

Terminalia arjuna is a traditional Ayurvedic herb that has recently been described to be effective for heart failure in a controlled clinical study [116]. The dosage is 500 mg every 8 h of the extract from its bark. The study documents a very promising effect of the plant in the case of severe and refractory heart failure with improvements to NYHA class II.

17.4.3 Tricks of the Trade

Undoubtedly, the plant most used in the case of heart failure is the hawthorn with excellent results when associated with ginseng, which enhances its tonic properties. To avoid hawthorn's "opposite effect" it is better to use it in the form of glycerine macerate (GM): using the gems, in fact, the action seems to be more "regulatory" compared with its leaves and flowers. For example: hawthorn tincture lowers blood pressure, whereas hawthorn GM rules it (that is, in the case of low blood pressure, it tends to raise the blood pressure a little). Hawthorn tincture works on tachycardia, whereas hawthorn GM also works on bradycardia. In addition, hawthorn MG can safely be combined with drugs.

Another great remedy that is used in the naturopathic field for both the prevention and treatment of infarction, heart failure, and for rhythm disturbances (angina, arrhythmias, extrasystoles, extrasystoles with mitral valve prolapse) is the dietary supplement *magnesium-potassium-bromelain*: 1 tablet three times a day. *Bromelain* is an enzyme derived from the pineapple stem and has a significant anti-inflammatory action on vascular walls combined with a lipid-lowering effect. To obtain good results, it should be taken for at least 6 months.

17.5 Bioenergetics (Acupuncture)

Acupuncture, modulating sympathetic activity, may be useful for people with heart failure [117, 118]. A pilot study of acupuncture reported intriguing results documenting a marked improvement in the 6-min walk test in subjects with stable NYHA class II to III heart failure on appropriate medical therapy compared with controls [119]. More research is needed to establish the precise rules for the application of this method in the context of CHF.

17.6 Mind–Body Therapies

In the clinical CHF context, the mind–body therapies play an important role in growing success. In particular, they seem to be very useful in combating depression that often accompanies the life of patients with heart failure [120, 121]. Depression is an independent negative prognostic factor in CHF and even alone can determine inflammation [122, 123], oxidative stress, and endothelial dysfunction with possible myocardial ischemia, leading to increased morbidity and mortality [10–12]. Numerous studies describe that an appropriate reduction in stress, in patients with CHF, causes a relief of depression and anxiety [124] with an improvement in risk profile and cardiovascular disease progression and outcomes [125–131]. Specifically, are seen an improvement of the autonomic balance and of the levels of circulating neurotransmitters [132], an increase in cardiac output and a decrease in peripheral resistance [133], and an increase in exercise capacity, a decrease in hospitalizations, with improvement of symptoms [134]. The techniques that can be applied in a program of care for a patient with CHF are: biofeedback [133], mindfulness meditation [135], and transcendental meditation [134]; other studies regarding the beneficial effect of mind–body therapies involve freeze-frame stress management [136], relaxation response training [137, 138], tai chi [139, 140], and behavioral changes [141].

17.7 Pharmaceuticals, Biomechanical therapy, Surgery

According to international cardiological guidelines, all patients with heart failure should be started on some combination of angiotensin-converting enzyme inhibitor, angiotensin receptor blocker, beta-blocker, and aldosterone antagonists, which all have a positive impact on mortality related to heart failure [1, 12]. Diuretics act by decreasing the preload, lessening the cardiac workload, and the most commonly used are loop diuretics, such as furosemide, which are especially beneficial once congestion has developed. Isosorbide dinitrate and hydralazine are useful for the treatment of heart failure in African–Americans (who do not appear to respond as favorably to ACE inhibitors or beta-blockers).

The acute setting may require the infusion of inotropes, ultrafiltration, or aortic counterpulsation.

The most significant recent change in the conventional medical treatment of CHF is the increased reliance on device therapy (cardiac resynchronization therapy and implantable cardioverter defibrillators) and left ventricular assist devices. For indications for their use, see Camm et al., McMurray et al., and Tarzia et al. [1, 142–144]. Heart transplantation remains the gold standard in the case of refractory heart failure.

17.8 Future Therapies

Future therapies under study for heart failure [145, 146] treatment involve: calcium sensitizers, continuous-flow left ventricular assist devices, cytokine inhibitors, endothelin receptor blockers, erythropoiesis-stimulating proteins, fish oils, free fatty acid oxidation inhibitors, gene expression (miRNA), matrix metalloproteinase inhibitors, modified natriuretic peptides, nitric oxide–enhancing therapy, phosphodiesterase-III inhibitors, ribose, statin therapy, stem and progenitor cell transplantation, taurine, and vasopressin antagonists.

References

1. Camm AJ, Thomas F, Luscher PWS (2009) ESC textbook of cardiovascular medicine, 2nd edn. Oxford Med: 1–1398
2. Uddin N, Patterson JH (2007) Current guidelines for treatment of heart failure: 2006 update. Pharmacotherapy 27:12S–17S
3. Young JB (1995) Contemporary management of patients with heart failure. Med Clin North Am 79:1171–1190
4. Packer M (1992) The neurohormonal hypothesis: a theory to explain the mechanism of disease progression in heart failure. J Am Coll Cardiol 20:248–254
5. Packer M (1993) How should physicians view heart failure? The philosophical and physiological evolution of three conceptual models of the disease. Am J Cardiol 71:3C–11C
6. Francis GS, Goldsmith SR, Levine TB, Olivari MT, Cohn JN (1984) The neurohumoral axis in congestive heart failure. Ann Intern Med 101:370–377
7. Rakel D (2012) Integrative medicine, 3rd edn. Elsevier, Amsterdam
8. Lloyd-Jones D et al (2010) Heart disease and stroke statistics—2010 update: a report from the American Heart Association. Circulation 121:e46–e215
9. Bleumink GS et al (2004) Quantifying the heart failure epidemic: prevalence, incidence rate, lifetime risk and prognosis of heart failure. The Rotterdam Study. Eur Heart J 25:1614–1619
10. Dal Lin C et al (2015) Coronary microvascular and endothelial function regulation: crossroads of psychoneuroendocrine immunitary signals and quantum physics [Part A]. J Integr Cardiol 1:132–163
11. Dal Lin C et al (2015) Coronary microvascular and endothelial function regulation: crossroads of psychoneuroendocrine immunitary signals and quantum physics [Part B]. J Integr Cardiol 1:164–188
12. Dal Lin C et al (2015) Coronary microvascular and endothelial function regulation: crossroads of psychoneuroendocrine immunitary signals and quantum physics [Part C]. J Integr Cardiol 1:189–209
13. Coats AJ, Adamopoulos S, Meyer TE, Conway J, Sleight P (1990) Effects of physical training in chronic heart failure. Lancet 335:63–66
14. Oka RK et al (2000) Impact of a home-based walking and resistance training program on quality of life in patients with heart failure. Am J Cardiol 85:365–369
15. Dimopoulos S et al (2006) Effects of exercise rehabilitation program on heart rate recovery in patients with chronic heart failure. Eur J Cardiovasc Prev Rehabil 13:67–73
16. Jónsdóttir S, Andersen KK, Sigurosson AF, Sigurosson SB (2006) The effect of physical training in chronic heart failure. Eur J Heart Fail 8:97–101
17. O'Connor CM et al (2009) Efficacy and safety of exercise training in patients with chronic heart failure: HF-ACTION randomized controlled trial. JAMA 301:1439–1450
18. Tabet J-Y et al (2008) Absence of exercise capacity improvement after exercise training program: a strong prognostic factor in patients with chronic heart failure. Circ Heart Fail 1:220–226

19. Taylor RS et al (2014) Exercise-based rehabilitation for heart failure. Cochrane Database Syst Rev 4: CD003331
20. Taylor RS et al (2015) Home-based versus centre-based cardiac rehabilitation. Cochrane Database Syst Rev 8:CD007130
21. Pizzorno JE, Murray MT (2013) Textbook of natural medicine, 4th edn. Elsevier, Amsterdam
22. Koenig HG et al (1997) Attendance at religious services, interleukin-6, and other biological parameters of immune function in older adults. Int J Psychiatry Med 27:233–250
23. Levin JS (1996) How prayer heals: a theoretical model. Altern Ther Health Med 2:66–73
24. Oman D, Reed D (1998) Religion and mortality among the community-dwelling elderly. Am J Public Health 88:1469–1475
25. Waldfogel S (1997) Spirituality in medicine. Prim Care 24:963–976
26. Fitchett G et al (2004) Religious struggle: prevalence, correlates and mental health risks in diabetic, congestive heart failure, and oncology patients. Int J Psychiatry Med 34:179–196
27. Beery TA, Baas LS, Fowler C, Allen G (2002) Spirituality in persons with heart failure. J Holist Nurs 20:5–25, quiz 26–30
28. Bekelman DB et al (2009) Symptom burden, depression, and spiritual well-being: a comparison of heart failure and advanced cancer patients. J Gen Intern Med 24:592–598
29. Westlake C, Dracup K (2001) Role of spirituality in adjustment of patients with advanced heart failure. Prog Cardiovasc Nurs 16:119–125
30. Vollman MW, LaMontagne LL, Wallston KA (2009) Existential well-being predicts perceived control in adults with heart failure. Appl Nurs Res 22:198–203
31. Gottlieb SS et al (1990) Prognostic importance of the serum magnesium concentration in patients with congestive heart failure. J Am Coll Cardiol 16:827–831
32. Gottlieb SS (1989) Importance of magnesium in congestive heart failure. Am J Cardiol 63:39G–42G
33. Cohen N et al (2000) Metabolic and clinical effects of oral magnesium supplementation in furosemide-treated patients with severe congestive heart failure. Clin Cardiol 23:433–436
34. Cohen N et al (2003) Serum magnesium aberrations in furosemide (frusemide) treated patients with congestive heart failure: pathophysiological correlates and prognostic evaluation. Heart 89:411–416
35. Oladapo OO, Falase AO (2000) Serum and urinary magnesium during treatment of patients with chronic congestive heart failure. Afr J Med Sci 29:301–303
36. Crippa G, Sverzellati E, Giorgi-Pierfranceschi M, Carrara GC (1999) Magnesium and cardiovascular drugs: interactions and therapeutic role. Ann Ital di Med interna organo Uff della Soc Ital di Med interna 14:40–45
37. Zenuk C et al (2003) Thiamine deficiency in congestive heart failure patients receiving long term furosemide therapy. Can J Clin Pharmacol 10:184–188
38. Chen MF, Chen LT, Gold M, Boyce HW (1996) Plasma and erythrocyte thiamin concentrations in geriatric outpatients. J Am Coll Nutr 15:231–236
39. Leslie D, Gheorghiade M (1996) Is there a role for thiamine supplementation in the management of heart failure? Am Heart J 131:1248–1250
40. Mendoza CE, Rodriguez F, Rosenberg DG (2003) Reversal of refractory congestive heart failure after thiamine supplementation: report of a case and review of literature. J Cardiovasc Pharmacol Ther 8:313–316
41. Arsenian MA (1997) Carnitine and its derivatives in cardiovascular disease. Prog Cardiovasc Dis 40:265–286
42. Nakagawa T, Sunamori M, Suzuki A (1994) The myocardial distribution and plasma concentration of carnitine in patients with mitral valve disease. Surg Today 24:313–317
43. Pierpont ME et al (1989) Myocardial carnitine in end-stage congestive heart failure. Am J Cardiol 64:56–60
44. Suzuki Y et al (1982) Myocardial carnitine deficiency in chronic heart failure. Lancet 1:116
45. Regitz V, Shug AL, Fleck E (1990) Defective myocardial carnitine metabolism in congestive heart failure secondary to dilated cardiomyopathy and to coronary, hypertensive and valvular heart diseases. Am J Cardiol 65:755–760
46. Corr PB, Gross RW, Sobel BE (1984) Amphipathic metabolites and membrane dysfunction in ischemic myocardium. Circ Res 55:135–154
47. Paulson DJ, Traxler J, Schmidt M, Noonan J, Shug AL (1986) Protection of the ischaemic myocardium by L-propionylcarnitine: effects on the recovery of cardiac output after ischaemia and reperfusion, carnitine transport, and fatty acid oxidation. Cardiovasc Res 20:536–541
48. Tassani V, Cattapan F, Magnanimi L, Peschechera A (1994) Anaplerotic effect of propionyl carnitine in rat heart mitochondria. Biochem Biophys Res Commun 199:949–953
49. Di Lisa F, Menabò R, Siliprandi N (1989) L-propionyl-carnitine protection of mitochondria in ischemic rat hearts. Mol Cell Biochem 88:169–173
50. Ferrari R et al (1992) Prolonged propionyl-L-carnitine pre-treatment of rabbit: biochemical, hemodynamic and electrophysiological effects on myocardium. J Mol Cell Cardiol 24:219–232
51. Sethi R, Wang X, Ferrari R, Dhalla NS (2004) Improvement of cardiac function and beta-adrenergic signal transduction by propionyl L-carnitine in congestive heart failure due to myocardial infarction. Coron Artery Dis 15:65–71
52. Cherchi A et al (1985) Effects of L-carnitine on exercise tolerance in chronic stable angina: a multicenter, double-blind, randomized, placebo

controlled crossover study. Int J Clin Pharmacol Ther Toxicol 23:569–572
53. Brevetti G et al (1988) Increases in walking distance in patients with peripheral vascular disease treated with L-carnitine: a double-blind, cross-over study. Circulation 77:767–773
54. Jeejeebhoy F et al (2002) Nutritional supplementation with MyoVive repletes essential cardiac myocyte nutrients and reduces left ventricular size in patients with left ventricular dysfunction. Am Heart J 143:1092–1100
55. Rizos I (2000) Three-year survival of patients with heart failure caused by dilated cardiomyopathy and L-carnitine administration. Am Heart J 139:S120–S123
56. Ferrari R et al (2004) Therapeutic effects of L-carnitine and propionyl-L-carnitine on cardiovascular diseases: a review. Ann N Y Acad Sci 1033:79–91
57. Mancini M, Rengo F, Lingetti M, Sorrentino GP, Nolfe G (1992) Controlled study on the therapeutic efficacy of propionyl-L-carnitine in patients with congestive heart failure. Arzneimittelforschung 42:1101–1104
58. Caponnetto S et al (1994) Efficacy of L-propionylcarnitine treatment in patients with left ventricular dysfunction. Eur Heart J 15:1267–1273
59. Anand I et al (1998) Acute and chronic effects of propionyl-L-carnitine on the hemodynamics, exercise capacity, and hormones in patients with congestive heart failure. Cardiovasc Drugs Ther 12:291–299
60. Pucciarelli G et al (1992) The clinical and hemodynamic effects of propionyl-L-carnitine in the treatment of congestive heart failure. Clin Ter 141:379–384
61. Nakamura Y et al (1982) Protection of ischaemic myocardium with coenzyme Q10. Cardiovasc Res 16:132–137
62. Crane FL, Navas P (1997) The diversity of coenzyme Q function. Mol Aspects Med 18[Suppl]:S1–S6
63. Frei B, Kim MC, Ames BN (1990) Ubiquinol-10 is an effective lipid-soluble antioxidant at physiological concentrations. Proc Natl Acad Sci U S A 87:4879–4883
64. Folkers K, Vadhanavikit S, Mortensen SA (1985) Biochemical rationale and myocardial tissue data on the effective therapy of cardiomyopathy with coenzyme Q10. Proc Natl Acad Sci U S A 82:901–904
65. Langsjoen PH, Vadhanavikit S, Folkers K (1985) Response of patients in classes III and IV of cardiomyopathy to therapy in a blind and crossover trial with coenzyme Q10. Proc Natl Acad Sci U S A 82:4240–4244
66. Langsjoen PH, Folkers K (1990) Long-term efficacy and safety of coenzyme Q10 therapy for idiopathic dilated cardiomyopathy. Am J Cardiol 65:521–523
67. Langsjoen PH, Langsjoen AM (1999) Overview of the use of CoQ10 in cardiovascular disease. Biofactors 9:273–284
68. Soja AM, Mortensen SA (1997) Treatment of congestive heart failure with coenzyme Q10 illuminated by meta-analyses of clinical trials. Mol Aspects Med 18[Suppl]:S159–S168
69. Langsjoen PH et al (1990) Pronounced increase of survival of patients with cardiomyopathy when treated with coenzyme Q10 and conventional therapy. Int J Tissue React 12:163–168
70. Baggio E, Gandini R, Plancher AC, Passeri M, Carmosino G (1994) Italian multicenter study on the safety and efficacy of coenzyme Q10 as adjunctive therapy in heart failure. CoQ10 Drug Surveillance Investigators. Mol Aspects Med 15 Suppl: s287–s294
71. Watson PS et al (1999) Lack of effect of coenzyme Q on left ventricular function in patients with congestive heart failure. J Am Coll Cardiol 33:1549–1552
72. Khatta M et al (2000) The effect of coenzyme Q10 in patients with congestive heart failure. Ann Intern Med 132:636–640
73. Chopra RK, Goldman R, Sinatra ST, Bhagavan HN (1998) Relative bioavailability of coenzyme Q10 formulations in human subjects. Int J Vitam Nutr Res Int Zeitschrift für Vitamin- und Ernährungsforschung J Int Vitaminol Nutr 68:109–113
74. Greenberg S, Frishman WH (1990) Co-enzyme Q10: a new drug for cardiovascular disease. J Clin Pharmacol 30:596–608
75. Folkers K et al (1990) Lovastatin decreases coenzyme Q levels in humans. Proc Natl Acad Sci U S A 87:8931–8934
76. Mortensen SA, Leth A, Agner E, Rohde M (1997) Dose-related decrease of serum coenzyme Q10 during treatment with HMG-CoA reductase inhibitors. Mol Aspects Med 18[Suppl]:S137–S144
77. Ghirlanda G et al (1993) Evidence of plasma CoQ10-lowering effect by HMG-CoA reductase inhibitors: a double-blind, placebo-controlled study. J Clin Pharmacol 33:226–229
78. Lamperti C et al (2005) Muscle coenzyme Q10 level in statin-related myopathy. Arch Neurol 62:1709–1712
79. Langsjoen PH, Langsjoen AM (2003) The clinical use of HMG CoA-reductase inhibitors and the associated depletion of coenzyme Q10. A review of animal and human publications. Biofactors 18:101–111
80. Spigset O (1994) Reduced effect of warfarin caused by ubidecarenone. Lancet 344:1372–1373
81. Zhou Q, Zhou S, Chan E (2005) Effect of coenzyme Q10 on warfarin hydroxylation in rat and human liver microsomes. Curr Drug Metab 6:67–81
82. Rector TS et al (1996) Randomized, double-blind, placebo-controlled study of supplemental oral L-arginine in patients with heart failure. Circulation 93:2135–2141
83. Hambrecht R et al (2000) Correction of endothelial dysfunction in chronic heart failure: additional effects of exercise training and oral L-arginine supplementation. J Am Coll Cardiol 35:706–713

84. Lerman A, Burnett JC, Higano ST, McKinley LJ, Holmes DR (1998) Long-term L-arginine supplementation improves small-vessel coronary endothelial function in humans. Circulation 97:2123–2128
85. Adams MR et al (1997) Oral L-arginine improves endothelium-dependent dilatation and reduces monocyte adhesion to endothelial cells in young men with coronary artery disease. Atherosclerosis 129:261–269
86. Bocchi EA et al (2000) L-arginine reduces heart rate and improves hemodynamics in severe congestive heart failure. Clin Cardiol 23:205–210
87. Doutreleau S et al (2005) Chronic but not acute oral L-arginine supplementation delays the ventilatory threshold during exercise in heart failure patients. Can J Appl Physiol Rev Can Physiol Appl 30:419–432
88. Bednarz B, Jaxa-Chamiec T, Gebalska J, Herbaczyńska-Cedro K, Ceremuzyński L (2004) L-arginine supplementation prolongs exercise capacity in congestive heart failure. Kardiol Pol 60:348–353
89. Watanabe G, Tomiyama H, Doba N (2000) Effects of oral administration of L-arginine on renal function in patients with heart failure. J Hypertens 18:229–234
90. Fontanive P et al (2009) Effects of L-arginine on the Minnesota Living with Heart Failure Questionnaire quality-of-life score in patients with chronic systolic heart failure. Med Sci Monit 15:CR606–CR611
91. Lonn E et al (2005) Effects of long-term vitamin E supplementation on cardiovascular events and cancer: a randomized controlled trial. JAMA 293:1338–1347
92. Chagan L, Ioselovich A, Asherova L, Cheng JWM (2002) Use of alternative pharmacotherapy in management of cardiovascular diseases. Am J Manag Care 8:270–285, quiz 286–288
93. Graham JD (1939) Crataegus oxyacantha in hypertension. Br Med J 2:951–953
94. Schüssler M, Hölzl J, Fricke U (1995) Myocardial effects of flavonoids from Crataegus species. Arzneimittelforschung 45:842–845
95. (2010) Crataegus oxyacantha (Hawthorn). Monograph. Altern Med Rev 15:164–167
96. Al Makdessi S, Sweidan H, Dietz K, Jacob R (1999) Protective effect of Crataegus oxyacantha against reperfusion arrhythmias after global no-flow ischemia in the rat heart. Basic Res Cardiol 94:71–77
97. Visioli F, Borsani L, Galli C (2000) Diet and prevention of coronary heart disease: the potential role of phytochemicals. Cardiovasc Res 47:419–425
98. Tongda X, Li D, Jiang D (2012) Targeting cell signaling and apoptotic pathways by luteolin: cardioprotective role in rat cardiomyocytes following ischemia/reperfusion. Nutrients 4:2008–2019
99. Mahmood ZA, Sualeh M, Mahmood SBZ, Karim MA (2010) Herbal treatment for cardiovascular disease the evidence based therapy. Pak J Pharm Sci 23:119–124
100. Firenzuoli F (2009) Fitoterapia. Elsevier, Guida all'uso clinico delle piante medicinali
101. Pratt C (2010) Alternative prevention and treatment of cardiovascular disease, part 2. Prim Care 37:339–366
102. Holubarsch CJ, Colucci WS, Meinertz T, Gaus W, Tendera M (2000) Survival and prognosis: investigation of Crataegus extract WS 1442 in congestive heart failure (SPICE)--rationale, study design and study protocol. Eur J Heart Fail 2:431–437
103. Holubarsch CJF, Colucci WS, Meinertz T, Gaus W, Tendera M (2008) The efficacy and safety of Crataegus extract WS 1442 in patients with heart failure: the SPICE trial. Eur J Heart Fail 10:1255–1263
104. Pittler MH, Guo R, Ernst E (2008) Hawthorn extract for treating chronic heart failure. Cochrane Database Syst Rev:CD005312
105. Daniele C, Mazzanti G, Pittler MH, Ernst E (2006) Adverse-event profile of Crataegus spp.: a systematic review. Drug Saf 29:523–535
106. Pittler MH, Schmidt K, Ernst E (2003) Hawthorn extract for treating chronic heart failure: meta-analysis of randomized trials. Am J Med 114:665–674
107. Schmidt U, Kuhn U, Ploch M, Hübner WD (1994) Efficacy of the Hawthorn (Crataegus) preparation LI 132 in 78 patients with chronic congestive heart failure defined as NYHA functional class II. Phytomedicine 1:17–24
108. Weikl A et al (1996) Crataegus Special Extract WS 1442. Assessment of objective effectiveness in patients with heart failure (NYHA II). Fortschr Med 114:291–296
109. Leuchtgens H (1993) Crataegus Special Extract WS 1442 in NYHA II heart failure. A placebo controlled randomized double-blind study. Fortschr Med 111:352–354
110. Tauchert M, Gildor A, Lipinski J (1999) High-dose Crataegus extract WS 1442 in the treatment of NYHA stage II heart failure. Herz 24:465–474, discussion 475
111. Degenring FH, Suter A, Weber M, Saller R (2003) A randomised double blind placebo controlled clinical trial of a standardised extract of fresh Crataegus berries (Crataegisan) in the treatment of patients with congestive heart failure NYHA II. Phytomedicine 10:363–369
112. Zick SM, Gillespie B, Aaronson KD (2008) The effect of Crataegus oxycantha Special Extract WS 1442 on clinical progression in patients with mild to moderate symptoms of heart failure. Eur J Heart Fail 10:587–593
113. Zick SM, Vautaw BM, Gillespie B, Aaronson KD (2009) Hawthorn Extract Randomized Blinded Chronic Heart Failure (HERB CHF) trial. Eur J Heart Fail 11:990–999
114. Furey A, Tassell M, Kingston R, Gilroy D, Lehane M (2010) Hawthorn (Crataegus spp.) in the treatment of cardiovascular disease. Pharmacogn Rev 4:32
115. Tankanow R et al (2003) Interaction study between digoxin and a preparation of hawthorn (Crataegus oxyacantha). J Clin Pharmacol 43:637–642

116. Bharani A, Ganguly A, Bhargava KD (1995) Salutary effect of Terminalia Arjuna in patients with severe refractory heart failure. Int J Cardiol 49:191–199
117. Middlekauff HR (2004) Acupuncture in the treatment of heart failure. Cardiol Rev 12:171–173
118. Middlekauff HR et al (2002) Acupuncture inhibits sympathetic activation during mental stress in advanced heart failure patients. J Card Fail 8:399–406
119. Kristen AV et al (2010) Acupuncture improves exercise tolerance of patients with heart failure: a placebo-controlled pilot study. Heart 96:1396–1400
120. Guck TP, Elsasser GN, Kavan MG, Barone EJ (2003) Depression and congestive heart failure. Congest Heart Fail 9:163–169
121. Watson K, Summers KM (2009) Depression in patients with heart failure: clinical implications and management. Pharmacotherapy 29:49–63
122. Ferketich AK, Ferguson JP, Binkley PF (2005) Depressive symptoms and inflammation among heart failure patients. Am Heart J 150:132–136
123. Jiang W et al (2000) Relationship of depression to increased risk of mortality and rehospitalization in patients with congestive heart failure. Arch Intern Med 161:1849–1856
124. Echols MR, Jiang W (2011) Clinical trial evidence for treatment of depression in heart failure. Heart Fail Clin 7:81–88
125. Luskin FM et al (1998) A review of mind-body therapies in the treatment of cardiovascular disease Part 1: Implications for the elderly. Altern Ther Health Med 4:46–61
126. Spence JD, Barnett PA, Linden W, Ramsden V, Taenzer P (1999) Lifestyle modifications to prevent and control hypertension. 7. Recommendations on stress management. Canadian Hypertension Society, Canadian Coalition for High Blood Pressure Prevention and Control, Laboratory Centre for Disease Control at Health Canada. CMAJ 160:S46–S50
127. Kulkarni S, O'Farrell I, Erasi M, Kochar MS (1998) Stress and hypertension. WMJ 97:34–38
128. Jain D et al (1998) Effects of mental stress on left ventricular and peripheral vascular performance in patients with coronary artery disease. J Am Coll Cardiol 31:1314–1322
129. Dembroski TM, MacDougall JM, Costa PT, Grandits GA (1989) Components of hostility as predictors of sudden death and myocardial infarction in the Multiple Risk Factor Intervention Trial. Psychosom Med 51:514–522
130. Gallacher JE, Yarnell JW, Sweetnam PM, Elwood PC, Stansfeld SA (1999) Anger and incident heart disease in the Caerphilly study. Psychosom Med 61:446–453
131. Seskevich J, Gabert H, Charles A, Cuffe MS (2005) Helping patients with heart failure manage stress. Nursing (Lond) 35(23)
132. Curiati JA et al (2005) Meditation reduces sympathetic activation and improves the quality of life in elderly patients with optimally treated heart failure: a prospective randomized study. J Altern Complement Med 11:465–472
133. Moser DK, Dracup K, Woo MA, Stevenson LW (1997) Voluntary control of vascular tone by using skin-temperature biofeedback-relaxation in patients with advanced heart failure. Altern Ther Health Med 3:51–59
134. Jayadevappa R et al (2007) Effectiveness of transcendental meditation on functional capacity and quality of life of African Americans with congestive heart failure: a randomized control study. Ethn Dis 17:72–77
135. Sullivan MJ et al (2009) The Support, Education, and Research in Chronic Heart Failure Study (SEARCH): A mindfulness-based psychoeducational intervention improves depression and clinical symptoms in patients with chronic heart failure. Am Heart J 157:84–90
136. Luskin F, Reitz M, Newell K, Quinn TG, Haskell W (2002) A controlled pilot study of stress management training of elderly patients with congestive heart failure. Prev Cardiol 5:168–172
137. Chang B-H et al (2005) A relaxation response randomized trial on patients with chronic heart failure. J Cardiopulm Rehabil 25:149–157
138. Chang B-H et al (2004) Relaxation response for Veterans Affairs patients with congestive heart failure: results from a qualitative study within a clinical trial. Prev Cardiol 7:64–70
139. Yeh GY et al (2004) Effects of tai chi mind-body movement therapy on functional status and exercise capacity in patients with chronic heart failure: a randomized controlled trial. Am J Med 117
140. Yeh GY, Wayne PM, Phillips RS (2008) T'ai Chi exercise in patients with chronic heart failure. Med Sport Sci 52:195–208
141. Shively M et al (2005) Effect of behavioral management on quality of life in mild heart failure: a randomized controlled trial. Patient Educ Couns 58:27–34
142. McMurray JJV et al (2012) ESC Guidelines for the diagnosis and treatment of acute and chronic heart failure 2012: The Task Force for the Diagnosis and Treatment of Acute and Chronic Heart Failure 2012 of the European Society of Cardiology Developed in collaboration with the Heart. Eur Heart J 33:1787–1847
143. Tarzia V et al (2014) Surgical implantation of the CardioWest Total Artificial Heart. Ann Cardiothorac Surg 3:624–625
144. Tarzia V et al (2014) Jarvik 2000: evolution of surgical implantation from conventional to minimally invasive technique. Ann Cardiothorac Surg 3:621–623
145. Jackevicius CA et al (2009) High-impact articles related to the management of heart failure: 2008 update. Pharmacotherapy 29:82–120
146. Tang WHW, Francis GS (2010) The year in heart failure. J Am Coll Cardiol 55:688–696

Integrated Approach to Arrhythmias 18

Carlo Dal Lin, Marco Silvestro, Raffaele Migliorini, Francesco Tona, and Massimo Fioranelli

18.1 Introduction

A crucial prerequisite for an effective treatment of arrhythmias and cardiac conduction disturbances is the accurate identification of the specific rhythm disorder, with the identification of the clinical picture associated with it and the definition of precise, safe, and effective therapeutic targets [1].

The clinical pictures fall into two broad categories: those that cause acute and transient electrophysiological abnormalities and those that, being chronic, provide the substrate for persistent or recurrent arrhythmias. In the first case, we find acute myocardial ischemia and the early stages of infarction, electrolyte disturbances, and the pro-arrhythmic action of certain drugs.

The second category includes chronic ischemic heart disease, cardiomyopathies, and the anatomical substrates for supraventricular arrhythmias.

Cardiac rhythm disorders may be aggravated by hemodynamic, electrolyte, and metabolic changes and respiratory diseases that must be corrected to obtain an effective therapeutic response. The therapeutic strategy depends on the presence and the characteristics of the symptoms and the potential morbidity and mortality. Some arrhythmias can be very annoying to patients, but they do not affect the long-term prognosis, whereas others with mild symptoms or those who are completely asymptomatic are burdened with a poor prognosis.

The standard 12-lead electrocardiogram and extended recording are the most readily available tools for diagnosis. In some cases, to achieve the diagnosis, it may be necessary to resort to vagal maneuvers or the administration of certain drugs (adenosine, verapamil). Recording devices activated by the patient can be used in the case of arrhythmias that occur infrequently; implantable recorders are useful if long periods of monitoring are required. The exercise test is useful to frame the arrhythmias induced by physical stress (especially ventricular premature beats and ventricular tachycardia), for the diagnosis of ischemic heart disease, to assess a dysfunction of the sinus node or the atrioventricular node, to evaluate the pro-arrhythmic effects of certain medications, or to assess the accessory pathway's refractory period in Wolff–Parkinson–White syndrome. In Tables 18.1 and 18.2 some practical information is reported to frame the symptoms and stratify the risk for patients with arrhythmia and possible criteria for a specialist assessment of the patient.

When a surface electrocardiogram is not sufficient, invasive studies can be useful: electrophysiological intracavitary study allows accurate

C. Dal Lin, M.D. (✉) • M. Silvestro, N.D. • R. Migliorini, M.D. • F. Tona, M.D., Ph.D.
Department of Cardiological, Thoracic and Vascular Sciences, Padua University Medical School, Padova, Italy
e-mail: carlodallin@libero.it

M. Fioranelli, M.D.
Department of Nuclear Physics, Sub-Nuclear and Radiation, Guglielmo Marconi University, Rome, Italy

M. Fioranelli (ed.), *Integrative Cardiology*, DOI 10.1007/978-3-319-40010-5_18

Table 18.1 Historical features of importance in the evaluation of the patient

1. Which arrhythmia is present?
2. Does the arrhythmia cause symptoms?
3. Does the arrhythmia have prognostic significance?
4. Is the problem life-threatening?
5. Does the patient require hospital admission or extensive testing?
6. Is specialist consultation required, and, if so, how urgently?
7. Is treatment required?

Source: modified from Rakel [3]

Table 18.2 Reasons for referral to a specialist

• Resuscitated ventricular fibrillation
• Sustained ventricular tachycardia
• Atrial fibrillation that is difficult to control or refractory to standard therapies
• Nonsustained ventricular tachycardia
• Symptomatic supraventricular tachycardia that is difficult to control
• Sinus bradycardia (sick sinus syndrome, tachy-brady syndrome)
• Second-degree atrioventricular block
• Unexplained ventricular ectopy in an athlete or in a symptomatic patient
• Syncope with a suspected arrhythmic mechanism
• Patients with devices (pacemakers, implantable defibrillators) who are unstable
• Uncontrolled rhythm problems

Source: Modified from Rakel [3]

mapping of arrhythmias and of therapeutic maneuvers of ablation. Defibrillators and pacemakers have the ability to record arrhythmic events that can then be analyzed by a doctor.

The treatment of arrhythmias has become very complex and ranges from the use of some simple principles of lifestyle to specialist drug therapies and invasive catheter-based or surgical procedures. A detailed description of specific treatments for these conditions is not within the scope of this chapter. According to Graboys (cited in Devries and Dalen [2]), key concepts to keep in mind in arrhythmia management are the following: "try simple measures first before considering drug therapy. Be the patient's advocate. Minimize tests, especially invasive tests in the elderly. Maintain a sense of humor and optimism." Let us focus on some concepts that underlie an integrative approach to patients with arrhythmias (Fig. 18.1).

18.2 Lifestyle

Lifestyle is of paramount importance in the case of arrhythmias [4–6]. Cigarette smoking and other forms of nicotine are harmful and exacerbate the risk of sudden death and arrhythmias of all types [5, 7]. Moreover, the combination of alcohol and nicotine intake tends to trigger arrhythmias [3].

18.3 Diet

Arrhythmias could develop from changes in diet or from comorbid eating disorders. Gastric distension following a large meal can trigger a vagally mediated atrial fibrillation, hypotension, and bradycardia [1]. Excessive caffeine, theophylline, and theobromine present in coffee, tea, and chocolate may cause ectopic beats [8–13]; alcohol may determine atrial fibrillation and ventricular ectopy [14–17], high levels of sodium (strengthens the effects of catecholamines favoring ventricular ectopy [18–23]), trans-fats (contained in doughnuts, fried foods, and artificial cheese such as in processed pizza) [24, 25], and severe fluctuations in blood sugar levels; food allergies [26] are also potential dietary triggers of cardiac arrhythmias.

Omega-3 fatty acids, albeit without proven anti-arrhythmic effects [27], improve outcomes [28, 29], especially in combination with a low dose of alcohol consumption [30–32].

Active ingredients found in some plants, such as *ephedra*, *ambrotose*, or *ginkgo*, can even cause lethal arrhythmias [3, 33, 34].

Diet is an important factor to be considered in patients receiving warfarin to optimize the values of the International Normalized Ratio, as there are many drug, food, and herbal interactions to control.

Finally, many arrhythmias are caused by dehydration [1]. Thus, the patient's hydration status should be checked, as many people (and

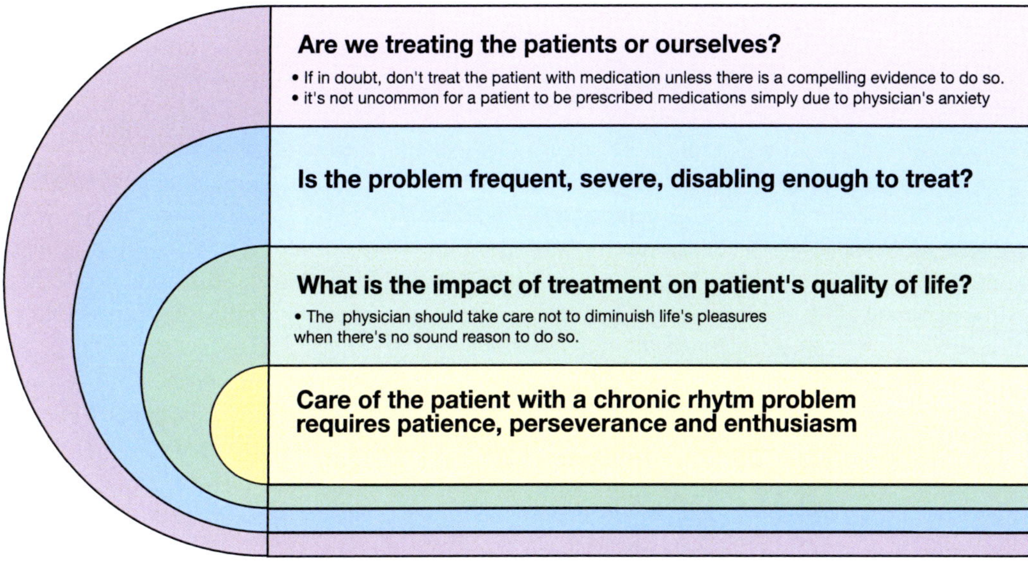

Fig. 18.1 Principles to guide treatment according to Graboys and Lown [116]. Modified from Devries and Dalen [2]

especially those with a heart disease or taking diuretics) are chronically dehydrated.

18.4 Supplements

Supplementation with *coenzyme Q10* (100–300 = m/day) determines a reduction of ventricular and atrial extrasystoles and atrial fibrillation paroxysms [35].

L-carnitine (3 g/day), improving energy processes in mitochondria and thus the myocardial performance, may be useful in preventing some atrial and ventricular arrhythmias; the precise mechanisms by which this occurs have not yet been well clarified [36–39].

Supplementation of *calcium* and *magnesium* has an anti-arrhythmic effect: in fact, the magnesium, in addition to slowing the atrioventricular conduction, acts as a "membrane stabilizer," decreasing the arrhythmic mechanism of "triggered activity" and the number of arrhythmic episodes related to it [23], and decreasing the risk for sudden death [40]. Data concerning magnesium and atrial fibrillation are conflicting [41, 42].

A key electrolyte in arrhythmic processes is *potassium* and its values must be kept at adequate and physiological levels for both preventive and therapeutic goals [1]. Particular attention should be paid to patients with a possible physiological and anatomical substrate for arrhythmias (such as ischemic heart disease or long QT syndrome) and those who take medications that could lead to a potassium deficiency (such as diuretics) [1].

Although high *copper* values are associated with worsening atherosclerosis, its supplementation (4 mg/day) could decrease ventricular extrasystoles [21]. Excess *zinc* determines copper deficiency and worsens arrhythmic activity, in addition to a *selenium* deficiency. In the latter case, there is no evidence for selenium supplementation with an anti-arrhythmic result [18, 43].

Omega-3 fatty acids have an anti-arrhythmic effect [44–48] (especially on premature ventricular beats [49, 50]), because they affect the activities of calcium and potassium ion channels [51]. This effect improves outcomes [52–54] in patients with heart disease (especially higher risk patients [55]), decreases the risk of sudden death in the case of ischemic heart disease [51, 56], and tends to reduce defibrillator shocks in patients with implantable cardioverter defibrillators (ICDs) [57]. Administration of omega-3 may be useful [58] in the case of atrial fibrillation [59–63] (especially after cardiac surgery, albeit with some conflicting evidence [64, 65]) and in the treatment of depression [66, 67], which is an important prognostic factor in cases of heart attack and a trigger for arrhythmias [68–70]. Omega-3 fatty acids are available in various forms, not only fish oil [71]. Some studies related to the use of omega-3 have failed to demonstrate an effect, probably because patients were already receiving optimal drug therapy [72].

We must pay close attention to certain toxins present in some supplements such as dioxins, polychlorinated biphenyls, polybrominated diphenyl ethers, and chlorinated pesticides [73].

An anti-arrhythmic effect of *vitamin D* has been described in sick sinus syndrome [74] and a favorable action of *vitamin C* in the treatment of atrial fibrillation [75–79], probably through its anti-oxidant and anti-inflammatory effects.

18.5 Exercise

Regular aerobic exercise with moderate effort is good for the cardiovascular system and this also applies to the treatment of rhythm disorders [1]. Indeed, exercise increases vagal tone and decreases the circulating levels of catecholamines and sensitivity to their effect. Attention should be paid to patients with malignant arrhythmias that could be aggravated by exercise. These patients should be monitored by specialists.

18.6 Mind–Body Therapy and Acupuncture

As William Harvey wrote in 1628 [80]: "every affection of the mind that is attended with either pain or pleasure, hope or fear, is the cause of an agitation whose influence extends to the heart". Perceived stress is a key factor in triggering the cascade of psycho-neuro-endocrine immunitary sequelae that can cause several adverse cardiovascular events, including some rhythm disorders [68–70].

As suggested by Graboys [81]: "I frequently ask the patient precisely when his or her symptoms began which may allow us to identify a 'trigger' which defines and unlocks the problem without the use of medications."

Mind–body techniques, and in particular, the practice of yoga and meditation, play a well-positioned role in the treatment of arrhythmias [82–84], as they are able to favorably alter the autonomic function of the practitioners [85], reducing the risk of ventricular fibrillation in high-risk patients or the number of arrhythmias in ICD carriers [84, 86–89]. The practice of yoga is very useful in the treatment of atrial fibrillation (especially if paroxysmal), as it reduces the paroxysms considerably [84, 90].

Even biofeedback [91–95] and psychosocial therapy [96] appear to reduce the number, frequency, and severity of palpitations related to arrhythmias, increase the heart rate variability, and decrease the risk of arrhythmic death.

Acupuncture can be considered a therapeutic option in patients with atrial fibrillation [97, 98], but it should for now be avoided in patients with a defibrillator, as it could trigger inappropriate shocks of the device [99].

18.7 Phytomedicine: A Perspective Solution for Arrhythmias

Many of the anti-arrhythmic drugs commonly in use are derived from plants. To cite a few examples: quinidine from cinchona bark; lidocaine, amiodarone from khellin present in *Ammi visnaga*, or digoxin from foxglove [100].

In nature, there are other phytoelements with anti-arrhythmic properties.

Ciwujia or Siberian ginseng (*Acanthopanax senticosus* Harms) extract reduces malignant arrhythmias (ventricular tachycardia and fibrillation) [101, 102].

Angelica and *Ginkgo biloba* may protect against arrhythmias occurring during myocardial ischemia and reperfusion [103, 104]. Licorice root has an anti-arrhythmic effect [105, 106].

Traditionally, motherwort (4–5 g/day) is useful for treating palpitations, because its principles (bufenolide, glycosides (stachydrine), and alkaloids) have a mild beta-blocking effect [3]. However, no randomized controlled trials have been performed using motherwort.

Khella (*Ammi visnaga*), in addition to having anti-angina properties, has significant anti-arrhythmic effects, as it is the original substance from which a very potent anti-arrhythmic drug, amiodarone, was derived [107–109].

Hyperoside (vitexin, rhamnose), rutin, and oligomeric procyanidins contained in hawthorn berries (160–900 mg in water–ethanol extract) can be used to treat atrial fibrillation [102], reducing the risk for sudden death, and helps to treat patients with heart failure [110].

Rhodiola produces some anti-arrhythmic effects [111], as it is able to increase the ventricular fibrillation threshold through the stimulation of kappa-opioid receptors [3] and by affecting intracellular calcium signaling [112].

The possibility of refractory ventricular tachycardia in the case of herbal aconite tea poisoning should be considered [113].

In the treatment of palpitations, herbs with a sedative effect can be useful (30 drops, 2–3 times daily, aqueous mixture of fluid extracts of *Crataegus oxyacantha*, *Passiflora incarnata* 25 mL in equal parts; or one tablet, three times daily of a mixture of *Lavandula officinalis* 50 mg, *Valeriana officinalis* 200 mg; *Melissa officinalis* as a mother tincture 20–30 drops 2–4 times a day, in the case of hyperthyroidism) [114].

Ethanol extracts of the plant *Sophora flavescens Ait.* reduce cardiac arrhythmias (ventricular tachycardia) induced by coronary artery ligation in rats, and by aconitine infusion in mice, suggesting their potential clinical use for anti-arrhythmic treatment [115].

Many other plants (garlic, agrimony, celery, ginger, berberine, corkwort, *Stephania tetrandra* root, astragalus, *Fissistigma glaucescens,* Xin Bao, Bu Xin, Yu Zhu, and Mai Dong), particularly used in the context of traditional Chinese medicine, possess anti-arrhythmic and cardioprotective activity, but there is a lack of scientific evidence for the reproducibility of their effects and their precise dosage to describe a potential use in the Western medical system.

Traditionally, the mild form of brady-arrhythmias can benefit from the use of coffee or dry extract of guarana (10% caffeine) 500 mg/tablets, 1–2 capsules before breakfast and lunch [116].

At the present time, however, the data are not definitive enough to recommend treatment with any of these herbal therapies for a specific form of arrhythmia.

18.8 Tricks of the Trade

Currently, natural remedies are effective in the management of palpitations related to stress and anxiety. In this scenario, it may be useful to resort to *linden, valerian*, or *passionflower*. It is possible to use the dietary supplement *potassium-magnesium-bromelain* mentioned in Chap. 17.

References

1. Camm AJ, Luscher TF, Serruys PW (2009) ESC textbook of cardiovascular medicine, 2nd edn. Oxford University Press, Oxford
2. Devries S, Dalen J (2011) Integrative cardiology. Oxford University Press, Oxford
3. Rakel D (2012) Integrative medicine, 3rd edn. Elsevier, Amsterdam
4. Løchen ML (1991) The Tromsø Study: associations between self-reported arrhythmia, psychological conditions, and lifestyle. Scand J Prim Health Care 9:265–270
5. Hinkle LE, Thaler HT, Merke DP, Renier-Berg D, Morton NE (1988) The risk factors for arrhythmic death in a sample of men followed for 20 years. Am J Epidemiol 127:500–515
6. Albert CM et al (1999) Moderate alcohol consumption and the risk of sudden cardiac death among US male physicians. Circulation 100:944–950
7. McCarty MF (1996) Fish oil may be an antidote for the cardiovascular risk of smoking. Med Hypotheses 46:337–347
8. Mehta A, Jain AC, Mehta MC, Billie M (1997) Caffeine and cardiac arrhythmias. An experimental study in dogs with review of literature. Acta Cardiol 52:273–283
9. Chou T (1992) Wake up and smell the coffee. Caffeine, coffee, and the medical consequences. West J Med 157:544–553

10. Myers MG, Harris L (1990) High dose caffeine and ventricular arrhythmias. Can J Cardiol 6:95–98
11. Mukamal KJ, Alert M, Maclure M, Muller JE, Mittleman MA (2006) Tea consumption and infarct-related ventricular arrhythmias: the determinants of myocardial infarction onset study. J Am Coll Nutr 25:472–479
12. Mattioli AV, Bonatti S, Zennaro M, Melotti R, Mattioli G (2008) Effect of coffee consumption, lifestyle and acute life stress in the development of acute lone atrial fibrillation. J Cardiovasc Med (Hagerstown) 9:794–798
13. Conen D et al (2010) Caffeine consumption and incident atrial fibrillation in women. Am J Clin Nutr 92:509–514
14. Dobmeyer DJ, Stine RA, Leier CV, Greenberg R, Schaal SF (1983) The arrhythmogenic effects of caffeine in human beings. N Engl J Med 308:814–816
15. Donnerstein RL, Zhu D, Samson R, Bender AM, Goldberg SJ (1998) Acute effects of caffeine ingestion on signal-averaged electrocardiograms. Am Heart J 136:643–646
16. Koskinen P, Kupari M, Leinonen H (1990) Role of alcohol in recurrences of atrial fibrillation in persons less than 65 years of age. Am J Cardiol 66:954–958
17. Rigou DG, Pichel G, Fasah L (1990) Ventricular arrhythmia in young university students without evidence of heart disease. Medicina (B Aires) 50:47–51
18. Lehr D (1994) A possible beneficial effect of selenium administration in antiarrhythmic therapy. J Am Coll Nutr 13:496–498
19. Lumme JA, Jounela AJ (1989) The effect of potassium and potassium plus magnesium supplementation on ventricular extrasystoles in mild hypertensives treated with hydrochlorothiazide. Int J Cardiol 25:93–97
20. Tsuji H, Venditti FJ, Evans JC, Larson MG, Levy D (1994) The associations of levels of serum potassium and magnesium with ventricular premature complexes (the Framingham Heart Study). Am J Cardiol 74:232–235
21. Spencer JC (1979) Direct relationship between the body's copper/zinc ratio, ventricular premature beats, and sudden coronary death. Am J Clin Nutr 32:1184–1185
22. Hardarson T, Kristinsson A, Skúladóttir G, Asvaldsdóttir H, Snorrason SP (1989) Cod liver oil does not reduce ventricular extrasystoles after myocardial infarction. J Intern Med 226:33–37
23. Bashir Y et al (1993) Effects of long-term oral magnesium chloride replacement in congestive heart failure secondary to coronary artery disease. Am J Cardiol 72:1156–1162
24. Lemaitre RN et al (2002) Cell membrane trans-fatty acids and the risk of primary cardiac arrest. Circulation 105:697–701
25. Zaloga GP, Harvey KA, Stillwell W, Siddiqui R (2006) Trans fatty acids and coronary heart disease. Nutr Clin Pract 21:505–512
26. De Luca L, Cinque C, Chiummariello S, Berni Canani R (1990) Cardiac involvement in food allergy. Study of cardiac activity by Holter monitoring in 12 allergic children during food challenge. Pediatr Med Chir 12:139–145
27. Leaf A, Xiao YF, Kang JX, Billman GE (2003) Prevention of sudden cardiac death by n-3 polyunsaturated fatty acids. Pharmacol Ther 98:355–377
28. Siddiqui RA, Harvey KA, Ruzmetov N, Miller SJ, Zaloga GP (2009) n-3 fatty acids prevent whereas trans-fatty acids induce vascular inflammation and sudden cardiac death. Br J Nutr 102:1811–1819
29. Yamagishi K et al (2008) Fish, omega-3 polyunsaturated fatty acids, and mortality from cardiovascular diseases in a nationwide community-based cohort of Japanese men and women the JACC (Japan Collaborative Cohort Study for Evaluation of Cancer Risk) Study. J Am Coll Cardiol 52:988–996
30. Renaud S, Lanzmann-Petithory D (2002) Dietary fats and coronary heart disease pathogenesis. Curr Atheroscler Rep 4:419–424
31. Di Giuseppe R et al (2009) Alcohol consumption and n-3 polyunsaturated fatty acids in healthy men and women from 3 European populations. Am J Clin Nutr 89:354–362
32. De Leiris J, Besse S, Boucher F (2010) Diet and heart health: moderate wine drinking strengthens the cardioprotective effects of fish consumption. Curr Pharm Biotechnol 11:911–921
33. Nazeri A et al (2009) Arrhythmogenicity of weight-loss supplements marketed on the Internet. Heart Rhythm 6:658–662
34. Haller CA, Benowitz NL (2000) Adverse cardiovascular and central nervous system events associated with dietary supplements containing ephedra alkaloids. N Engl J Med 343:1833–1838
35. Langsjoen PH, Langsjoen AM (1999) Overview of the use of CoQ10 in cardiovascular disease. Biofactors 9:273–284
36. Lango R, Smolenski RT, Narkiewicz M, Suchorzewska J, Lysiak-Szydlowska W (2001) Influence of L-carnitine and its derivatives on myocardial metabolism and function in ischemic heart disease and during cardiopulmonary bypass. Cardiovasc Res 51:21–29
37. Arsenian MA (1997) Carnitine and its derivatives in cardiovascular disease. Prog Cardiovasc Dis 40:265–286
38. Mondillo S et al (1995) Therapy of arrhythmia induced by myocardial ischemia. Association of L-carnitine, propafenone and mexiletine. Clin Ter 146:769–774
39. Najafi M, Garjani A, Maleki N, Eteraf Oskouei T (2008) Antiarrhythmic and arrhythmogenic effects of L-carnitine in ischemia and reperfusion. Bull Exp Biol Med 146:210–213
40. Chiuve SE, Korngold EC, Januzzi JL, Lou GM, Albert CM (2011) Plasma and dietary magnesium and risk of sudden cardiac death in women. Am J Clin Nutr 93:253–260

41. Onalan O et al (2007) Meta-analysis of magnesium therapy for the acute management of rapid atrial fibrillation. Am J Cardiol 99:1726–1732
42. Chu K, Evans R, Emerson G, Greenslade J, Brown A (2009) Magnesium sulfate versus placebo for paroxysmal atrial fibrillation: a randomized clinical trial. Acad Emerg Med 16:295–300
43. Godwin KO (1965) Abnormal electrocardiograms in rats fed a low selenium diet. Q J Exp Physiol Cogn Med Sci 50:282–288
44. Billman GE, Hallaq H, Leaf A (1994) Prevention of ischemia-induced ventricular fibrillation by omega 3 fatty acids. Proc Natl Acad Sci U S A 91:4427–4430
45. Xiao YF, Kang JX, Morgan JP, Leaf A (1995) Blocking effects of polyunsaturated fatty acids on Na^+ channels of neonatal rat ventricular myocytes. Proc Natl Acad Sci U S A 92:11000–11004
46. Kang JX, Leaf A (1995) Prevention and termination of beta-adrenergic agonist-induced arrhythmias by free polyunsaturated fatty acids in neonatal rat cardiac myocytes. Biochem Biophys Res Commun 208:629–636
47. Leaf A (1995) Omega-3 fatty acids and prevention of ventricular fibrillation. Prostaglandins Leukot Essent Fatty Acids 52:197–198
48. Hallaq H, Sellmayer A, Smith TW, Leaf A (1990) Protective effect of eicosapentaenoic acid on ouabain toxicity in neonatal rat cardiac myocytes. Proc Natl Acad Sci U S A 87:7834–7838
49. Sellmayer A, Witzgall H, Lorenz RL, Weber PC (1995) Effects of dietary fish oil on ventricular premature complexes. Am J Cardiol 76:974–977
50. Geelen A et al (2005) Effects of n-3 fatty acids from fish on premature ventricular complexes and heart rate in humans. Am J Clin Nutr 81:416–420
51. Hallaq H, Smith TW, Leaf A (1992) Modulation of dihydropyridine-sensitive calcium channels in heart cells by fish oil fatty acids. Proc Natl Acad Sci U S A 89:1760–1764
52. Chung MK (2004) Vitamins, supplements, herbal medicines, and arrhythmias. Cardiol Rev 12:73–84
53. Holub DJ, Holub BJ (2004) Omega-3 fatty acids from fish oils and cardiovascular disease. Mol Cell Biochem 263:217–225
54. Mozaffarian D (2008) Fish and n-3 fatty acids for the prevention of fatal coronary heart disease and sudden cardiac death. Am J Clin Nutr 87:1991S–1996S
55. Marik PE, Varon J (2009) Omega-3 dietary supplements and the risk of cardiovascular events: a systematic review. Clin Cardiol 32:365–372
56. Burr ML et al (1989) Effects of changes in fat, fish, and fibre intakes on death and myocardial reinfarction: diet and reinfarction trial (DART). Lancet 2:757–761
57. Raitt MH et al (2005) Fish oil supplementation and risk of ventricular tachycardia and ventricular fibrillation in patients with implantable defibrillators: a randomized controlled trial. JAMA 293:2884–2891
58. Kowey PR, Reiffel JA, Ellenbogen KA, Naccarelli GV, Pratt CM (2010) Efficacy and safety of prescription omega-3 fatty acids for the prevention of recurrent symptomatic atrial fibrillation. JAMA 304:2363
59. Christensen JH (2003) n-3 fatty acids and the risk of sudden cardiac death. Emphasis on heart rate variability. Dan Med Bull 50:347–367
60. Monahan KD, Wilson TE, Ray CA (2004) Omega-3 fatty acid supplementation augments sympathetic nerve activity responses to physiological stressors in humans. Hypertension 44:732–738
61. Holguin F et al (2005) Cardiac autonomic changes associated with fish oil vs soy oil supplementation in the elderly. Chest 127:1102–1107
62. Mozaffarian D (2004) Fish intake and risk of incident atrial fibrillation. Circulation 110:368–373
63. Sarrazin J-F et al (2007) Reduced incidence of vagally induced atrial fibrillation and expression levels of connexins by n-3 polyunsaturated fatty acids in dogs. J Am Coll Cardiol 50:1505–1512
64. Calò L et al (2005) N-3 Fatty acids for the prevention of atrial fibrillation after coronary artery bypass surgery: a randomized, controlled trial. J Am Coll Cardiol 45:1723–1728
65. Saravanan P et al (2010) Omega-3 fatty acid supplementation does not reduce risk of atrial fibrillation after coronary artery bypass surgery: a randomized, double-blind, placebo-controlled clinical trial. Circ Arrhythm Electrophysiol 3:46–53
66. Mozaffarian D (2005) Interplay between different polyunsaturated fatty acids and risk of coronary heart disease in men. Circulation 111:157–164
67. Ander BP et al (2004) Dietary flaxseed protects against ventricular fibrillation induced by ischemia-reperfusion in normal and hypercholesterolemic Rabbits. J Nutr 134:3250–3256
68. Dal Lin C et al (2015) Coronary microvascular and endothelial function regulation: crossroads of psychoneuroendocrine immunitary signals and quantum physics [Part A]. J Integr Cardiol 1:132–163
69. Dal Lin C et al (2015) Coronary microvascular and endothelial function regulation: crossroads of psychoneuroendocrine immunitary signals and quantum physics [Part B]. J Integr Cardiol 1:164–188
70. Dal Lin C et al (2015) Coronary microvascular and endothelial function regulation: crossroads of psychoneuroendocrine immunitary signals and quantum physics [Part C]. J Integr Cardiol 1:189–209
71. Platt R (2000) Current concepts in optimum nutrition for cardiovascular disease. Prev Cardiol 3:83–87
72. Rauch B et al (2010) OMEGA, a randomized, placebo-controlled trial to test the effect of highly purified omega-3 fatty acids on top of modern guideline-adjusted therapy after myocardial infarction. Circulation 122:2152–2159

73. Bushkin-Bedient S, Carpenter DO (2010) Benefits versus risks associated with consumption of fish and other seafood. Rev Environ Health 25:161–191
74. Kessel L (1990) Sick sinus syndrome cured by vitamin D? Geriatrics 45:83–85
75. Carnes CA et al (2001) Ascorbate attenuates atrial pacing-induced peroxynitrite formation and electrical remodeling and decreases the incidence of postoperative atrial fibrillation. Circ Res 89:E32–E38
76. Korantzopoulos P et al (2005) Oral vitamin C administration reduces early recurrence rates after electrical cardioversion of persistent atrial fibrillation and attenuates associated inflammation. Int J Cardiol 102:321–326
77. Eslami M et al (2007) Oral ascorbic acid in combination with beta-blockers is more effective than beta-blockers alone in the prevention of atrial fibrillation after coronary artery bypass grafting. Tex Heart Inst J 34:268–274
78. Papoulidis P et al (2011) The role of ascorbic acid in the prevention of atrial fibrillation after elective on-pump myocardial revascularization surgery: a single-center experience—a pilot study. Interact Cardiovasc Thorac Surg 12:121–124
79. Rodrigo R et al (2010) Use of vitamins C and E as a prophylactic therapy to prevent postoperative atrial fibrillation. Int J Cardiol 138:221–228
80. Harvey W (2001) On the motion of the heart and blood in animals. Vol. 38 Part 3. The Harvard Classics. P.F. Collier Son, New York. 1909–1914; Bartleby.com. (1628)
81. Graboys TB (1984) Stress and the aching heart. N Engl J Med 311:594–595
82. Alexander CN, Robinson P, Orme-Johnson DW, Schneider RH, Walton KG (1994) The effects of transcendental meditation compared to other methods of relaxation and meditation in reducing risk factors, morbidity, and mortality. Homeost Heal Dis 35:243–263
83. Zamarra JW, Schneider RH, Besseghini I, Robinson DK, Salerno JW (1996) Usefulness of the transcendental meditation program in the treatment of patients with coronary artery disease. Am J Cardiol 77:867–870
84. Kanmanthareddy A et al (2015) Alternative medicine in atrial fibrillation treatment-Yoga, acupuncture, biofeedback and more. J Thorac Dis 7:185–192
85. Cysarz D, Büssing A (2005) Cardiorespiratory synchronization during Zen meditation. Eur J Appl Physiol 95:88–95
86. Olex S, Newberg A, Figueredo VM (2013) Meditation: should a cardiologist care? Int J Cardiol 168:1805–1810
87. Barnes VA, Kapuku GK, Treiber FA (2012) Impact of transcendental meditation on left ventricular mass in African American adolescents. Evid Based Complement Alternat Med 2012(923153)
88. Walton KG, Schneider RH, Nidich S (2004) Review of controlled research on the transcendental meditation program and cardiovascular disease. Risk factors, morbidity, and mortality. Cardiol Rev 12:262–266
89. Ospina MB et al (2007) Meditation practices for health: state of the research. Evid Rep Technol Assess 155:1–263
90. Lakkireddy D et al (2013) Effect of yoga on arrhythmia burden, anxiety, depression, and quality of life in paroxysmal atrial fibrillation: The YOGA my heart study. J Am Coll Cardiol 61:1177–1182
91. Weiss T (1977) Biofeedback training for cardiovascular dysfunctions. Med Clin North Am 61:913–928
92. Johnston D (1978) Clinical applications of biofeedback. Br J Hosp Med 20:561–566
93. Silver BV, Blanchard EB (1978) Biofeedback and relaxation training in the treatment of psychophysiological disorders: or are the machines really necessary? J Behav Med 1:217–239
94. Janssen K (1983) Treatment of sinus tachycardia with heart-rate feedback. J Behav Med 6:109–114
95. Vaitl D (1984) 'One need not be a fakir or guru.' Biofeedback as an interdisciplinary research technic. Fortschr Med 102:541–544
96. Cowan MJ, Pike KC, Budzynski HK (2001) Psychosocial nursing therapy following sudden cardiac arrest: impact on two-year survival. Nurs Res 50:68–76
97. Lomuscio A, Belletti S, Battezzati PM, Lombardi F (2011) Efficacy of acupuncture in preventing atrial fibrillation recurrences after electrical cardioversion. J Cardiovasc Electrophysiol 22:241–247
98. VanWormer AM, Lindquist R, Sendelbach SE (2008) The effects of acupuncture on cardiac arrhythmias: a literature review. Hear Lung J Acute Crit Care 37:425–431
99. Lau E, Birnie D, Lemery R, Tang A, Green M (2005) Acupuncture triggering inappropriate ICD shocks. Europace 7:85–86
100. Benson H, McCallie DP (1979) Angina pectoris and the placebo effect. N Engl J Med 300:1424–1429
101. Tian BJ, Gao TL, Song ZL (1989) Effects of ciwujia (Acanthopanax senticosus Harms) on reperfusion-induced arrhythmia and action potential alterations in the isolated rat heart. Zhongguo Zhong Yao Za Zhi 14:493–512
102. Miller LG (1998) Herbal medicinals: selected clinical considerations focusing on known or potential drug-herb interactions. Arch Intern Med 158:2200–2211
103. Shen J et al (1998) Effects of EGb 761 on nitric oxide and oxygen free radicals, myocardial damage and arrhythmia in ischemia-reperfusion injury in vivo. Biochim Biophys Acta 1406:228–236
104. Zhuang XX (1991) Protective effect of Angelica injection on arrhythmia during myocardial ischemia reperfusion in rat. Zhong Xi Yi Jie He Za Zhi 11:360–361
105. Chen R, Yuan C (1991) Experimental anti-arrhythmic effects of zhigancao (prepared licorice) injection. Zhongguo Zhong Yao Za Zhi 16:617–619

106. Klepser TB, Klepser ME (1999) Unsafe and potentially safe herbal therapies. Am J Health Syst Pharm 56:125–138; quiz 139–41
107. Rauwald HW, Brehm O, Odenthal KP (1994) The involvement of a $Ca^{2þ}$ channel blocking mode of action in the pharmacology of Ammi visnaga fruits. Planta Med 60:101–105
108. Balbaa SI, Zaki AY, Abdel-Wahab SM (1968) A micro-method for the estimation of khellin in presence of other constituents of Ammi visnaga fruits. Planta Med 16:329–334
109. Chen M, Stohs SJ, Staba EJ (1969) The biosynthesis of radioactive khellin and visnagin from C14-acetate by Ammi visnaga plants. Planta Med 17:319–327
110. Holubarsch CJF, Colucci WS, Meinertz T, Gaus W, Tendera M (2008) The efficacy and safety of Crataegus extract WS 1442 in patients with heart failure: the SPICE trial. Eur J Heart Fail 10:1255–1263
111. Maslov LN et al (2009) Antiarrhythmic activity of phytoadaptogens in short-term ischemia-reperfusion of the heart and postinfarction cardiosclerosis. Bull Exp Biol Med 147:331–334
112. Zhang D-L, Zhang Y-T, Yin J-J, Zhao B-L (2004) Oral administration of Crataegus flavonoids protects against ischemia/reperfusion brain damage in gerbils. J Neurochem 90:211–219
113. Lowe L, Matteucci MJ, Schneir AB (2005) Herbal aconite tea and refractory ventricular tachycardia. N Engl J Med 353:1532
114. Firenzuoli F (2009) Fitoterapia. Guida all'uso clinico delle piante medicinali. Elsevier, Milan
115. Dai S, Chan MY, Lee SS, Ogle CW (1986) The antiarrhythmic effects of Sophora flavescens Ait in rats and mice. Am J Chin Med 14:119–123
116. Graboys TB, Lown B (1983) Coffee, arrhythmias, and common sense. N Engl J Med 308:835–837

Integrated Approach to Oncological Supportive Medicine

19

Bruno Pironi, Massimo Bonucci, Maria Grazia Roccia, and Massimo Fioranelli

New anticancer therapies have led to a long life expectancy for many patients; however, treatment-related comorbidities have become an issue for long-term cancer survivors. Cardiac toxicity is one of the most feared side effects of anticancer agents; thus the gain in life expectancy due to anticancer therapy may be countered by increased mortality owing to cardiac problems.

The type and duration of cancer treatment still play an important role in determining cardiovascular (CV) injury or toxicity. CV toxicity can be caused by:

1. Direct injury to or death of cardiac myocytes
2. Stimulation of myocardial fibrosis
3. Provocation of stress-induced myocardial ischemia via endothelial dysfunction
4. Vascular injury
5. Myocardial and/or pericardial inflammation
6. Arrhythmogenic or conduction abnormalities
7. Autonomic dysfunction
8. Valvular disease
9. Exacerbation of known CV risk factors (e.g., hypertension, accelerated atherosclerosis, or Raynaud's syndrome) [1–3]

The most frequent clinical syndromes correlated with this effect are heart failure, pericarditis and myocarditis, arrhythmias, sudden death, cardiogenic shock, thrombosis, and myocardial ischemia (Table 19.1).

In addition to traditional cardiotoxic agents, such as anthracyclines or radiation-related heart disease, newer therapies including tyrosine kinase inhibitors [4–6] and even therapies that are not necessarily classified as "chemotherapy" may also promote CV disease or events. For example, the administration of hormone deprivation therapies, which have dramatically reduced cancer recurrence and improved survival in women with breast cancer and men with prostate cancer, is now increasingly associated with CV events [7, 8].

Obviously, a chemotherapeutic agent can induce CV toxicity through multiple mechanisms and change their effect in relation to the combination of the antiblastic therapy.

In Table 19.1 the CV effect of a single agent is described, and we analyze the most common clinical syndrome related to its CV toxicity (Table 19.2).

B. Pironi
MG Vannini hospital, Rome, Italy

M. Bonucci • M.G. Roccia
Guglielmo Marconi University, Rome, Italy

M. Fioranelli (✉)
Department of Nuclear Physics, Sub-Nuclear and Radiation, MG Vannini Hospital, Rome, Italy
e-mail: massimo.fioranelli@gmail.com

M. Fioranelli (ed.), *Integrative Cardiology*, DOI 10.1007/978-3-319-40010-5_19

Table 19.1 Cardiovascular effect of a single chemotherapeutic agent

Class	Examples	Cancers treated	Cardiotoxicity
Anthracyclines	Doxorubicin, epirubicin	Acute leukemia, Hodgkin's and non-Hodgkin's lymphoma, breast cancer	Acute: HF, arrhythmias, QT changes Chronic (dose-dependent): HF nonreversible
Alkylating agents	Cyclophosphamide	Blood, breast, endometrial, bladder cancer	Reversible HF, pericardial effusion, arrhythmias
Antimicrotubule agent	Paclitaxel, docetaxel	Breast and ovarian cancer, Kaposi's sarcoma, prostate and bladder cancer, gastric adenocarcinoma	Bradycardia, myocardial ischemia, syncope, LV dysfunction, ventricular arrhythmias
Antimetabolites	Cisplatin, 5-fluorouracil	Solid tumors (lung, colon, breast)	Myocardial ischemia, myocardial infarction, arrhythmias
Vinca alkaloids	Vincristine, vinblastine	Leukemia, lymphoma	Myocardial ischemia
Tyrosine kinase-inhibiting antibodies	Trastuzumab, bevacizumab, rituximab, alemtuzumab	Breast and lung cancer, metastatic colorectal cancer, lymphomas, leukemias, transplant rejection	Reversible LV dysfunction, venous thrombosis, systemic hypertension
Small-molecule tyrosine kinase inhibitors	Imatinib, sorafenib, lapatinib, sunitinib	Renal cell cancer, lung and pancreatic cancer, leukemia	LV dysfunction, myocardial infarction, pericardial effusion, HF
Others	Tamoxifen, arsenic trioxide, retinoic acid, thalidomide	Breast cancer, multiple myeloma, melanoma, metastatic renal cell carcinoma	Deep-vein thrombosis, pulmonary embolism, stroke, myocarditis

HF heart failure, *LV* left ventricular

Table 19.2 Common clinical syndromes related to chemotherapeutic agents

Drugs associated with CHF	Anthracycline Cyclophosphamide Tyrosine kinase-inhibiting antibodies
Drugs associated with ischemia or thromboembolism	Antimetabolites Antimicrotubule agent Cisplatin Thalidomide
Drugs associated with hypertension	Bevacizumab Cisplatin Sorafenib
Hemorrhagic myocarditis (rare)	Cyclophosphamide
Bradyarrhythmias	Paclitaxel
Raynaud's phenomenon	Vinblastine
QT prolongation	Arsenic trioxide
Pulmonary fibrosis	Methotrexate

19.1 Congestive Heart Failure

For Left ventricular dysfunction means a global decrease in LVEF or more severe in the septum; symptoms of congestive heart failure (CHF) include decline of the left ventricular ejection fraction (LVEF) at least 5% to less than 55% with signs or symptoms of CHF, or at least 10 to 55% without signs or symptoms [9, 10]. The most common form of cardiotoxicity is anthracycline-related CHF.

19.1.1 Anthracycline Cardiotoxicity

Doxorubicin cardiotoxicity varies from 4 to 36% depending on the dose; epirubicin and idarubicin have a lower incidence of CHF.

Free radical formation is generally accepted as the main mechanism; apoptosis also plays a prominent role in the myocardial cell loss that has been demonstrated in such cases. Risk factors for AC are high, single intravenous dose; time of drug infusion <30 min; history of previous irradiation; use of other concomitant agents such as cyclophosphamide, trastuzumab, and paclitaxel; female gender; and young or old age.

There is an acute effect with a transient decline in myocardial contractility after infusion and a chronic progressive effect presenting as dilated cardiomyopathy is typically manifested as clinical heart failure or subclinical decline in myocardial function, and may present early, within 1 year of the termination of chemotherapy, or late-delayed, becoming evident beyond 1 year post-treatment. The chronic cardiomyopathy is related to myocardial necrosis and vacuolization, caused by the suppression of the synthesis of DNA, RNA, proteins, and transcription factors. Reduced protein expression results in disruption of sarcomeric proteins and myofilaments. Anthracycline also alters the adenylyl cyclase activity and calcium homeostasis disrupting the dynamic regulation of cardiac function [11–13].

19.1.2 Trastuzumab (Biological Therapies)

This is a monoclonal antibody that binds to the extracellular domain of HER2 (human epidermal growth factor receptor 2), inhibiting signal transduction. The HER2 gene is overexpressed in 15–20% of breast cancer cases, with overproduction of HER2.

The treatment with this type of therapy results in higher rates of cardiac dysfunction if combined with a high dose of anthracyclines (>300 mg/m^2).

The cardiotoxicity is related to the role of HER2 in cardiomyocyte survival and development [14, 15]: the cellular level overexpression of HER2 and/or neuregulin (NRG)-mediated activation of the HER2/HER4 signaling pathway protect against oxidative stress and prevent apoptosis. High serum levels of HER2 have been detected in individuals with chronic HF [16, 17] and clinical trials have shown that administration of recombinant human NRG-1 improves cardiac function in chronic HF and is well tolerated [18]. Thus, although cardiac stress leads to increased HER2 expression and HER2/HER4 activation by NRG, for example, during anthracycline therapy with pressure overload, inhibition of HER2 by trastuzumab induces ventricular dysfunction, developing dilated cardiomyopathy. The concomitant use of trastuzumab and anthracyclines increases ROS levels, and creates an oxidative stress that causes overexpression of angiotensin II, which inhibits the action of NRG and its binding to HER, blocking anti-apoptotic pathways. Moreover, the Ang II, through activation of NADPH oxidase, produces superoxide anion radicals (potent ROS; Fig. 19.1).

The incidence of cardiotoxicity was evaluated in several studies and the highest incidence was registered in association with anthracycline (>20%) [19, 20].

19.1.3 Tyrosine Kinase Inhibitors (Biological Therapies)

Tyrosine kinase inhibitors (TKIs) are small-molecule targeted therapeutics that are directed against specific molecules and signaling pathways [21]. The drugs in this class are similar; they differ in their specific targets or combination of targets and thus result in a variety of toxicities.

For example, CHF caused by sunitinib may be related to mitochondrial damage in cardiomyocytes or activation of apoptosis and interference in cellular metabolism. CHF related to the use of lapatinib may be a result of HER2 inhibition [22].

19.2 Systemic Hypertension

The principal mechanism involved is the inhibition of vascular endothelial growth factor (VEGF) by anti-angiogenic cancer drugs (i.e., bevacizumab, sunitinib, and sorafenib), which lead to endothelial cell dysfunction and defects within the vascular lining, resulting in activation of tissue factor, thus leading to an increased risk for thromboembolism. In addition, inhibition of VEGF may cause a reduction in nitric oxide and prostacyclin, which promotes vasoconstriction and increases peripheral vascular resistance [21, 22].

The incidence of hypertension in clinical trials ranged from 7 to 36%. Pre-existing hypertension is an important risk factor for severe hypertensive sequelae in cancer patients, and aggressive

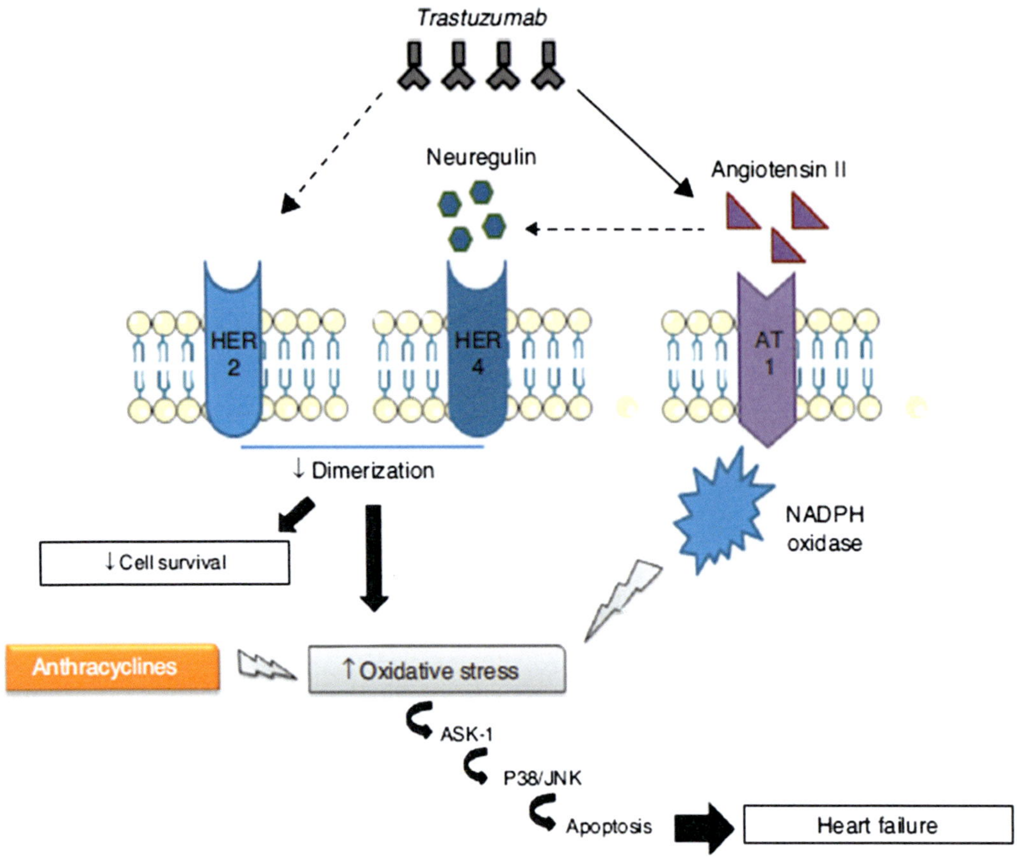

Fig. 19.1 Mechanism of action of trastuzumab

antihypertensive medication before and during treatment with anti-angiogenic drugs is essential [23–25].

19.3 Myocardial Ischemia: Fluoropyrimidines

The pathogenesis of cardiotoxicity is unknown; the mechanisms involved are probably coronary vasospasm, arterial thromboembolic events, arteritis, interaction with the coagulation system, and direct toxicity on myocardium, such as the accumulation of metabolites that interfere with cellular metabolism and apoptosis leading to inflammatory lesions that could mimic myocarditis. Clinical presentations are stable angina, and myocardial infarction more often in patients with pre-existing coronary atherosclerosis. The drugs particularly involved are fluoropyrimidines (such as 5-fluorouracil), bevacizumab, anti-microtubule agents (paclitaxel and docetaxel), tyrosine kinase inhibitors (sorafenib and sunitinib), and the Vinca alkaloids vincristine and vinorelbine [6, 26]

Toxicity appears to be dose-dependent and infusion-rate-dependent. The percentage of clinical presentation for angina is 45%, for myocardial infarction 22%, for arrhythmias 23%, for acute pulmonary edema 5%, for cardiac arrest 1.4%, and for pericarditis 2%, with a mortality rate of 2.2–13% in the literature [27].

19.4 Arrhythmias

The chemotherapeutic agents known to cause arrhythmias are anthracyclines (doxorubicin and epirubicin), anti-microtubule agents (paclitaxel and docetaxel), antimetabolites (capecitabine, 5-flurouracil, and gemcitabine), alkylating agents (cisplatin and cyclophosphamide), tyrosine kinase inhibitors (trastuzumab and cetuximab), arsenic trioxide, thalidomide, and interleukin 2.

The most frequent arrhythmia registered is atrial fibrillation with to unknown and variable incidence related to treatments. Cancer itself causes arrhythmias independently of pre-existing risk factors that obviously increase morbidity (advanced age, radiotherapy of the heart, the presence of amyloid infiltration, and any underlying conduction system disturbance) [28].

19.5 Thromboembolism

Venous thromboembolism is a leading cause of death in cancer patients and is associated with the use of anti-angiogenic drugs, thalidomide, lenalidomide, bevacizumab, and hormone therapy such as tamoxifen. The thrombogenic mechanism of these drugs involves direct action on endothelial cells and increased platelet aggregation.

19.6 Radiotherapy

Another type of anticancer therapy is radiation, which is administered in about 50% of patients with cancer. The groups of patients in which radiation-associated cardiac injuries are of clinical importance are those with curable malignancies (mainly Hodgkin's lymphoma and early-stage breast cancer, lung, and esophageal cancer) irradiated at a relatively younger age; thus, there is enough time to develop clinically significant late cardiac injury. The extent of cardiotoxicity depends mainly on radiation dose, the area of the heart exposed, and the particular technique applied. Risk factors for radiation-associated heart damage include dose >30–35 Gy, a large volume of irradiated heart, younger age at exposure, longer time since exposure, use of cytotoxic chemotherapy, endocrine therapy or trastuzumab, and the presence of other risk factors such as diabetes, hypertension, dyslipidemia, obesity, and smoking [29].

The mechanism of cardiotoxicity is likely secondary to the generation of reactive oxygen species, which disrupt DNA strands and lead to vascular endothelial damage, and inflammation, which leads to fibrosis [30, 31].

RT heart injury can cause various cardiac syndromes such as the following:

- Arteritis of the endothelium of coronary arteries, which can cause premature coronary artery disease and atherosclerosis mainly in the left anterior descending and right coronary artery, 10–15 years after RT.
- Acute pericarditis and symptomatic (hemodynamic compromise with constriction or tamponade) or asymptomatic chronic pericardial effusion usually appear 6–12 months following RT.
- Myocarditis and congestive heart failure due to nonspecific diffuse interstitial fibrosis.
- Valvular stenosis and regurgitation mainly of mitral and aortic valves.
- Fibrosis of the conduction system and disturbed heart rate and complete or incomplete heart block.

19.7 Monitoring and Non-Invasive Diagnosis

Patients undergoing anticancer therapy should follow standard guidelines for reducing CV risk, such as blood pressure control, lipid-level reduction, smoking cessation, and lifestyle modifications.

Baseline clinical evaluation, ECG evaluation, and periodic monitoring of cardiac function with echocardiography are considered according to the type of patients and chemotherapeutic treatment.

There are recent research initiatives suggesting the possible utility of non-invasive imaging technologies for identifying subclinical CV injury in those receiving treatment for and surviving cancer.

19.7.1 Role of Echocardiography

In addition to evaluating LV structure, echocardiography provides information on both systolic function and diastolic function; also, recent techniques have become available to measure myocardial deformation, including LV strain, strain rate, or twist and torsion that may provide a new understanding regarding the early stages of the pathophysiology of cardiac dysfunction upon receipt of cancer treatment [32, 33]. Moreover, echocardiography provides additional information about valvular function and pericardial fluid/physiology that might occur after cancer treatment.

The m-mode, Doppler, and 2D and 3D information is useful, not only for diagnosing a cardiac injury, but also often to predict the cardiotoxicity. For example, some studies have shown that LV diastolic properties, such as a decrease in the E/A ratio, or prolongation of IVRT, or the deceleration time of early diastolic filling, can predict doxorubicin-induced LV systolic dysfunction [34]. Some authors demonstrated that a reduction of more than 10% of global and regional longitudinal and radial strain in the first weeks of treatment with anthracycline and trastuzumab predicts the later development of a reduction of LVEF 6 months after the initiation of these therapies [32, 35] with a sensitivity of 78% and specificity of 79%, and a negative predictive value of 93%.

Other studies try to determine the prognostic utility of other echocardiographic measures, such as the twist and torsion of the LV in those treated for cancer, and this may be the expression of myo-filament disorganization and cardiomyocyte necrosis.

19.7.2 Role of Cardiovascular Magnetic Resonance Imaging

Cardiovascular magnetic resonance (CMR) imaging gives information about cardiac and vascular anatomy, tissue characteristics (presence of fibrosis, inflammation, injury, etc.), left and right ventricular systolic or diastolic function, blood flow, and myocardial perfusion or metabolism for the purposes of understanding the etiology of LV systolic or diastolic dysfunction. For this reason, the American College of Cardiology/American Heart Association recognize CMR imaging as a method of identifying CV dysfunction after treatment for cancer and have incorporated it across research studies to define the pathophysiology of cancer treatment-related CV toxicity. By CMR imaging the presence and severity of morphological and functional abnormalities of the LV or RV myocardium can be identified and understood, determining the underlying etiology (e.g., ischemic versus non-ischemic disease) of LV or RV dysfunction, and identifying prognostic factors related to patient outcomes. CMR offers more accurate assessment of function and morphology than most available imaging modalities, providing reliable volumetric data with high diagnostic image quality in nearly all patients. Table 19.3 displays quantitative and qualitative parameters, each of which can be used as

Table 19.3 Cardiovascular magnetic resonance imaging-derived parameters in patients with suspected heart failure

	Parameters
Systolic function	LV and RV end-diastolic volume and indices
	LV and RV end-systolic volume and indices
	LV and RV stroke volume and ejection fraction
	Cardiac output and cardiac index
	Regional and global measures of myocardial strain
Morphology	LV mass and indices
	Mean and maximum myocardial wall thickness
	Assessment of pericardium
Wall stress	End-systolic wall stress
Diastolic function	Circumferential strain and strain rate
	End-diastolic forward flow in pulmonary veins
	E/A ratio
Reversible acute injury	Edema
Irreversible injury	Myocardial fibrosis

diagnostic markers or descriptors in patients with suspected heart failure [36].

19.7.3 Role of Cardiovascular Computed Tomography

Cardiovascular CT may be useful for evaluating the pericardium of patients who received radiation or surgical treatments; to identify abnormal thickening and calcification of the pericardium; and to measure coronary artery calcium or directly visualize the coronary arteries. There are currently insufficient data to recommend the routine use of coronary CT angiography or calcium scoring in patients who underwent high-dose radiation therapy. In addition, the presence of coronary artery calcification before treatment for cancer has not been shown to predict future CV risk upon receipt of chemotherapy, tyrosine kinase inhibitors, or radiation therapy.

19.7.4 Role of Nuclear Medicine Imaging

Today, equilibrium radionuclide angiography (ERNA) is used to measure LV function through determination of the LV ejection fraction (LVEF). LV diastolic function is often assessed using radioisotope-based techniques. Count–time curves, the peak filling rate (PFR), the PFR normalized to stroke volume, and time-to-peak filling rate are detected with planar equilibrium radionuclide ventriculography (ERNV). For example, a reduction in these ERNV measures of LV diastolic function correlates with the simultaneous decreases in LVEF, suggesting an impairment of systolic and diastolic function during anthracycline therapy [37, 38]

19.7.5 Role of Biomarkers

Early identification of patients at risk for cardiotoxicity represents a primary goal for cardiologists and oncologists; we know the usefulness of LVEF monitoring in patients who have undergone chemotherapy, but it is not specific and sensitive enough to predict damage, because it permits the identification of cardiac damage only after the onset of cardiac dysfunction. An alternative diagnostic strategy is the use of troponin and cardiac peptides in the early detection of cardiotoxicity in clinical practice. Measurement of EF may underestimate actual cardiac damage, because patients may experience subtle changes in cardiac function not detected on imaging studies. Serum cardiac biomarkers, such as N-terminal prohormone brain natriuretic peptide and/or troponin, may also play a role in the detection of cardiac damage, but further investigation is needed to classify their predictive value.

The mechanisms responsible for troponin release after chemotherapy are still being defined. Results of many studies support the non-ischemic etiology of the serum troponin increase after chemotherapy [39]. Furthermore, the persistence of cTnI elevation, observed in some studies, 1 month or more after the end of chemotherapy, suggests the occurrence of a release pattern different from ischemic injury [40]. In acute coronary syndromes, indeed, troponin typically returns to baseline within 10 days and is associated with, not followed by, ventricular dysfunction [41].

Troponin determination detects the presence of cardiotoxicity very early, before impairment of cardiac function, and can be revealed by any other diagnostic technique. Immediately after the last dose of chemotherapy, determination of troponin allows for the discrimination of patients at a high risk for cardiotoxicity from patients at low risk; among patients with positive troponin values, persistence of the increase 1 month after the last administration of chemotherapy is related to an 85% probability of major cardiac events within the first year of follow-up [39, 42, 43], whereas a persistently negative troponin test result can identify, with a predictive negative value of 99%, patients with the lowest risk for cardiotoxicity (Fig. 19.2).

Although the role of Tn is clear, for the cardiac natriuretic peptides (CNPs), such as B-type natriuretic peptide (BNP) and the amino-terminal

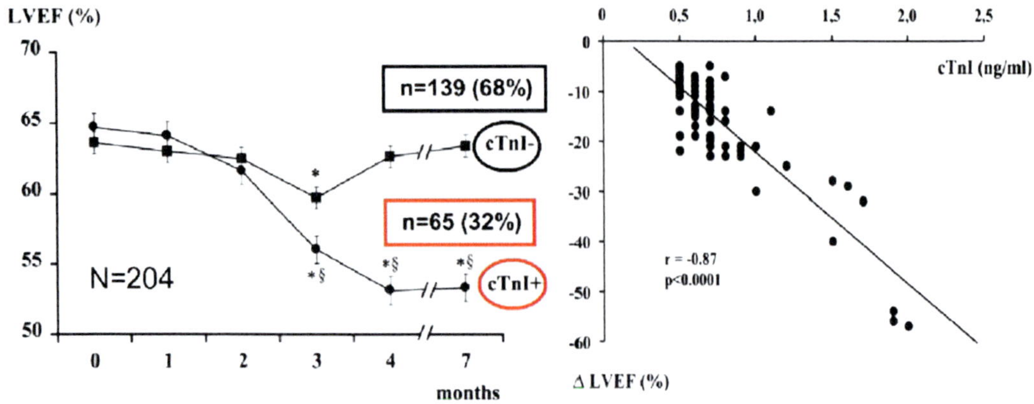

Fig. 19.2 Left ventricular dysfunction predicted by early troponin I release after high-dose chemotherapy. Cardinale et al. [42]

fragment of its precursor (NT-proBNP), it is not the same thing. They represent efficient markers of ventricular dysfunction as they are rapidly produced and secreted by the heart in response to ventricular wall distention. There are no definitive results regarding the role of CNPs in assessing cardiotoxicity in clinical practice.

19.8 Treatment and Prevention

Drugs used to treat heart failure have also shown promise in the prevention of chemotherapy-induced cardiotoxicity; early detection of cardiotoxicity is of crucial importance ineffectively preventing or treating patients in a phase in which the disease is still reversible. Jensen, in some studies, considered around 108 patients with anthracycline cardiomyopathy only, who had symptoms of heart failure. Forty-six patients (43%) were treated with digitalis and diuretics, and 32 patients (30%) were treated with different angiotensin-converting enzyme inhibitor (ACEIs; enalapril in most cases); among them, only 13 patients received ACEIs as a first treatment. Finally, only 5 patients (5%) were treated with beta-blockers alone (carvedilol in most cases), and only 25 patients (23%) received a combination of both these classes of drugs. Therefore, no clear evidence can be obtained from these findings in terms of defining the best therapeutic strategy for this CMP [44–47].

A study of 50 patients randomly assigned to receive prophylactic carvedilol or placebo before anthracycline chemotherapy found that beta-blockers preserve EF [48]. Similar results were seen with nebivolol [49]. A larger randomized trial that included 473 patients demonstrated that enalapril may also help prevent cardiotoxicity; however, the mean age was 45 years, and the benefits in the elderly are not known [43].

Cardinale et al. [50] demonstrated that early treatment is particularly critical in asymptomatic patients. Indeed, most responders were either asymptomatic or had a low New York Heart Association (NYHA) functional class at the time of HF therapy initiation (Fig. 19.3).

Preventing AC-induced cardiotoxicity while treating the malignancy remains the ultimate goal of therapy; cardiac function should also be monitored in patients receiving potentially cardiotoxic chemotherapy to detect early cardiac abnormalities while they are still reversible.

Indeed, the American College of Cardiology and the American Heart Association recommend routine echocardiography at baseline and recurrent re-evaluation [51].

We can say that for a correct treatment a prevention of cardiotoxicity is useful:

– Periodic monitoring (every 12 weeks) of cardiac function with echocardiography

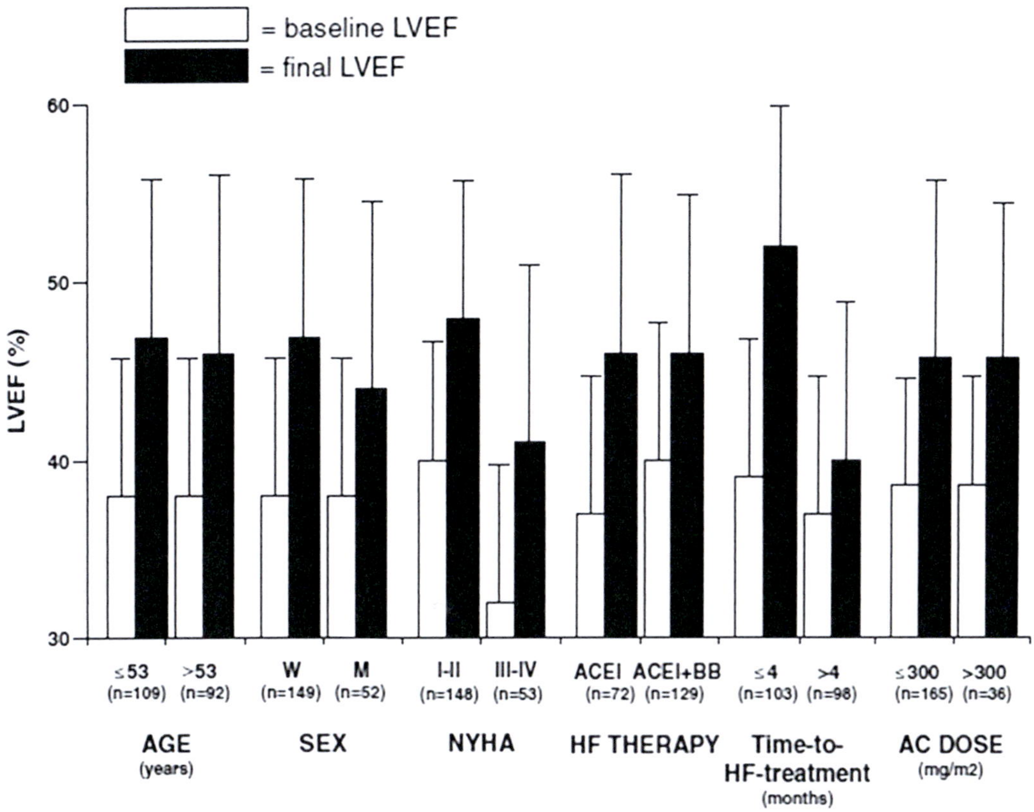

Fig. 19.3 Left ventricular ejection fraction (*LVEF*) before (baseline) and after (final) heart failure (*HF*) therapy in various subgroups of patients. For age, time-to-HF treatment, and anthracycline (*AC*) dose, patients were stratified according to the median value. $p<0.001$ for all comparisons. *ACEI* angiotensin-converting enzyme inhibitor, *BB* beta-blocker, *M* men, *NYHA* New York Heart Association, *W* women

(especially for anthracyclines and their derivates, or monoclonal antibodies) [III, A].

- Assessment of baseline systolic and diastolic cardiac function with echocardiography should be conducted before treatment with monoclonal antibodies [III, A] or anthracyclines and their derivates in patients aged >60 years, or with CV risk factors such as hypertension, hypercholesterolemia, diabetes, and obesity.
- LVEF reduction of 20% from baseline despite normal function or LVEF decline <50% necessitates reassessment or discontinuation of therapy and further frequent clinical and echocardiographic checks. In these patients, even if asymptomatic, aggressive medical therapy is mandatory, especially if the neoplasia could have a long-term survival; it consists of ACE inhibitors and beta-blockers.
- A predictive role for biomarkers of cardiotoxicity caused by cancer therapy is not well defined enough to include them as routine screening measurements. Nevertheless, persistent increases in cardiac troponin I or BNP concentrations seem to identify patients at risk for cardiotoxicity.

Regarding the role of therapy in preventing the effect of asymptomatic cardiotoxicity, which may leave the heart vulnerable to added stressors, we received significant information from the PRADA randomized study that assessed whether the angiotensin receptor blocker candesartan, the beta-blocker metoprolol, or a combination of the two can prevent a reduction in LVEF, as measured by CMR imaging in patients receiving adjuvant oncological therapy for early breast cancer. The reduction of EF assessed by CMR imaging was 2.6% in the placebo group and 0.6% in the candesartan group. Such a statistically significant difference was not found in the metoprolol group, which, unlike the candesartan, did not show any benefit in the prevention of the reduction of the EF [52].

19.9 New Perspectives: Nutrigenomics

One of the most simple but important considerations is that chronic inflammation is related to cancer induction, with evidence of activation of inflammatory genes and genes controlling cell growth factors, angiogenesis, and cytokine/chemokine regulation [53, 54]. The carcinogenic conditions are obesity, hyperglycemia, autoimmune diseases, persistent infections caused by some viruses such as human papilloma (cervical carcinoma), herpes virus (lymphoma), hepatitis B and C (hepatocarcinoma), cytomegalovirus (glioblastoma), and *Helicobacter pylori* (gastric cancer). All these conditions produce cancer, inducing a chronic inflammation [55].

Nutrigenomics is a multidisciplinary science that manages to combine genetics with nutrition, trying to play an active role. Using a combination of agents or a multitargeted approach could theoretically permit the administration of the lowest active dose of each agent and therefore lower the potential for adverse side effects. Phytochemicals are known to inhibit a number of diverse targets. Cancer cell growth is driven by multiple signaling pathways, a multistep process by which cancer cells acquire characteristics of unlimited proliferation potential, lack of response to growth signals, and resistance to cell death. Identifying the most important players or biomarkers in carcinogenesis has been difficult because of the heterogeneity of cancer and the constantly changing cancer genome. For example, tumors that are drug-sensitive can at the same time develop drug-resistant mutations [56, 57].

Selected anticancer natural products, such as mixed tocopherols, curcumin, quercetin, vitamin C, and resveratrol, without interference with conventional treatment, have powerful anti-oxidant/anti-inflammatory activity. Polyphenolics, for example, may protect against various chronic degenerative diseases such as cancer or CV disease [58].

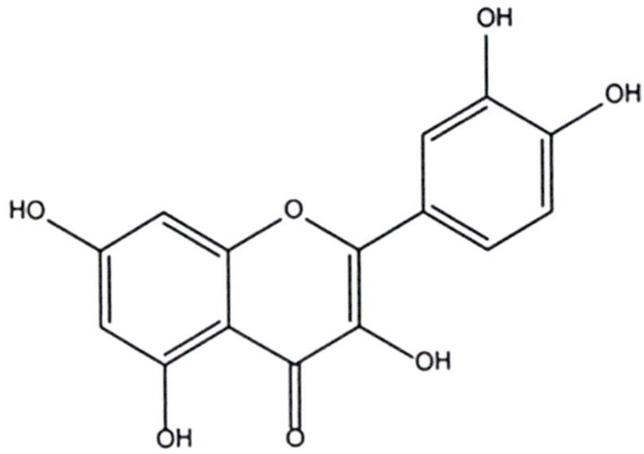

Fig. 19.4 Formula for quercetin

Quercetin (3,3′,4′,5,7-pentahydroxyflavone) (Fig. 19.4) is an important dietary flavonoid present in red onions, apples, berries, citrus fruits, tea, and red wine [59], and exhibits anti-oxidant, anti-inflammatory, anti-obesity, and anticancer properties. Quercetin has received increasing attention as a pro-apoptotic flavonoid with specific, and almost exclusive, effects on tumor cells rather than normal, non-transformed cells [60]. Another effect with an unclear mechanism, demonstrated by Arçari et al. [61], is related to weight reduction and the regulation of the expression of genes related to in vitro adipogenesis.

The anticancer effect and "chemopreventer" role with the modulation of cancer cell apoptosis were confirmed by Zhao et al. [62], demonstrating in liver cancer cells the inhibition of FASN (animal fatty acid synthase) causing HepG2 cell (human liver cancer) apoptosis.

Resveratrol (Fig. 19.5): is produced by plants as a defense mechanism in response to fungal diseases, stress, and UV radiation; the primary dietary sources of resveratrol are grapes and peanuts. Resveratrol exhibits anticancer properties by inhibiting cell proliferation, inducing apoptosis, decreasing angiogenesis, and causing cell cycle arrest in several cancer cell lines.

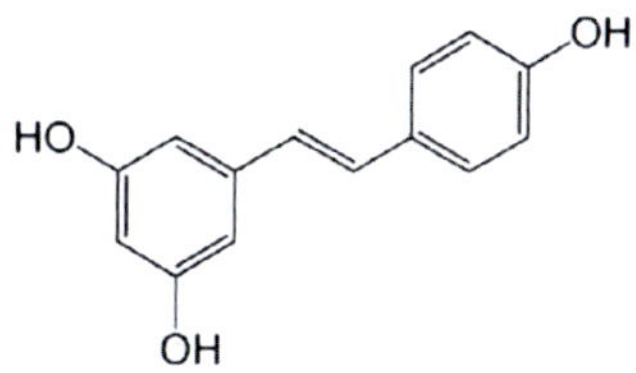

Fig. 19.5 Formula for resveratrol

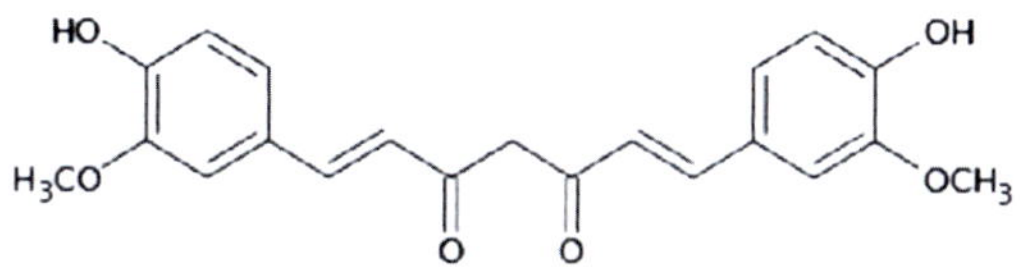

Fig. 19.6 Curcumin formula

It induces apoptosis through the induction of p53 phosphorylation and also suppresses AP1 and cyclooxygenase 2 activities, leading to cancer cell death [63]. In several cancer cell lines within different phases, the combination of resveratrol and quercetin exhibited a synergistic antiproliferative effect, for example, in MOLT-4 leukemia cells, decreasing the percentage of cells in the S phase and increasing the percentage of cells in the G0/G1 phase, which is consistent with the inhibition of the progression from the G0/G1 to the S phase [64, 65].

In some recent studies the effect of curcumin (Fig. 19.6) was analyzed, a polyphenol responsible for the yellow color of turmeric, one of the main components of the spice "curry". Curcumin is potentially beneficial in the treatment of metabolic diseases and diabetes mellitus, and in the prophylaxis of CV diseases such as atherosclerosis, cardiac hypertrophy, and remodeling. Although few clinical studies investigating the direct effects of curcumin on the CV system are available at days, promising experimental evidence has shown potential in the management and prevention of heart diseases. Antioxidant compounds, like curcumin, may have cardioprotective effects during the chemotherapeutic treatment (for example, with adriamycin). In a study conducted in murine models, administration of high doses of curcumin (200 mg/kg within 7 days, previously up to 2 days after treatment with adriamycin) was associated with a significant reduction of the cardiotoxic effect of chemotherapy.

The therapeutic effects of curcumin were studied in particular in the prevention and treatment of neoplastic and inflammatory pathological conditions [66, 67]. Curcumin is well tolerated when taken at high doses (up to 12 g per day). Although few clinical studies are designed to study the direct effects of curcumin on the CV system, the first experimental evidence suggests the potential preventive and protective role in heart disease.

The number of the known biological functions of ascorbic acid vitamin C is continually expanding. Its principal effect is the autoxidation producing hydrogen peroxide (H_2O_2). In the presence of catalytic metals this oxidation is accelerated [68].

Recent pharmacokinetic data indicate that intravenous (i.v.) administration of ascorbate bypasses the tight control of the gut producing highly elevated plasma levels; ascorbate at very high levels can act as a prodrug to deliver a significant flux of H_2O_2 to tumors.

Plants and most animals synthesize ascorbate from glucose. In primitive fish, amphibians, and reptiles, ascorbate synthesis takes place in kidney, whereas the liver is the site of synthesis in mammals.

In human and animal tissues, the highest concentrations of ascorbate are in the adrenal and pituitary glands (Table 19.4) [69]. Ascorbate is a physiological reductant in the dopamine β-hydroxylase-catalyzed reaction that converts dopamine to norepinephrine in the chromaffin granules of adrenal medulla. It is important as a reducing agent to maintain iron in the ferrous state.

Epidemiological evidence suggests that vitamin C-rich foods play a protective role against the development of cancer; plasma concentrations of ascorbate have been shown to be inversely associated with cancer risk [70]. A possible explanation is related to the [71] demonstration that some cancer cells have increased sensitivity to ascorbate-induced cytotoxicity compared with normal cells. In a complementary study, Du et al. [72, 73] demonstrated that

Table 19.4 Ascorbate content of human tissues

Tissue	Ascorbate (mmol/kg wet tissue)	Ascorbate (mM)
Adrenal glands	1.7–2.3	
Pituitary gland	2.3–2.8	
Liver	0.8–1	
Spleen	0.8–1	
Pancreas	0.8–1	
Kidneys	0.28–0.85	
Skeletal muscle	0.17–0.23	
Brain	0.74–0.85	
Placenta	0.23–0.72	
Plasma (healthy)		0.04–0.08
Red blood cell		0.04–0.06
Neutrophil		1.2
Lymphocyte		4.0
Monocyte		3.2
Platelet		3.7
Cerebral spinal fluid		0.15–0.25
Neuron		10
Glial cells		1
Lens		2.5–3.4
Corneal epithelium		12.5
Aqueous humor		0.4–1.1
Alveolar macrophage		0.32
Bronchoalveolar lavage		0.04–0.06
Saliva		0.04–0.05

pancreatic cancer cells are more sensitive to pharmacological concentrations of ascorbate than their normal cell counterparts. The difference in sensitivity between normal and cancer cells toward ascorbate may be due to low levels of anti-oxidant enzymes and high endogenous levels of ROS in cancer cells [74]. The relatively lower activities of catalase, glutathione peroxidase, and peroxiredoxins in cancer cells could potentially contribute to the less efficient removal of H_2O_2 and increased sensitivity to ascorbate-induced cytotoxicity.

19.10 Conclusion

The majority of the natural products found to have powerful and versatile anticancer effects have shown a very wide margin of safety. The newer techniques, such as nanosizing and microencapsulation with phospholipids, have greatly improved both gut absorption and bioavailability. Combination with dietary programs designed to utilize what we now know about the anticancer effects of various foods can greatly improve the prevention and treatment of cancers.

It can be seen that conventional anticancer therapy has extremely high toxicity and treatment concentrations are often close to fatal systemic toxic effects. The natural products are powerful anticancer agents when used alone and significantly improve conventional chemotherapy and radiation therapy treatments; the use of these valuable agents is currently reasonable, both as cancer preventatives and in the treatment of established cancers.

References

1. Gharib MI, Burnett AK (2002) Chemotherapy-induced cardiotoxicity: current practice and prospects of prophylaxis. Eur J Heart Fail 4:235–242
2. Pai VB, Nahata MC (2000) Cardiotoxicity of chemotherapeutic agents: incidence, treatment and prevention. Drug Saf 22:263–302
3. Kongbundansuk S, Hundley WG (2014) Noninvasive imaging of cardiovascular injury related to the treatment of cancer. JACC Cardiovasc Imaging 7 (8):824–838
4. Grenier MA, Lipshultz SE (1998) Epidemiology of anthracycline cardiotoxicity in children and adults. Semin Oncol 25 [4 Suppl 10]:72–85
5. Lipshultz SE, Alvarez JA, Scully RE (2008) Anthracycline associated cardiotoxicity in survivors of childhood cancer. Heart 94:525–533
6. Yeh ET, Tong AT, Lenihan DJ et al (2004) Cardiovascular complications of cancer therapy: diagnosis, pathogenesis and management. Circulation 109:3122–3131
7. Raschi E, Vasina V, Ursino MG et al (2010) Anticancer drugs and cardiotoxicity: insights and perspectives in the era of targeted therapy. Pharmacol Ther 125:196–218
8. Seidman AD, Berry D, Cirrincione C et al (2008) Randomized phase III trial of weekly compared with every-3-weeks paclitaxel for metastatic breast cancer, with trastuzumab for all HER-2 overexpressors and random assignment to trastuzumab or not in HER-2 nonoverexpressors: final results of Cancer and Leukemia Group B protocol 9840. J Clin Oncol 26:1642–1649
9. Seidman A, Hudis C, Pierri MK et al (2002) Cardiac dysfunction in the trastuzumab clinical trials experience. J Clin Oncol 20:1215–1221

10. Adao R (2013) Gilles de Keulenaer Cardiotoxicity associated with cancer therapy: pathophysiology and prevention. Rev Port Cardiol 32(5):395–409
11. Takahashi S, Denvir MA, Harder L et al (1998) Effects of in vitro and in vivo exposure to doxorubicin (adriamycin) on caffeine-induced Ca^{2+} release from sarcoplasmic reticulum and contractile protein function in 'chemically-skinned' rabbit ventricular trabeculae. Jpn J Pharmacol 76:405–413
12. Lebrecht D, Kokkori A, Ketelsen UP et al (2005) Tissue-specific mtDNA lesions and radical-associated mitochondrial dysfunction in human hearts exposed to doxorubicin. J Pathol 207:436–444
13. Fu M, Matoba M, Liang QM et al (1994) Properties of G-protein modulated receptor-adenylyl cyclase system in myocardium of spontaneously hypertensive rats treated with adriamycin. Int J Cardiol 44:9–18
14. Lee KF, Simon H, Chen H et al (1995) Requirement for neuregulin receptor erbB2 in neural and cardiac development. Nature 378:394–398
15. Zhao YY, Sawyer DR, Baliga RR et al (1998) Neuregulins promote survival and growth of cardiac myocytes. Persistence of ErbB2 and ErbB4 expression in neonatal and adult ventricular myocytes. J Biol Chem 273:10261–10269
16. Lemmens K, Doggen K, de Keulenaer GW (2007) Role of neuregulin-1/ErbB signaling in cardiovascular physiology and disease: implications for therapy of heart failure. Circulation 116:954–960
17. Perik PJ, de Vries EG, Gietema JA et al (2007) Serum HER2 levels are increased in patients with chronic heart failure. Eur J Heart Fail 9:173–177
18. Jabbour A, Hayward CS, Keogh AM et al (2011) Parenteral administration of recombinant human neuregulin-1 to patients with stable chronic heart failure produces favourable acute and chronic haemodynamic responses. Eur J Heart Fail 13:83–92
19. Bowles EJ, Wellman R, Feigelson HS et al (2012) Risk of heart failure in breast cancer patients after anthracycline and trastuzumab treatment: a retrospective cohort study. J Natl Cancer Inst 104:1293–1305
20. Chavez-MacGregor M, Zhang N, Buchholz TA et al (2013) Trastuzumab-related cardiotoxicity among older patients with breast cancer. J Clin Oncol 31:4222–4228
21. Arora A, Scholar EM (2005) Role of tyrosine kinase inhibitors in cancer therapy. J Pharmacol Exp Ther 315:971–979
22. Yeh ET, Bickford CL (2009) Cardiovascular complications of cancer therapy: incidence, pathogenesis, diagnosis, and management. J Am Coll Cardiol 53:2231–2247
23. Yang JC, Haworth L, Sherry RM et al (2003) A randomized trial of bevacizumab, an anti-vascular endothelial growth factor antibody, for metastatic renal cancer. N Engl J Med 349:427–434
24. Hurwitz H, Fehrenbacher L, Novotny W et al (2004) Bevacizumab plus irinotecan, fluorouracil, and leucovorin for metastatic colorectal cancer. N Engl J Med 350:2335–2342
25. Sandler A, Gray R, Perry MC et al (2006) Paclitaxel-carboplatin alone or with bevacizumab for non-small cell lung cancer. N Engl J Med 355:2542–2550
26. Anderson JL, Adams CD, Antman EM et al. (2007) ACC/AHA 2007 guidelines for the management of patients with unstable angina/non ST-elevation myocardial infarction: a report of the American College of Cardiology/American Heart Association Task Force on Practice Guidelines (Writing Committee to Revise the 2002 Guidelines for the Management of Patients With Unstable Angina/Non ST-Elevation Myocardial Infarction): developed in collaboration with the American College of Emergency Physicians, the Society for Cardiovascular Angiography and Interventions, and the Society of Thoracic Surgeons: endorsed by the American Association of Cardiovascular and Pulmonary Rehabilitation and the Society for Academic Emergency Medicine. Circulation 116: e148–304.
27. Saif MW, Shah MM et al (2009) Fluoropyrimidine-associated cardiotoxicity: revisited. Expert Opin Drug Saf 8:191
28. Guglin M, Aljayeh M, Saiyad S et al (2009) Introducing a new entity: chemotherapy-induced arrhythmia. Europace 11:1579–1586
29. Bovelli DG (2010) Plataniotis cardiotoxicity of chemotherapeutic agents and radiotherapy-related heart disease: ESMO Clinical Practice Guidelines. Ann Oncol 21 [Suppl 5]:v277–v282. doi:10.1093/annonc/mdq200
30. Clarke M, Collins R, Darby S et al (2005) Effects of radiotherapy and of differences in the extent of surgery for early breast cancer on local recurrence and 15-year survival: an overview of the randomised trials. Lancet 366:2087–2106
31. Curigliano G, Cardinale D, Suter T et al (2012) Cardiovascular toxicity induced by chemotherapy, targeted agents and radiotherapy: ESMO Clinical Practice Guidelines. Ann Oncol 23:vii155–vii166
32. Sawaya H, Sebag IA, Plana JC et al (2011) Early detection and prediction of cardiotoxicity in chemotherapy-treated patients. Am J Cardiol 107:1375–1380
33. Biswas M, Sudhakar S, Nanda NC et al (2013) Two and three-dimensional speckle tracking echocardiography: clinical applications and future directions. Echocardiography 30:88–105
34. Tassan-Mangina S, Codorean D, Metivier M et al (2006) Tissue Doppler imaging and conventional echocardiography after anthracycline treatment in adults: early and late alterations of left ventricular function during a prospective study. Eur J Echocardiogr 7:141–146
35. Stoodley PW, Richards DA, Hui R et al (2011) Two dimensional myocardial strain imaging detects changes in left ventricular systolic function

immediately after anthracycline chemotherapy. Eur J Echocardiogr 12:945–952
36. Hundley WG, Bluemke DA, Finn JP et al (2010) ACCF/ACR/AHA/NASCI/SCMR 2010 expert consensus document on cardiovascular magnetic resonance: a report of the American College of Cardiology Foundation Task Force on Expert Consensus Documents. J Am Coll Cardiol 55:2614–2662
37. Hesse B, Lindhardt TB, Acampa W et al (2008) EANM/ESC guidelines for radionuclide imaging of cardiac function. Eur J Nucl Med Mol Imaging 35:851–885
38. Cottin Y, Touzery C, Coudert B et al (1995) Impairment of diastolic function during short-term anthracycline chemotherapy. Br Heart J 73:61–64
39. Cardinale D, Sandri MT, Colombo A et al (2004) Prognostic value of troponin I in cardiac risk stratification of cancer patients undergoing high-dose chemotherapy. Circulation 109:2749–2754
40. Lipshultz SE, Rifai N, Sallan SE et al (1997) Predictive value of cardiac troponin T in pediatric patients at risk for myocardial injury. Circulation 96:2641–2648
41. Newby LK, Christenson RH, Ohman EM et al (1998) Value of serial troponin T measures for early and late risk stratification in patients with acute coronary syndromes. Circulation 98:1853–1859
42. Cardinale D, Sandri MT, Martinoni A et al (2000) Left ventricular dysfunction predicted by early troponin I release after high dose chemotherapy. J Am Coll Cardiol 36:517–522
43. Cardinale C, Colombo A, Sandri MT et al (2006) Prevention of high-dose chemotherapy-induced cardiotoxicity in high risk patients by angiotensin-converting enzyme inhibition. Circulation 114:2474–2481
44. Jensen BV, Skovsgaard T, Nielsen SL (2002) Functional monitoring of anthracycline cardiotoxicity: a prospective, blinded, long-term observational study of outcome in 120 patients. Ann Oncol 13:699–709
45. Jensen BV, Nielsen SL, Skovsgaard T (1996) Treatment with angiotensin converting-enzyme inhibitor for epirubicin-induced dilated cardiomyopathy. Lancet 347:297–299
46. Noori A, Lindenfeld J, Wolfel E, Ferguson D, Bristow MR, Lowes BD (2000) Beta-blockade in adriamycin-induced cardiomyopathy. J Card Fail 6:115–119
47. Saini J, Rich MW, Lyss AP (1987) Reversibility of severe left ventricular dysfunction due to doxorubicin cardiotoxicity. Report of three cases. Ann Intern Med 106:814–816
48. Kalay N, Basar E, Ozdogru I et al (2006) Protective effects of carvedilol against anthracycline-induced cardiomyopathy. J Am Coll Cardiol 48:2258–2262
49. Kaya MG, Ozkan M, Gunebakmaz O et al (2013) Protective effects of nebivolol against anthracycline induced cardiomyopathy: a randomized control study. Int J Cardiol 167:2306–2310
50. Cardinale D, Colombo A (2010) Anthracycline-induced cardiomyopathy clinical relevance and response to pharmacologic therapy. J Am Coll Cardiol 55(3):213–220
51. Cheitlin MD, Armstrong WF, Aurigemma GP et al (2003) ACC/AHA/ ASE 2003 guideline update for the clinical application of echocardiography: summary article: a report of the American College of Cardiology/American Heart Association Task Force on Practice Guidelines (ACC/AHA/ASE Committee to Update the 1997 Guidelines for the Clinical Application of Echocardiography). J Am Coll Cardiol 42:954–970
52. Heck SL, Gulati G et al (2012) Rationale and Design of the Prevention of Cardiac Dysfunction during an Adjuvant Breast Cancer Therapy (PRADA) Trial. Cardiology 123:240–247
53. Kono Y, Kawakami S, Higuchi Y, Yasashita F, Hashida M (2014) In vitro evaluation of inhibitory effects of nuclear factor-kappaB activity by small interfering RNA on pro-tumor characteristics of M2-like macrophages. Biol Pharm Bull 37:137–144
54. Kortylewski M, Kujawski M, Wang T, Wei S, Zhang S, Pilon-Thomas S et al (2005) Inhibiting STAT3 signaling in the hematopoietic system elicits multicomponent antitumor immunity. Nat Med 11:1314–1321
55. Reya T, Morrison SJ, Clarke MF, Weissman IK (2001) Stem cells, cancer, and cancer stem cells. Nature 414:105–111
56. Luo J, Solimini NL, Elledge SJ (2009) Principles of cancer therapy: oncogene and non-oncogene addiction. Cell 136:823–837
57. Kobayashi S et al (2005) EGFR mutation and resistance of non-small-cell lung cancer to gefitinib. N Engl J Med 352:786–792
58. Saiko P, Szakmary A, Jaeger W, Szekeres T (2008) Resveratrol and its analogs: defense against cancer, coronary disease and neurodegenerative maladies or just a fad? Mut Res 658:68–94
59. Erlund I (2004) Review of the flavonoids quercetin, hesperetin, and naringenin. Dietary sources, bioactivities, bioavailability, and epidemiology. Nutr Res 24:851–874
60. Du G, Lin H, Wang M et al (2010) Quercetin greatly improved therapeutic index of doxorubicin against 4T1 breast cancer by its opposing effects on HIF-1α in tumor and normal cells. Cancer Chemother Pharmacol 65:277–287
61. Arçari DP, Santos JC, Gambero A, Ribeiro ML (2013) The in vitro and in vivo effects of yerba mate *(Ilex paraguariensis)* extract on adipogenesis. Food Chem 141:809–815
62. Zhao P et al (2014) Quercetin inhibits fatty acid synthase. Oncol Lett 8:765–769
63. Zykova TA et al (2008) Resveratrol directly targets COX-2 to inhibit carcinogenesis. Mol Carcinog 47:797–805

64. Juan ME, Wenzel U, Daniel H, Planas JM (2008) Resveratrol induces apoptosis through ROS-dependent mitochondria pathway in HT-29 human colorectal carcinoma cells. J Agric Food Chem 56:4813–4818
65. Mertens-Talcott SU, Bomser JA, Romero C, Talcott ST, Percival SS (2005) Ellagic acid potentiates the effect of quercetin on p21waf1/cip1, p53, and MAP-kinases without affecting intracellular generation of reactive oxygen species in vitro. J Nutr 135:609–614
66. Goel A, Kunnumakkara AB, Aggarwal BB (2008) Curcumin as "Curecumin": from kitchen to clinic. Biochem Pharmacol 75(4):787–809
67. Duvoix A, Blasius R, Delhalle S et al (2005) Chemopreventive and therapeutic effects of curcumin. Cancer Lett 223(2):181–190
68. Bielski BHJ (1982) Chemistry of ascorbic acid radicals. In: Seib PA, Tolbert BM (eds) Ascorbic acid: chemistry, metabolism, and uses, vol 200. American Chemical Society, Washington DC, pp 81–100
69. Hornig D (1975) Distribution of ascorbic acid, metabolites and analogues in man and animals. Ann N Y Acad Sci 258:103–118
70. Gonzalez CA, Riboli E (2010) Diet and cancer prevention: contributions from the European Prospective Investigation into Cancer and Nutrition (EPIC) study. Euro J Cancer 46:2555–2562
71. Chen Q, Espey MG, Sun AY, Pooput C, Kirk KL, Krishna MC, Khosh DB, Drisko J, Levine M (2008) Pharmacologic doses of ascorbate act as a prooxidant and decrease growth of aggressive tumor xenografts in mice. Proc Natl Acad Sci U S A 105:11105–11109
72. Du J, Martin SM, Levine M, Wagner BA, Buettner GR, Wang SH, Taghiyev AF, Du C, Knudson CM, Cullen JJ (2010) Mechanisms of ascorbate-induced cytotoxicity in pancreatic cancer. Clin Cancer Res 16:509–520
73. Du J et al (2012) Ascorbic acid, Chemistry, biology and the treatment of cancer. Biochim Biophys Acta 1826(2):443–457
74. Oberley LW (2005) Mechanism of the tumor suppressive effect of MnSOD overexpression. Biomed Pharmacother 59:143–148

20 Heart and Skin: The Paradigm of Cytokine-Mediated Cardiovascular Metabolic Disease in Psoriasis

Torello Lotti

20.1 Introduction

All organs and biological systems are controlled and managed by a continuous information exchange driven by cytokines, neuropeptides, neurohormones, growth factors, and other signaling molecules [1, 2].

These mediators therefore play a key role in the maintenance of homeostatic parameters and, consequently, in determining the state of health or disease, both considered as expressions of the fluctuation of the levels of these substances. Furthermore, the cross-talk breakdown induced by an imbalance in the signaling molecules is a fundamental factor for the onset of inflammatory, allergic, autoimmune, and neoplastic diseases [1–4].

A detailed analysis of all axis components leads to a new insight into the biological functions of the body, in accordance with the psycho-neuro-endocrine immunology (PNEI) principles [1, 2, 5–8]. Skin homeostasis and skin diseases are among the most complex and fascinating models of PNEI (Fig. 20.1).

T. Lotti (✉)
University of Rome "G.Marconi", Rome, Italy

Institute of Dermatology, Florence, Italy

World Health Academy Dermatology, Zurich, Switzerland
e-mail: professor@torellolotti.it; http://csrmr.unimarconi.it/

20.2 Psoriasis

Psoriasis is a common, chronic, relapsing, inflammatory skin disease affecting up to 3% of the world's population [9, 10].

Up to 90% of patients with psoriasis have plaque psoriasis or psoriasis vulgaris, characterized by the presence of raised, well-demarcated, erythematous oval plaques with adherent silvery scales involving mainly the elbows, knees, scalp, and rima ani.

The scales are a result of a hyperproliferative epidermis (increased mitotic rate of basal keratinocytes) with premature maturation of keratinocytes and incomplete cornification, together with retention of nuclei in the stratum corneum (parakeratosis). As a result, the epidermis is thickened (acanthosis), with elongated rete ridges.

In the dermis, a dermal inflammatory infiltrate of dendritic cells, macrophages, and T cells in the dermis and neutrophils can be observed.

Last, an increased number of tortuous capillaries that reach the skin surface through a markedly thinned epithelium are often present [11].

Substantial advances have recently been made in elucidating the molecular mechanisms of psoriasis, and new efficacious drugs have been introduced for the treatment of this disease. However, major issues remain unresolved, including the primary nature of the disease, the immune cause of the inflammatory process, the

M. Fioranelli (ed.), *Integrative Cardiology*, DOI 10.1007/978-3-319-40010-5_20

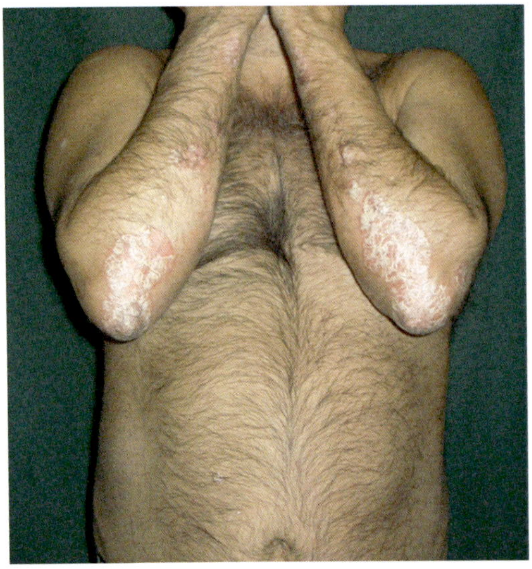

Fig. 20.1 Plaque psoriasis in a patient who is mildly overweight

relevance of cutaneous and systemic factors, and the role of genetic and environmental influences on disease initiation, progression, and response to therapy [11].

Psoriasis is well known to be associated with a high degree of morbidity. Patients' quality of life is severely compromised; they are embarrassed about the appearance of their skin, and they have reduced levels of employment and income [10, 12, 13].

The costs of the disease and long-term therapy have a major impact on healthcare systems and on society in general [10, 12, 13].

20.3 Immune Imbalance in Psoriasis

Regarding the immunopathogenesis of psoriasis, the presence of an immune imbalance (characterized by an altered ratio between specific cytokines released by T helper (Th) 1/Th17 and Treg/Th2 lymphocyte subsets) is considered a key etiological factor [1, 2, 9, 14]. Various immune cell types play an important role, particularly CD4+ Th17 and Th1 cells. Together with CD4+ T cells, other T-cell subsets (Th22 and Th21) and CD8+ T cells infiltrating the epidermis represent the major source of interferon-γ, interleukin (IL)-17, IL-22, and tumor necrosis factor (TNF)-α [14].

In psoriatic lesional skin, a large number of these cytokines is observed. In addition, dendritic cell–derived cytokines (IL-23, IL-20, TNF-α) and keratinocyte-derived cytokines and chemokines (i.e., CXCL8, CXCL1, CCL20, IL-36) offer a relevant contribution to psoriatic lesional skin formation [1, 9, 14].

20.4 Psoriasis: Implications Beyond the Skin

20.4.1 Articular, Nail, and Mucosal Involvement

Psoriasis is important to the clinician because it has treatment implications beyond the care of skin lesions. It represents a model for studies of mechanisms in chronic inflammation processes. Psoriasis is associated with a decreased quality of life and with severe comorbidities [10].

Psoriatic arthritis is an inflammatory form, commonly associated with cutaneous psoriasis in up to 42% of cases. Many patients suffer from psoriasis several years before developing arthritis. More rarely, arthritis precedes psoriasis, or the initial presentation includes arthritis and psoriasis together. The severity and involvement of arthritis is rarely related to the course and clinical presentation of the skin disease [11, 14].

Nail psoriasis, presenting as pitting, oil spots, ridging, onycholysis, and subungual hyperkeratosis, is reported in up to 55% of adult psoriatic patients, and this psoriasis involvement is highly connected to psoriatic arthritis, with an association in up to 80% of cases.

Psoriatic lesions may also involve the oral and genital mucosae. The tongue in particular can be affected, showing benign migratory geographic features [11].

20.4.2 Psoriasis Comorbidities

There is increasing evidence that psoriasis has many immunological and metabolic associations that may play a role in disease in other organ systems. Epidemiological studies have demonstrated an association between psoriasis and noncutaneous diseases such as tonsillitis, Crohn's disease, obesity, heart diseases, and chronic alcoholism. Patients with psoriasis are at an increased risk for developing cardiovascular (CV) disease and metabolic syndrome compared with controls without psoriasis [14–37].

Recently, the International Psoriasis Council led an initiative to better define the association between various cardiometabolic comorbidities and psoriasis, focusing on the association of psoriasis with a higher risk of myocardial infarction, stroke, and metabolic syndrome [14, 35].

Metabolic syndrome is characterized by central obesity, atherogenic dyslipidemia, hypertension, and glucose intolerance. Obesity is a common comorbidity of psoriasis. Multiple studies have demonstrated that patients with psoriasis are more likely overweight (BMI: 25 kg/m^2 and <30 kg/m^2) or obese (BMI: 30 kg/m^2) compared with patients without psoriasis [14, 25].

Together with an increase in the BMI, psoriatic patients have significantly higher concentrations of triglycerides and total cholesterol, in addition to higher concentrations of low-density lipoprotein and very low-density lipoprotein cholesterol: all of these factors are established and well-known risk factors for cardiovascular disease [14, 24, 33–35].

Lastly, psoriasis is also associated with impaired glucose tolerance and type 2 diabetes. Psoriatic patients are more likely than healthy individuals to demonstrate insulin resistance when challenged with oral glucose (Fig. 20.1) [14, 24, 33–35].

20.5 Psoriasis and Heart Comorbidities

Whether because of the high incidence of metabolic syndrome or because of systemic inflammation, an important association between psoriasis and heart comorbidities has been reported [14–23]. Increased rates of concurrent CV disease, including hypertension, diastolic dysfunction, and heart failure have been noted in patients with psoriasis.

Epidemiological studies reported the association with shorter life expectancy, frequently attributable to CV events. Although an increased prevalence of CV events, such as myocardial infarction, stroke, ventricular dysfunction, and atherosclerosis, has been reported among psoriatic patients, psoriasis likely plays an independent role in the increased CV risk. This could be at least partly explained by the chronic systemic inflammatory state [32].

In fact, evidence is accumulating with regard to the improvement of early subclinical vascular alterations and CV morbidity and mortality by treatment with anti-inflammatory drugs, such as anti-TNF-α and methotrexate [29–32].

20.6 Evidence to Support an Association Between Psoriasis and Cardiometabolic Diseases

The inflammatory state that characterizes psoriasis and cardiometabolic diseases, e.g., obesity and atherosclerosis, recognizes a potentially shared pathophysiology involving immune activation of T helper cell (Th)-1, Th-17, regulatory T cell, and inflammatory cytokine signaling, such as TNF-a, IL-6, IL-8, IL-17, L-22, IL-36, and chemokines CCL-2 and CXC-1, -3, -10 [14, 32, 33].

The common pathophysiology potentially explains common treatment strategies and response to treatments [29–32].

With increased evidence and definition of cardiometabolic comorbidities in patients with psoriasis, there has been a growing interest from the dermatology community in elucidating the link and the common pathogenesis of psoriasis and cardiometabolic diseases [14]. Furthermore, there is a need for the stratification of the diseases according to valuable biomarkers.

Biomarkers are crucial within the context of stratified medicine in the diagnosis of diseases, the evaluation of systemic involvement, and therapy for "systemic" psoriasis.

Furthermore, novel, cheap, and non- or low-invasive techniques will be fundamental in the identification and quantification of systemic involvement.

20.7 Low-Dose Cytokines for the Treatment of Psoriasis

Low-dose cytokine treatment is aimed at correcting the psoriatic immune imbalance, characterized by the hyperproduction of Th1/Th17 cytokines. A multicenter, double-blind, placebo-controlled clinical study [34] described the efficacy of specific low-dose cytokines (IL-4, IL-10, and IL-11, at a concentration of 10 fg/mL, GUNA., Milan, Italy) for the 8-month treatment of psoriasis vulgaris. The study evaluated the effectiveness on the extension of psoriatic lesions (measured using the Psoriasis Area Severity Index [PASI]) and the improvement in the quality of life (with the use of the Dermatology Life Quality Index [DLQI]). The study reported a significant reduction of psoriasis extension (PASI) together with an improvement in the quality of life (DLQI). No adverse event was reported during the whole trial. Similarly, an observational study [9] evaluated the pharmacological activity of the treatment based on the use of UVA-1 laser therapy with or without the co-administration of low-dose cytokines (interleukin [IL]-4, IL-10) and anti-IL-1 antibodies in patients affected by psoriasis vulgaris (LOTTI). The co-administration of low-dose cytokines in combination with a UVA-1 laser was shown to be more effective in ameliorating psoriasis skin involvement (PASI) in comparison with UVA-1 laser alone.

20.8 Conclusion: Management of a Patient Affected by Systemic Psoriasis

It is well known among insiders that it is always more important to consider and treat a patient with skin psoriasis as a patient with a systemic immune inflammatory disease, with well-characterized skin involvement. The sequence of events is not known. Many cytokines are involved: in Table 20.1, some of these and their effects on the skin and dermal vessels are reported [7, 40]. This may suggest that inflammation does precede the diseases and, later, specific organ inflammation, psoriasis, and atherosclerosis develop.

Nowadays, the systemic association is common, and a more precise definition of systemic pathogenesis and involvement of psoriasis is needed.

New biological drugs have been introduced with success into the clinical management of skin and the involvement of articular psoriasis.

Low-dose cytokines have provided significant improvement in various skin diseases by restoring the immune balance, altered by a deregulated cytokine synthesis. The preliminary positive results induce the researchers to highlight innovative strategies for the treatment of dermatological diseases characterized by an immune Th1/Th17–Treg/Th2 imbalance such as psoriasis. The association between psoriasis and systemic comorbidities reflects a systemic immune imbalance.

Further studies are needed to confirm the role of low-dose cytokines in the treatment of psoriasis, together with the analysis of skin and systemic involvement.

Table 20.1 Main activities of mediators and their receptors on the cutaneous cells and immune system

Mediator	Receptors	Sources, receptors expressed mainly by	Remarks
Acetylcholine	Nicotinergic and muscarinergic acetylcholine receptors	Nerves, endothelium, mast cells, fibroblasts, melanocytes	• Mediates itching in atopic dermatitis • mAChR3 is probably involved in itching • Regulates keratinocyte proliferation, adhesion, migration, and differentiation
Adenosine triphosphate (ATP)	Purinergic P2 receptors (ionotropic P2XRs or metabotropic P2YRs)		• Involved in neurogenic inflammation • Induces release of IL-6, IL-8, MCP-1 • Increases expression of ICAM-1
Calcitonin gene-related peptide (CGRP) (and adrenomedullin, ADM)	CGRP receptor-calcitonin-like receptor/receptor activity modifying protein 1 (CL-R/RAMP1) ADM-receptor-CL-R/RAMP2 or CL-R/RAMP3	CGRP: sensory nerve fibers CGRP receptor: keratinocytes	CGRP • Involved in pain transmission (central but not peripheral) and in the prolongation of pruritus latency following SP injection (inhibitory effect on itching) • Increase in CGRP fibers in itchy skin diseases • Important mediator of neurogenic vasodilatation ("wheal-and-flare" reaction) • Stimulates adhesion of leukocytes and monocytes to endothelial cells • Stimulates TNF-α and IL-8 release from mast cells • Modulates (inhibition) the cutaneous macrophage and Langerhans cell functions • Has a mitogenic effect on endothelial cells and keratinocytes • Induces mast cells to release histamine and pro-inflammatory mediators such as TNF-α and IL-8
Catecholamines	Adrenergic receptors (AR): α, β	Released by nerve fibers, keratinocytes, melanocytes. Receptors by natural killer cells, monocytes, T cells	• Suppresses IL-12 production and increases IL-10 release in dendritic cells (DCs) • Augments T-cell production • Inhibits TNF-α release from monocytes • Modulates keratinocyte differentiation

(continued)

Table 20.1 (continued)

Mediator	Receptors	Sources, receptors expressed mainly by	Remarks
			• Regulates melanogenesis • β_2 receptors mediate α-MSH central inhibition of skin inflammation
Corticotropin-releasing hormone (CRH; see also opioids and pro-opiomelanocortin)	CRH-R1 and -R2	CRH-R1: keratinocytes, mast cells; CRH-R2: bone marrow mast cells	• Release of histamine, cytokines, TNF-α, VEGF from mast cells • CRH-R1 downregulation upon stress and infection • CRH-R2 mRNA induced by IL-4 in mast cells • High expression of CRH-R1 in urticaria and lichen simplex • Stimulates fibroblast proliferation and inhibits keratinocyte proliferation • Stimulates corticosterone production in fibroblasts • Regulates pigmentation
Endocannabinoids	Cannabinoid receptors (CB1, CB2)	Released by nerves, T cells, macrophages Receptors on nerves, mast cells, macrophages, keratinocytes, skin appendages	• Antipruritic effects at the periphery; antinociceptive and antihyperalgesic • Inhibit cytokines of innate and adaptive immune responses, downregulate release of IL-1, TNF-α, and CXCL8, and upregulate IL-10 • Suppress TH1-cell activity and increase TH2-cell activity; decrease production of IFN-γ and IL-12 and expression of IL-12R; increase IL-4 production • Have protective effect during sepsis • Attract human eosinophils, B cells, DCs, increased in HIV • Lipopolysaccharides stimulate release of cannabinoids from macrophages and DCs • CB2 reduces cutaneous edema
Endothelin (ET)	Endothelin receptors (ETA, ETB)	Nerves, endothelium, mast cells, fibroblasts, melanocytes	• Involved in burning and pruritus • Degraded by chymase via ETA • ET-1 induces TNF-α, and IL-6 production by mast cells

(continued)

Table 20.1 (continued)

Mediator	Receptors	Sources, receptors expressed mainly by	Remarks
			• Involved in tissue remodeling and fibrogenesis • ETB mediates upregulation of melanoma cell adhesion molecule
Interleukin-31	IL-31R (heterodimer)	Keratinocytes, sensory nerves	• Released during skin inflammation by T cells and macrophages • Induces release of inflammatory mediators from keratinocytes, induces itching • Causes skin barrier dysfunction
Kallikreins, proteases	Partly by proteinase-activated receptors (PARs, tryptic enzymes)	PAR1: keratinocytes, endothelial cells, mast cells, platelets PAR2: keratinocytes, endothelial cells, mast cells, nerves PAR4: T cells, mast cells, (macrophages?)	• Involved in angiogenesis, clearance of cytokines and pigmentation • pH affects serine protease activity in the epidermis • Kallikreins may be involved in systemic sclerosis • PAR1: platelet regulation; induces proliferation in keratinocytes • MMP-1 activates PAR1 • PAR2: involved in itching behavior in mice overexpressing epidermal kallikrein-7. Tryptase induces inflammation and itching by a neurogenic mechanism via PAR2 • Microbial proteases may induce pruritus and inflammation via PAR2
Neurokinin A (NKA) Substance P (SP) Hemokinin-1 (HK-1)	Tachykinin (neurokinin) receptor-1, -2, -3	Sensory nerve fibers, dermal microvascular endothelial cells, keratinocytes, B cells	SP • Increases blood vessel permeability • Induces microvascular endothelium adhesion molecules (ELAM-1) • Induces the "wheal-and-flare" reaction • Increases cutaneous fibrinolytic activity • Stimulates the activity of cutaneous mast cells (release of histamine and TNF-α) • Stimulates leukocytes chemotaxis

(continued)

Table 20.1 (continued)

Mediator	Receptors	Sources, receptors expressed mainly by	Remarks
			• Stimulates the activity of macrophages and neutrophils (e.g., increase in the H_2O_2 production) • Stimulates the mitogenesis of T cells • Stimulates the activity of keratinocytes • Is involved in central pain transmission • Tachykinins contribute to pain processing HK-1 • Expressed by T cells and macrophages • Involved in B-cell development and stimulates IFN-γ production in T cells NKA • Upregulation of keratinocyte nerve growth factor expression
Endovanilloids (heat, acidosis, eicosanoids, histamine, bradykinin, extracellular ATP, prostaglandins, various neurotrophins)	Activation of vanilloid receptor-1 (TRPV1) Sensitization of TRPV1 via activation of specific receptors	TRPV1 is expressed on sensory neurons, mast cells, epidermal, and hair follicle keratinocytes, Langerhans cells, smooth muscle, sebocytes	TRPV1 • Short-term TRPV1 activation: pain and itch induction • Depletes neuropeptides from sensory neurons. Long-term antipruritic effect of TRPV1 agonists (e.g., capsaicin): suspend interplay between sensory neurons and mast cells • Affects epidermal and hair follicle proliferation, differentiation, apoptosis, and cytokine release. Increased expression in epidermal keratinocytes of prurigo nodularis patients; induces neurogenic inflammation
Histamine	Histamine receptors (H1R, H4R)	Sensory nerve fibers, endothelial cells, T cells	• Induces pruritus by stimulating specific sensory fibers, whereas H1 and H2 antagonists reduce pruritus in numerous clinical trials • Induces plasma extravasation and vasodilatation; communicates with T cells via histamine receptors

(continued)

Table 20.1 (continued)

Mediator	Receptors	Sources, receptors expressed mainly by	Remarks
			• In mice, H3 antagonists induce scratching behavior, whereas H1 and H4 antagonists effectively suppress pruritus
Nerve growth factor (NGF), brain-derived neurotrophic factor (BDNF), neurotrophins (NT-3, NT-4)	Specific receptors Trk A: NGF; Trk B: NT-4, BDNF; Trk C: NT-3	Keratinocytes, mast cells, fibroblasts, eosinophils	NGF • NGF levels enhanced in atopic dermatitis (AD) • Induces tryptase release from mast cells • Inducible by histamine • Is upregulated during inflammation, stimulates mast cells, induces proliferation and differentiation of B cells, and stimulates neuronal cells • Trk A: enhanced in keratinocytes during inflammation BDNF • Increases eosinophil chemotaxis levels in AD and inhibits apoptosis NT-3, NT-4 • NT-3 inhibits inflammatory hyperalgesia in rats. NT-4: enhanced in AD and induces sprouting
Neuropeptide Y (NPY)	Neuropeptide Y receptor-1 and -2 (Y1, Y2)	Sensory nerves, keratinocytes	• Inhibits adenylyl cyclase, regulates blood flow, and stimulates vasoconstriction
Opioids	δ, k, μ Opioid receptors (partly receptor independent cell activation)	Sensory nerves, keratinocytes, T cells, B cells	• Antipruritic effects of μ-opioid antagonists (central effect) and k-opioid agonists (spinal cord level) • μ-opioid receptor upregulation in atopic dermatitis • Keratinocyte-derived β-endorphin induces peripheral analgesia • T cells express various opioid receptors and opioids induce T-cell chemotaxis • Inhibit B-cell IgG production via IL-6 modulation

(continued)

Table 20.1 (continued)

Mediator	Receptors	Sources, receptors expressed mainly by	Remarks
Pituitary adenylate cyclase activating polypeptide (PACAP)	PAC1R, PAC2R, PAC3R (and splice variants); also binds to VPAC1R and VPAC2R	Sensory and autonomic nerves, T cells, macrophages, keratinocytes, dermal microvascular endothelial cells, Merkel cells	• Potent vasodilator • Involved in flush, pain, neurodegeneration • Enhanced in psoriasis plaques • Downregulates capacity of APCs for antigen presentation: inhibits the induction of contact hypersensitivity by reducing LCs • In vitro it induces release of histamine from mast cells; downregulates release of IL-2, IL-6, TNF-α from T cells and macrophages • Early inflammation: it drives T cells into an anti-inflammatory response. Late inflammation: stimulates T-cell proliferation and differentiation into Th2 helper cells
Proopiomelanocortins (POMC gene) (endorphins, enkephalins, dynorphins, MSH, ACTH, lipotrophin; see also CRH, opioids)	Opioid receptors, MCR, ACTH-R, CRH-R	Melanocytes, keratinocytes, adnexal epithelial cells, endothelial cells, Langerhans cells, mast cells, fibroblasts, monocytes, and macrophages	• Upon cleavage by prohormone convertase (PC1, 2) POMC derived • Peptides mediate a variety of processes in skin α-Melanocyte-stimulating hormone (α-MSH) • Downregulates the costimulatory molecule CD86 on monocytes, macrophages, and neutrophils • Reduces the release of pro-inflammatory cytokines, including TNF-α, IL-1, and IL-8, and induces anti-inflammatory cytokines such as IL-10 • Influences the expression of the adhesion molecules, including E-selectin and vascular cell adhesion molecule-1 (VCAM-1) • Influences the release of other neuropeptides, such as VIP and CGRP

(continued)

Table 20.1 (continued)

Mediator	Receptors	Sources, receptors expressed mainly by	Remarks
Prostaglandins	Prostanoid (P) receptors (DP, EP, IP)	Sensory nerve fibers, keratinocytes	• PGE2 induces pain over itching in humans • PGD2 reduces IgE-mediated scratching in mice • PGE2 may potentiate edema in the skin • DP1 impedes TNF-α-induced migration of human Langerhans cells (LCs), inhibits the chemotactic responses of human LCs to chemokines, induces IL-10 production
Somatostatin (SST) (1–14, 1–28)	SST receptors 1–5	Skin: Merkel cells, sweat glands, Langerhans cells, keratinocytes, fibroblasts, macrophages	• In atopic skin, the expression of SST disappeared • Has inhibitory effects on T-cell proliferation • Antiproliferative on keratinocytes • Anti-inflammatory: downregulation of pro-inflammatory cytokines • SST receptors are upregulated in melanoma
Substance P			• Increases blood vessel permeability • Induces microvascular endothelium adhesion molecules (ELAM-1) • Induces the "wheal-and-flare" reaction • Increases cutaneous fibrinolytic activity • Stimulates the activity of cutaneous mast cells (release of histamine) • Stimulates leukocyte chemotaxis • Stimulates the activity of macrophages and neutrophils (e.g., increases the H_2O_2 production) • Stimulates the mitogenesis of T cells • Stimulates keratinocyte maturation
Vasoactive intestinal polypeptide (VIP)	VPAC1R, VPAC2R	Sensory and autonomic nerves, T cells, macrophages, keratinocytes, dermal microvascular endothelial cells, Merkel cells, smooth muscle cells	• Anti-inflammatory effects • Inhibits natural killer cell activity of large granular lymphocytes • Inhibits the migration of lymphocytes in vascular and connective tissues

(continued)

Table 20.1 (continued)

Mediator	Receptors	Sources, receptors expressed mainly by	Remarks
			• Inhibits T-cell response • Induces NO synthesis; upregulates IL-10 in DCs; downregulates TLR4 expression and TLR4-mediated chemokine generation • Downregulates IL-1, TNF-α, and MCP-1; anti-apoptotic in Th2 cells • Enhances monocyte migration in chemotaxis chambers • Participates in the "wheal-and-flare" reaction although mainly the histamine releases from mast cells • Stimulates the sweat secretion • Inhibits delayed-type hypersensitivity and prevents from graft-versus-host-disease • Induces pruritus and increases blood flow in human skin

From Lotti et al. [7] and modified from Roosterman et al. [40]

References

1. Lotti T, Hercogova J, Wollina U, Chokoeva AA, Zarrab Z, Gianfaldoni S, Roccia MG, Fioranelli M, Tchernev G (2015) Treating skin diseases according to the low dose medicine principles. Data and hypotheses. J Biol Regul Homeost Agents 29 [Suppl 1]: 47–51
2. Lotti T, Hercogova J, Wollina U, Chokoeva AA, Zarrab Z, Gianfaldoni S, Roccia MG, Fioranelli M, Tchernev G (2015) Psycho-neuro-endocrine-immunology and low dose cytokines therapy: principles and evidences for an innovative medical approach in acute and chronic inflammatory diseases. J Biol Regul Homeost Agents 29 [Suppl 1]:37–45
3. Ngoc PL, Gold DR, Tzianabos AO et al (2005) Cytokines, allergy, and asthma. Curr Opin Allergy Clin Immunol 5(2):161–166
4. Commins SP, Borish L, Steinke JW (2010) Immunologic messenger molecules: cytokines, interferons, and chemokines. J Allergy Clin Immunol 125 [Suppl 2]: S53–S72
5. Ader R, Cohen N (1993) Psychoneuroimmunology: conditioning and stress. Annu Rev Psychol 44:53–85
6. Ader R, Cohen N, Felten D (1995) Psychoneuroimmunology: interactions between the nervous system and the immune system. Lancet 345(8942):99–103
7. Lotti T, D'Erme AM, Hercogová J (2014) The role of neuropeptides in the control of regional immunity. Clin Dermatol 32(5):633–645
8. Reiche EM, Nunes SO, Morimoto HK (2004) Stress, depression, the immune system, and cancer. Lancet Oncol 5(10):617–625
9. Lotti T (2015) Successful combination treatment for psoriasis with phototherapy and low-dose cytokines: a spontaneous, retrospective observational clinical study. Hautarzt 66(11):849–854
10. Nestle FO, Kaplan DH, Barker J (2009) Psoriasis. N Engl J Med 361(5):496–509
11. Saraceno R, Chiricozzi A, Chimenti S (2015) Psoriasis. In: Katsambas A, Lotti T, Dessinioti C, D'Erme AM (eds) European handbook of dermatological treatments. Springer, Berlin, pp 797–816
12. Horn EJ, Fox KM, Patel V, Chiou CF, Dann F, Lebwohl M (2007) Association of patient-reported psoriasis severity with income and employment. J Am Acad Dermatol 57:963–971
13. Thomas J, Rolstad T, Margolis DJ (2004) Determinants of quality of life in patients with

psoriasis: a study from the US population. J Am Acad Dermatol 51:704–708
14. Shlyankevich J, Mehta NN, Krueger JG, Strober B, Gudjonsson JE, Qureshi AA, Tebbey PW, Kimball AB (2014) Accumulating evidence for the association and shared pathogenic mechanisms between psoriasis and cardiovascular-related comorbidities. Am J Med 127(12):1148–1153
15. Gelfand JM, Neimann AL, Shin DB, Wang X, Margolis DJ, Troxel AB (2006) Risk of myocardial infarction in patients with psoriasis. JAMA 296(14):1735–1741
16. Gelfand M, Dommasch ED, Shin DB, Azfar RS, Kurd SK, Wang X, Troxel AB (2009) The risk of stroke in patients with psoriasis. J Invest Dermatol 129(10):2411–2418
17. Friedewald VE, Cather JC, Gelfand JM, Gordon KB, Gibbons GH, Grundy SM, Jarratt MT, Krueger JG, Ridker PM, Stone N, Roberts WC (2008) AJC editor's consensus: psoriasis and coronary artery disease. Am J Cardiol 102(12):1631–1643
18. Mehta NN, Azfar RS, Shin DB, Neimann AL, Troxel AB, Gelfand JM (2010) Patients with severe psoriasis are at increased risk of cardiovascular mortality: cohort study using the general practice research database. Eur Heart J 31(8):1000–1006
19. Mehta NN, Yu Y, Pinnelas R, Krishnamoorthy P, Shin DB, Troxel AB, Gelfand JM (2011) Attributable risk estimate of severe psoriasis on major cardiovascular events. Am J Med 124(8):775.e1–775.e6
20. Prodanovich S, Kirsner RS, Kravetz JD, Ma F, Martinez L, Federman DG (2009) Association of psoriasis with coronary artery, cerebrovascular, and peripheral vascular diseases and mortality. Arch Dermatol 145(6):700–703
21. Armstrong AW, Gelfand JM, Boehncke WH, Armstrong EJ (2013) Cardiovascular comorbidities of psoriasis and psoriatic arthritis: a report from the GRAPPA 2012 annual meeting. J Rheumatol 40(8):1434–1437
22. Armstrong AW, Brezinski EA, Follansbee MR, Armstrong EJ (2014) Effects of biologic agents and other disease-modifying antirheumatic drugs on cardiovascular outcomes in psoriasis and psoriatic arthritis: a systematic review. Curr Pharm Des 20(4):500–512
23. Armstrong EJ, Harskamp CT, Armstrong AW (2013) Psoriasis and major adverse cardiovascular events: a systematic review and meta-analysis of observational studies. J Am Heart Assoc 2(2):e000062
24. Armstrong AW, Harskamp CT, Armstrong EJ (2013) Psoriasis and the risk of diabetes mellitus: a systematic review and meta-analysis. JAMA Dermatol 149(1):84–91
25. Armstrong AW, Harskamp CT, Armstrong EJ (2013) Psoriasis and metabolic syndrome: a systematic review and meta-analysis of observational studies. J Am Acad Dermatol 68(4):654–662
26. Gargiulo P, Marsico F, Parente A, Paolillo S, Cecere M, Casaretti L, Pellegrino AM, Formisano T, Fabiani I, Soricelli A, Trimarco B, Perrone-Filardi P (2014) Ischemic heart disease in systemic inflammatory diseases. An appraisal. Int J Cardiol 170(3):286–290
27. Ridker PM (2010) Psoriasis, inflammation, and vascular risk: a problem more than skin deep? Eur Heart J 31(8):902–904
28. Solomon DH, Massarotti E, Garg R, Liu J, Canning C, Schneeweiss S (2011) Association between disease-modifying antirheumatic drugs and diabetes risk in patients with rheumatoid arthritis and psoriasis. JAMA 305(24):2525–2531
29. Wu JJ, Poon KY, Channual JC, Shen AY (2012) Association between tumor necrosis factor inhibitor therapy and myocardial infarction risk in patients with psoriasis. Arch Dermatol 148(11):1244–1250
30. Ahlehoff O, Skov L, Gislason G, Gniadecki R, Iversen L, Bryld LE, Lasthein S, Lindhardsen J, Kristensen SL, Torp-Pedersen C, Hansen PR (2015) Cardiovascular outcomes and systemic anti-inflammatory drugs in patients with severe psoriasis: 5-year follow-up of a Danish nationwide cohort. J Eur Acad Dermatol Venereol 29(6):1128–1134
31. Ahlehoff O, Skov L, Gislason G, Lindhardsen J, Kristensen SL, Iversen L, Lasthein S, Gniadecki R, Dam TN, Torp-Pedersen C, Hansen PR (2013) Cardiovascular disease event rates in patients with severe psoriasis treated with systemic anti-inflammatory drugs: a Danish real-world cohort study. J Intern Med 273(2):197–204
32. Mosca S, Gargiulo P, Balato N, Di Costanzo L, Parente A, Paolillo S, Ayala F, Trimarco B, Crea F, Perrone-Filardi P (2015) Ischemic cardiovascular involvement in psoriasis: a systematic review. Int J Cardiol 178:191–199
33. Gisondi P, Cazzaniga S, Chimenti S, Giannetti A, Maccarone M, Picardo M, Girolomoni G, Naldi L, Psocare Study Group (2013) Metabolic abnormalities associated with initiation of systemic treatment for psoriasis: evidence from the Italian Psocare Registry. J Eur Acad Dermatol Venereol 27(1):e30–e41
34. Vena GA, Altomare G, Ayala F, Berardesca E, Calzavara-Pinton P, Chimenti S, Giannetti A, Girolomoni G, Lotti T, Martini P, Mazzaglia G, Peserico A, Puglisi Guerra A, Sini G, Cassano N, Cricelli C (2010) Incidence of psoriasis and association with comorbidities in Italy: a 5-year observational study from a national primary care database. Eur J Dermatol 20(5):593–598
35. Lotti T, Hercogova J, Prignano F (2010) The concept of psoriatic disease: can cutaneous psoriasis any longer be separated by the systemic comorbidities? Dermatol Ther 23(2):119–122
36. Hercogová J, Ricceri F, Tripo L, Lotti T, Prignano F (2010) Psoriasis and body mass index. Dermatol Ther 23(2):152–154

37. Pietrzak A, Brzozowska A, Lotti T, Mosiewicz J, Wysokiński A, Mieczkowska J, Hercogova J, Bartosińska J, Juszkiewicz-Borowiec M, Chodorowska G (2013) Future diagnosis, today's treatment – cardiomyopathy in the course of psoriasis: a case report. Dermatol Ther 26(6):489–492
38. Butcher M, Galkina E (2011) Current views on the functions of interleukin-17A-producing cells in atherosclerosis. Thromb Haemost 106(5):787–795
39. Roberti ML, Ricottini L, Capponi A, Sclauzero E, Vicenti P, Fiorentini E, Savoia C, Scornavacca G, Brazioli D, Gaio L, Giannetti R, Ignazzi C, Meloni G, Chinni LM (2014) Immunomodulating treatment with low dose interleukin-4, interleukin-10 and interleukin-11 in psoriasis vulgaris. J Biol Regul Homeost Agents 28(1):133–139
40. Roosterman D, Goerge T, Schneider SW, Bunnett NW, Steinhoff M (2006) Neuronal control of skin function: the skin as a neuroimmunoendocrine organ. Physiol Rev 86(4):1309–1379

MIX
Papier aus verantwortungsvollen Quellen
Paper from responsible sources
FSC® C105338

If you have any concerns about our products,
you can contact us on
ProductSafety@springernature.com

In case Publisher is established outside the EU,
the EU authorized representative is:
Springer Nature Customer Service Center GmbH
Europaplatz 3, 69115 Heidelberg, Germany

Printed by Libri Plureos GmbH
in Hamburg, Germany